Pediatric Nursing Care Plans

2nd edition

Marie Jaffe, R.N., M.S.
(deceased)

revised by:

Verna Hendricks-Ferguson, R.N., M.S.N., C.S.
Shawn Pohlman, R.N., M.S.N.
Pamela Simpson, R.N., R.N.C., M.S., I.B.C.L.C., W.H.N.P.
Laurie Sparks, R.N., M.S., C.P.N.P., Ph.D.(c)

Skidmore-Roth Publishing, Inc

SR
Skidmore-Roth

Editor: Molly Sullivan
Cover Design: Scott Matthews
Typesetting: Affiliated Executive Systems

Copyright 1993, 1998 by Skidmore-Roth Publishing, Inc.

ISBN 1-56930-057-7

Notice: The author(s) and the publisher of this volume have taken care to make certain all information is correct and compatible with the standards generally accepted at the time of publication.

Skidmore-Roth Publishing, Inc.
400 Inverness Drive South, Suite 260
Englewood, Colorado 80112

Introductory Remarks

The Second Edition

The health of children requires the necessity for the family/caretakers and all health personnel to become aware of the special physical, emotional, and psychological needs of this group. This enhances the good health that is needed to accommodate the rapidity of growth and development and multitude of internal and external factors that confront childhood regardless of who delivers the care to children; adequate nutrition, activity, safety, affection, and stimulation are effective means to promote good health.

Pediatric nursing promotes, restores, and maintains the health of children and the care plan is a written tool that identifies problem areas, and documents nursing activities in an individual manner to facilitate an ill child's journey to wellness or comfort a child's journey during a life threatening illness leading to death. These care plans cover common acute and chronic illnesses associated with the general age group of the infant from 1-12 months of age, the toddler from 1-3 years of age, the preschooler from 3-5 years of age, and the schoolager from 5-12 years of age. Conditions specific to the neonatal and adolescent have been excluded although some conditions with onset during the neonatal period and those continuing into adolescence are included. Emergency conditions and illnesses requiring acute care in an intensive care unit are also excluded.

I am grateful to and thank the publisher, Linda Skidmore-Roth, for the patience and support offered during the writing and development of this book.

Marie S. Jaffe

Using the Pediatric Care Plans

These plans have been developed to reflect physical and functional titles listed according to body systems or psychosocial problems of the hospitalized infant and child. Included are the most common acute and chronic problems and illnesses associated with children from 1 month of age through preadolescence. Each system includes an Overview of the general system, General physiological changes in structure and function associated with growth and development of children and Essential nursing diagnoses and care plans that are usually identified with a particular system. These essential nursing diagnosis and care plans may be cross-referenced with plans for conditions within the system or with plans for conditions within other systems if they apply. Each essential nursing diagnosis and care plan developed for a system includes:

- Nursing diagnosis as stated in the North American Nursing Diagnosis Association (NANDA) taxonomy

- All of the related factors or risk factors and the defining characteristics specific to each related factor that have a relationship with the conditions associated with the infant or child that could be applicable to any system

- Outcome criteria defining the expected general goal to be achieved

- Listing of interventions with rationales that include goal to be achieved

- Listing of interventions with rationales that include actions that may be performed for all of the related or risk factors identified for the diagnosis and applicable to any cross-referenced condition as well as the conditions included in the system

- Information, Instruction, Demonstration including interventions and rationales that pertain to the teaching function of the nurse that involve parent(s), family, and child according to educational background, age, and developmental level of the responsible persons

- Discharge or Maintenance Evaluation including specific actions and behaviors expected of the parent(s), family, and child as a result of the interventions planned to achieve the desired outcomes

Each condition within the system includes an introductory paragraph that provides information about the condition in relation to the infant and child; a Pathophysiological flow sheet depicting causative factors, pathology, resultant signs and systems, complications, and in some instances, treatments for resolution of the disorder; Medical care that lists possible medications prescribed for the condition(s) and drug action, diagnostic procedures, laboratory tests and expected results (The Medical care listing is not in order of priority as this may vary with individual children); Nursing care plan that includes the Essential nursing diagnoses with specific related factors or risks and defining characteristics as they relate to the condition and taken from the system that includes the essential diagnoses and plans used (these are referenced so that the developed plan may be used in this condition), followed by the Specific nursing diagnoses and their related or risk factors, defining characteristics followed by the same format as the essential diagnoses and care plans.

Since it is not uncommon for an infant or child to develop complications to an illness, more than one care plan may be used or combined with the plan for the presenting illness if appropriate, i.e., pneumonia is a complication of cystic fibrosis and both care plans may be helpful. It is hoped that the practitioner will find these plans to be flexible enough to accomplish this interrelationship among the nursing diagnoses and their related care options.

Table of Contents

Cardiovascular System

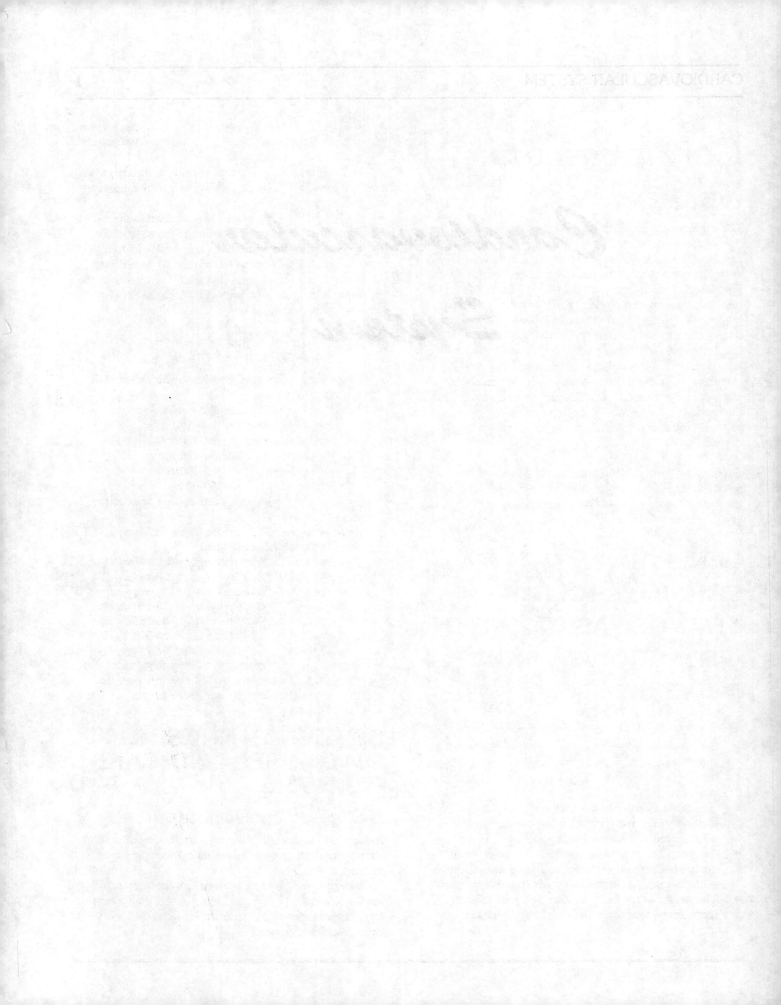

Cardiovascular System

The cardiovascular system includes a pumping structure (heart) and a network of vessels (arteries, veins, and capillaries), which work together to circulate oxygen and nutrients to all parts of the body. Any alterations in the function of these structures affect the well being of the infant/child and cause physical and psychosocial problems for both the affected child and family. Diseases of this system are classified as congenital heart defects (malformations of the heart structure) or acquired disorders (results of infectious process, autoimmune, or environmental responses). Each disorder and its associated changes in function determine the acuity or chronicity of the condition, limitations in growth and development patterns, and course of treatment (medical and/or surgical repair).

Shortly after birth, as fetal circulation is converted to a postnatal development of circulation and pumping action, the system functions within adult parameters as growth and development occurs.

GENERAL CARDIOVASCULAR CHANGES ASSOCIATED WITH GROWTH AND DEVELOPMENT

Heart and blood vessel structure

- Circulation at birth involves the closure of the fetal shunts (foremen ovale at birth, ductus arteriosus by the fourth day after birth, and eventually the ductus venosus).
- Size of the heart in the infant is larger in relation to total body size and occupies a larger space in the chest surrounded by the lungs.
- The heart lies at a transverse angle in infancy and gradually changes to a lower and more oblique angle as the lungs grow until maturity is reached.
- The weight of the heart doubles by 1 year of age, increases by four times the weight by 5 years of age.

- The walls of the ventricle are of equal thickness but become thicker on the left side as demand of peripheral circulation increases.
- Arteries and veins become longer as the body grows, and the walls of the vessels thicken as blood pressure increases.
- The apical pulse is located laterally and to the left of the fourth intercostal space and to the right of the midclavicular line in infants and small children; it changes laterally to the left of the fifth intercostal space and midclavicular line after 7 years of age; the point of maximal intensity (PHI) may be noted at these same areas.

Circulatory function and hemodynamics

- Blood pressure increases and pulse decreases with growth in heart size.
- Heart rate (pulse), resting and awake:

Infant-3 months:	100-180/min
3 months-2 years:	80-120/min
2-4 years:	80-110/min
4-school-aged:	75-100/min
Adolescents:	60-90/min

  Increases vary with age, sleep, resting or activity status.
- Pulse pressure 10-15 mm Hg during infancy; 20-50 mm Hg throughout childhood.
- Blood pressure (varies with age and position):

	Systolic (average)	Diastolic (average)
Infant	65-90 mm Hg	55-56 mm Hg
1-5 years	90-95 mm Hg	54-56 mm Hg
5-10 years	14-102 mm Hg	56-62 mm Hg
Over 10 years	102-121 mm Hg	62-70 mm Hg

- Highest internal pressure is in the left ventricle after birth as the pressure on the left side is higher than the pressure on the right side of the heart.

ESSENTIAL NURSING DIAGNOSES AND CARE PLANS

Decreased cardiac output

Related to: Mechanical factors — alterations in preload; alterations in afterload; alterations in inotropic changes in heart

Defining characteristics: Variations in hemodynamic readings (BP, CVP); hypovolemia; jugular vein distention; oliguria; decreased peripheral pulses; cold, clammy skin; crackles; dyspnea

Related to: Electrical factors — alterations in rate; alterations in rhythm; alterations in conduction

Defining characteristics: Arrhythmias, ECG changes, bradycardia, changes in contractility resulting from preload or afterload abnormalities

Related to: Structural factors

Defining characteristics: Murmurs, fatigue, cyanosis, pallor of skin and mucous membranes, dyspnea, clubbing, activity intolerance

Outcome Criteria

Return and/or maintenance of stable BP, pulse rate and rhythm; respiratory parameters within baseline levels; absence of arrhythmias

Interventions	Rationales
Assess cardiac output by monitor — heart rate (apica and peripheral pulses) for 1 minute, noting quality, rate, rhythm, intensity pulse deficiency; use radial site with gentle palpation in child over 2 years of age, and use apical site with stethoscope and correct size diaphragm in infant and young child; grade pulse on a range from 0 to +4	Cardiac output is the amount of blood pumped from the heart in 1 minute and is determined by multiplying the heart rate by the stroke volume (amount of blood ejected with 1 contraction), which depends on heart contractility, preload and afterload; pulse easily obliterated by compression
Assess blood pressure using proper size cuff; diaphragm on stethoscope of proper size; and aneroid or mercury instrument, Doppler method, or electronic device. Approximate cuff width sizes are 4-6 cm for infant, 8-9 cm for child 2-10 years of age; BP cuff bladder should completely encircle extremity circumference and cuff width should cover 2/3 of upper arm/thigh. Take BP of infant with infant supine; take child BP with child sitting and arm supported at heart level; sites for BP determinations may be (radial), leg (popliteal), or ankle (dorsalis pedis)	Doppler method transmits audible sounds through a transducer in the cuff caused by ultrasound frequency caused by blood flow in the artery; the use of ocillometry transmits pressure changes through the arterial wall to the pressure cuff which are detected by an indicator that prints out the readings for BP and pulse

Interventions	Rationales
Assess BP when infant/child is at rest	Crying or other activity can increase BP 5-10 mm Hg; BP elevations that are considered abnormal are: >110/70 in 3-6 year olds, >120/75 in 6-9 year olds, and >130/80 in 10-13 year olds
Assess existence of arrhythmias per ECG tracings	Device that measures and records the heart's electrical activity and provides information about heart rate and rhythm, hypertrophy, effects of electrolyte imbalances, conduction problems and cardiac ischemia
Administer cardiac glycosides, vasodilators; monitor for digoxin toxicity by symptoms of anorexia, nausea, vomiting, bradycardia, arrhythmias and digoxin level within 0.8-2.0 mcg/L range (therapeutic level) potassium level; take apical pulse for 1 minute before administering digoxin, and withhold if pulse below desired level for age of child	Vasodilators decrease pulmonary and systemic vascular resistance, which decrease afterload and BP; cardiac glycoside strengthens and decreases the heart rate, which decreases the workload of the heart by more efficient cardiac performance; decreased potassium level enhances risk for digoxin toxicity
Position for comfort and chest expansion in Fowler's, provide quiet environment, pace any activity to allow for rest	Promotes ease of breathing and rest; reduces stress and workload of the heart
Monitor temperature for increases	Pulse increased at rate of 8-10/minute with every degree of elevation on F scale
Attach cardiac monitor to infant/child if prescribed	Reveals changes in heart rate and respirations

Information, Instruction, Evaluation

Interventions	Rationales
Inform about heart condition's effect on pulse and blood pressure, and the need for rest and reduction of stress	Provides information to promote compliance with medical regimen and realization of importance of reducing workload of the heart
Instruct in correct taking of peripheral and apical pulses and when to take them	Encourages caretaker, parent(s) to correctly monitor changes in heart function
Instruct in administration of cardiac glycoside: form, dosage, how to take, frequency and time of day, to give 1 hour before or after feedings and not with food, to avoid second dose if child vomits, to avoid making up missed doses when less than 4 hours have passed, and to maintain careful records of administration and effects or adverse signs/symptoms	Ensures correct administration of cardiac glycoside to prevent toxicity and improve cardiac performance
Inform to report changes in pulse, blood pressure, digoxin toxicity, change in breathing pattern, edema, presence of infection	Allows for prompt treatment to prevent complications like dysrhythmias or heart failure
Instruct in application, settings and alarms in use of cardiac monitor	Monitoring may be advised and prescribed for cardiac and respiratory changes

Discharge or Maintenance Evaluation

- Vital signs maintained within baseline parameters for age and gender
- Compliance and accurate administration of medications with desired effect achieved
- Verbalizes signs and symptoms to report
- Provides stress-free environment with adequate rest for infant/child
- Adequate cardiac function maintained with urinary output, breathing, nutritional status, activity tolerance within normal parameters
- Absence of dysrhythmias noted on ECG

Fluid volume excess

Related to: Compromised regulatory mechanisms
Defining characteristics: Edema (periorbital usually but may be dependent on weight gain, effusion, shortness of breath, orthopnea, crackles, change in respiratory pattern (dyspnea, tachypnea), oliguria, specific gravity changes, altered electrolytes
Related to: Excessive sodium intake
Defining characteristics: Weight gain, edema, blood pressure changes (increased), oliguria, altered electrolytes, increase in preload, venous congestion

Outcome Criteria

Absence of fluid retention or overload, with I&0 and VS within baseline ranges

Interventions	Rationales
Assess presence of edema in periorbital tissue or dependent areas, such as extremities when standing; in sacrum and scrotum when in lying position; or generalized in an infant; neck vein distension in child	Increased sodium and water retention result in increased systemic vascular pressure and fluid overload, which lead to edema; gravity determines the site of dependent edema
Weigh daily BID or as needed on same scale, at same time, and with same clothing	Weight gain from fluid retention is an early sign of fluid retention
Assess for plueral effusion by presence of dyspnea, tachypnea, crackles, orthopnea, acites; for hepatomegaly by measuring abdominal girth	Indication of gross fluid retention which causes impaired organ function (pulmonary and system venous congestion) is associated with some cardiac or renal conditions
Assess for oliguria, increased specific gravity, electrolyte imbalances	Indicates decreased renal perfusion, which activates the renin-angiotensin and aldosterone mechanism, resulting in water, sodium, and potassium retention
Administer diuretic therapy early in the day (for child), and monitor resulting diuresis by accurate I&O and weight	Diuretics prevent resaborption of water, sodium and potassium by tubules in the kidneys, resulting in excretion of excess
Note and document I&O (including losses from	Intake and output ratio should normally be 2:1 or

Interventions	Rationales
breathing and diaphoresis) and intake from all fluids IV or orally taken with medications and meals; if child not toilet trained, weigh diaper to calculate output at 1 gm = 1 ml	1-2 ml/kg/h
Restrict fluid intake by removing availability of fluids; schedule over 24 hours with most given during the day hours, using small cups and allowing older child to keep track of daily amounts	Supports need for additional loss of fluid based on age and using possible limit of 65 ml/kg/24 hrs as a guideline
Limit sodium intake by removing salt shaker, foods high in salt	Sodium intake should be limited to 2 gm/day or 1-2 mEq/kg/24 hr as a guideline
Maintain bedrest, and position and support any edematous body parts; change position q2h or as needed; provide sheepskin, eggcrate mattress	Protects and supports edematous parts from pressure and trauma

Information, Instruction, Demonstration

Interventions	Rationales
Instruct in taking weights, noting and reporting gains and losses; and in measuring I&O, and reporting excessive outputs from diuretic therapy or decreases in comparison or intake	Monitors weight to determine fluid accumulation and I&O to prevent imbalances (fluid overload or dehydration)
Instruct and assist to develop low sodium menus, low potassium diet if needed; avoid: adding salt to foods, snack foods, bacon, lunch meats for sodium restriction; and bananas, orange juice, legumes, whole grains for potassium restriction	Acquaints caretaker and child with foods to restrict or eliminate from diet

Interventions	Rationales
Instruct in correct administration of diuretic early in the day for a child; include amount, frequency, side effects, and amount of output to expect in relation to intake	Promotes excretion of fluid to prevent accumulation
Instruct and assist to schedule fluid intake over 24 hours, with major portion administered during day hours	Promotes compliance if fluids are restricted

Discharge or Maintenance Evaluation

- Absence of edema, signs, and symptoms associated with fluid accumulation in organs
- Blood pressure, pulse, respirations within normal parameters for age and gender
- I&O ratio remains within normal amounts
- Weight maintained with absence of sudden increases or decreases
- Correct administration of prescribed medications with expected results
- Compliance with reduced fluid intake, and optimal scheduling of sodium and potassium intake unless potassium depleted with use of diuretics

Altered tissue perfusion: cardiopulmonary, cerebral, gastrointestinal, renal, peripheral

Related to: Interruption of arterial or venous flow, exchange problems, hypovolemia

Defining characteristics: Cardiopulmonary — BP and pulse changes, dyspnea, tachypnea, changes in ABGs, cyanosis, changes in cardiac output, ventilation perfusion imbalances, crackles

Cerebral — hanges in mentation, restlessness, lethargy

Gastrointestinal — vomiting, inability to digest and absorb nutrients, gastric distention

Renal — oliguria, anuria, periorbital edema, electrolyte imbalance

Peripheral — skin cold, mottled, or pale; decreased peripheral pulses

Outcome Criteria

Optimal circulatory function, with blood flow and provision of oxygen and nutrients to all body organs

Interventions	Rationales
Assess organ functional abilities in relation to disease and its effect on a particular system	Interrelationships of systems cause an overlapping of signs and symptoms associated with tissue perfusion causing changes in elimination, oxygenation, nutrition, and mental function
Assess pulse, blood pressure, presence of peripheral pulses, capillary refill time, skin color and temperature; oxygenation saturation as measured by pulse oximetry; urinary output, mentation, anorexia, gastric distention	Provides information about cardiac output, which, if decreased, will reduce blood flow and tissue perfusion
Provide O_2 by hood, cannula, or face mask, depending on age and at rate determined by ABGs	Provides oxygen to organs for proper functioning
Administer vasodilator, cardiac glycoside	Promotes cardiac output and slows and strengthens heart rate for a more efficient pump action and increased return flow of blood to the heart and decreased heart workload
Position change q2-4h to avoid pressure on susceptible body parts, perform ROM if needed	Promotes circulation and prevents breakdown of tissue from further perfusion decreases associated with pressure
Position in Fowler's at height of comfort if respiratory status compromised by pulmonary perfusion	Decreases blood volume returning to heart by pooling of blood in lower dependent parts of the body

Information, Instruction, Demonstration

Interventions	Rationales
Inform of causes of decreased circulation and its effect on body organs	Promotes understanding of condition and risk to organ function
Demonstrate positions that enhance comfort and circulation, such as cardiac chair or infant seat, which alleviate pressure on body parts; use of pillows to maintain Fowler's position	Promotes comfort and prevents tissue breakdown
Inform to avoid tight and restrictive clothing, such as belts, elastic waists on pajamas, diapers	Constricts circulation

Discharge or Maintenance Evaluation

- Return of VS to normal ranges for age and gender
- Organ function within normal parameters
- Extremities warm, normal color with equal palpable pulses
- ABGs within normal levels
- Resolution of hypoxemia
- Urinary output at baseline levels
- Absence of abdominal distention with adequate nutritional intake

Cardiac Catheterization

Cardiac catheterization is the insertion of a flexible catheter through a blood vessel (most often the femoral vein) into the heart for diagnostic and therapeutic purposes. It is usually combined with angiography when radiopaque contrast media is injected through the catheter and circulation is visualized on fluoroscopic monitors. Catheterization allows measurement of blood gases and pressures within chambers and great vessels; measurement of cardiac output; and detection of anatomical defects such as septal defects or obstruction to blood flow. Therapeutic, or interventional, cardiac catheterizations use balloon angioplasty to correct such defects as stenotic valves or vessels, aortic obstruction (particularly recoarctation of the aorta), and closure of patent ductus arteriosus.

MEDICAL CARE

Chest x-ray: to determine condition of lung fields and cardiac size.
EKG: to detect any cardiac conduction changes or abnormalities.
Complete blood count: to provide baseline data and assure the child is not in an infectious state.
Blood coagulation time: to provide baseline data for comparison after the procedure.
Type and crossmatch: obtained for interventional cardiac catheterizations since risk of hemorrhage is greater; not usually obtained for diagnostic procedures.
Analgesics: precatheterization sedation given on-call to the catheterization laboratory: meperidine (Demerol) IM, PO, midazolam (Versed) PO, chloral hydrate, PO, PR.
Intravenous fluids: IV access is essential for additional medications during catheterization and may be started on the nursing unit or after arrival at the laboratory. Ringers lactate or 5% Ringers lactate are routine.

NURSING CARE PLANS

Essential nursing diagnoses and plans associated with this procedure:

Fluid volume deficit (222)

Related to: NPO status, blood loss during the catheterization, and diuretic effect of the contrast media
Defining characteristics: Elevated temperature, increased heart rate and respiratory rate, decreased blood pressure, decreased skin turgor, pallor, dry mucous membranes

Pain (31)

Related to: Percutaneous puncture site, numerous needle sticks from local anesthesia during procedure, positioning during procedure
Defining characteristics: Crying, guarding or refusal to move, verbal expression of pain, increased heart rate and respiratory rate. Cardiac catheterization is described by most children as painful, but there should be minimal pain postcatheterization (puncture site described as sore). Severe pain needs further investigation

SPECIFIC DIAGNOSES AND CARE PLANS

Anxiety of parent(s) and child

Related to: Invasive, painful procedure, risk of harm, separation from parents, fear of needles, and fear of exposure
Defining characteristics: Apprehension, expressed concern over impending procedure. In children: increased motor activity, inattention, withdrawal, crying, clinging to parent(s), verbal protests

Outcome Criteria

Reduced parental and child anxiety

Interventions	Rationales
Assess parent(s) and child's understanding of catheterization and any special fears	Provides information on parent(s) and child's knowledge, misunderstanding and particular concerns; sources of anxiety for the parent(s) include fear and uncertainty over the procedure, fear of complications, guilt and anxiety over the child's pain, and uncertainty over the outcome; for the child, fears may include: fear of

Interventions	Rationales
	mutilation and death, separation from parent(s), fear of the unknown (if the first catheterization), or remembered fear and pain (if repeat catheterization)
Allow expression of fears, clarify any misconceptions or lack of knowledge	Allows parent(s) and child to express feelings and provides them correct, complete information
Encourage the child to take a familiar, comforting item (stuffed animal, pillow, taped music, etc.) with them to the laboratory	A familiar object provides comfort and security to the child experiencing unfamiliar events and surroundings
Encourage parents to accompany child to the laboratory and be with child immediately following the procedure	Children cope with stressful events best when in the presence of their parent(s)

Information, Instruction, Demonstration

Interventions	Rationales
Emotionally prepare the child using age-appropriate guidelines; use concrete explanations just prior to an event for younger children. Include information on what the child will experience through all senses (sights, smells, sounds, feel)	Age-appropriate information given to the child allows for greater understanding and reassurance; young children process information through all their senses and need to know what to expect to better cope
Explain reason for each pre- and post-catheterization procedure	Knowledge of rationale for all treatments provides greater understanding and acceptance
Inform parent(s) that the child may temporarily act differently at home: may need to stay close to parent(s), have nightmares, and be less independent; encourage parent(s) to comfort and reassure child, to allow child to "re-live"	Stressful events may cause the child to need extra reassurance and may cause a temporary regression in development as the child reverts to comfortable, familiar "safe" activities; children, like adults, have a need to re-play stressful

Interventions	Rationales
the experience through stories or play, and to accept temporary set-backs in development	events in order to understand and cope, and this is often accomplished through play activities
Inform parent(s) about, and demonstrate how to care for the child's catheterization site; leave steri-strips in place until they fall off, do not place child in a tub bath for 3 days, immediately report any bleeding, bruising, redness or swelling to physician	Information provides parent(s) the knowledge they need to feel comfortable and confident in caring for their child

Discharge or Maintenance Evaluation

- Expresses understanding of the procedure and all treatments
- Comfortable in expressing feelings
- Parent(s) express decreased anxiety
- Parent(s) verbalize care of puncture site and when to seek help
- Parent(s) express understanding that their child may need more attention for awhile and that this is normal

Risk for injury

Related to: Altered hemostasis and trauma from percutaneous puncture
Defining characteristics: Increased apical heart rate and decreased blood pressure, bleeding from catheterization site, bruising, decreased level of consciousness, presence of occult or frank blood in urine and stools

Outcome Criteria

No serious injury will occur

Interventions	Rationales
Obtain baseline laboratory values from precatheterization assessment	Provides comparative data for postcatheterization assessment
Assess vital signs (apical HR, respiratory rate and BP) every 15 minutes X 4, every 30 minutes X 3 hours, then every 4 hours	Changes in vital signs may indicate blood loss, and 15 with internal bleeding may be the first indicator

Interventions	Rationales
Maintain pressure dressing on catheterization site and check every 30 minutes for bleeding	Constant pressure on site is needed to prevent site; no bleeding, even oozing, should occur; if bleeding does occur, apply continuous direct pressure 1" above puncture site and notify physician immediately
Maintain bedrest for 6 hours postcatheterization	Bedrest prevents strain to catheterization site which otherwise might precipitate bleeding; a 45-degree head elevation and slight bend at the knees is acceptable; young children may be held by parents: this is beneficial in decreasing agitation

Information, Instruction, Demonstration

Interventions	Rationales
Inform parent(s) and child of need for frequent assessments and for bedrest	Promotes understanding and cooperation
Encourage parent(s) and child to engage in quiet activities; i.e., reading stories, music	Allows for expression and interaction without physical stress; provides distraction for comfort
Encourage parent(s) of infants and young children to hold their children as an acceptable alternative to resting in bed	Allows parent(s) to touch and comfort their child in a more normal manner; this decreases the child's agitation, thereby promoting more rest
Instruct parent(s) to immediately report any sign of bleeding	Increases close monitoring of the site

Discharge or Maintenance Evaluation

- Pressure dressing removed after 24 hours
- Steri-strips over puncture site intact
- Puncture site clean and dry; no oozing, redness or swelling
- Vital signs are stable

- Parent(s) verbalize need to continue to observe for bleeding at home and to apply pressure and report to physician if bleeding occurs

Altered tissue perfusion: (Peripheral)

Related to: Clot formation at puncture site
Defining characteristics: Cool, mottled appearance of involved extremity, decreased or absent pulses distal to catheterization site, pain, tingling or numbness in involved extremity

Outcome Criteria

Affected extremity will be pink, warm and well perfused

Interventions	Rationales
Assess temperature, color and capillary refill of affected extremity and assess distal pulses by palpation and Doppler every 15 minutes X 4, every 30 minutes x 3 hours, then every 4 hours	Clots form at puncture site and the child is at risk of the clots seriously obstructing distal blood and resulting in tissue damage. An infant weighing less than 10 Kg. and children receiving interventional catheterizations are at greater risk for harmful clot formation. Assessing the extremity frequently for adequate perfusion allows for early intervention as needed
Maintain bedrest with extremity straight or slight bend in knee (10 degrees) for 6 hours	Bedrest and slight, or no flexion, allows for greater blood flow and decreases risk of further trauma which could increase clot formation
Apply warmth to the opposite extremity	Improves circulation without causing risk of increased bleeding at site

Information, Instruction, Demonstration

Interventions	Rationales
Inform parent(s) and child of need for frequent assessment of vital signs and need for bedrest with extremity extension	Promotes understanding and cooperation

Discharge or Maintenance Evaluation

- Involved extremity warm, normal color, pulses present and equal
- No complaints of any pain, numbness or tingling in extremity
- Able to bear weight on affected extremity
- Child should be sponge-bathed or take showers (if age appropriate) for bathing for 3 days to prevent infection of site

Hyperthermia

Related to: Reaction to radiopaque contrast material used in catheterization
Defining characteristics: Elevated body temperature (38.0-39.0 degrees C) within a few hours of procedure

Outcome Criteria

Return to normal body temperature 8-12 hours after catheterization

Interventions	Rationales
Continue IV fluids while child is drowsy, and when fully awake, encourage PO intake	Increased fluid intake promotes more rapid excretion of the dye
Assess body temperature every hour X 6 hours and then routine	Provides information on which to take action
Administer age-appropriate doses to decrease fever with acetaminophen every 4 hours	Acetaminophen will help decrease fever and associated discomfort
Record hourly I&O	Assesses routine adequacy of fluid intake and elimination

Information, Instruction, Demonstration

Interventions	Rationales
Instruct parent(s) to encourage PO fluids; ask parent(s) about child's fluid preferences	Involving parent(s) in care increases the likelihood of achieving the goal; consulting parent(s) about preferences results in offering the most appropriate choices

Discharge or Maintenance Evaluation

- Body temperature normal
- Tolerating regular diet well
- Parent(s) verbalize need to report any increase in temperature to physician

Congenital Heart Defects

Congenital heart defects are abnormal malformations of the heart that involve the septums, valves, and large arteries. They are classified as acyanotic or cyanotic defects. Acyanotic defects occur when a left-to-right shunt is present allowing a mixture of oxygenated and unoxygenated blood to enter the systemic circulation. The most common consequences of these defects in children are growth retardation and congestive heart failure (CHF), although cyanosis may also occur.

Common cyanotic defects include tetralogy of Fallot and transposition of great vessels. Tetralogy of Fallot involves four defects that include pulmonic stenosis (PS), ventricular septal defect (VSD), right ventricular hypertrophy, and an aorta that overrides the VSD. Transposition of great vessels is a condition in which the aorta arises from the right ventricle instead of the left ventricle, and the pulmonary artery arises from the left ventricle instead of the right ventricle, causing a reversal of the normal position of these arteries.

Acyanotic defects include coarctation of aorta, patent ductus arteriosus and ventricular septal defect. Coarctation of the aorta is the narrowing of the aorta proximal to the ductus arteriosus (preductal), distal to the ductus arteriosus (postductal) or level with the ductus arteriosus (auxtaductal). The position of the narrowing during fetal development determines circulation to the lower body and development of collateral circulation. Patent ductus arteriosus is the failure of the structure needed for fetal circulation to close after birth. Ventricular septal defect is the incomplete development of the septum that separates the right and left ventricles, and it often accompanies other defects.

Congenital heart defects vary in severity, symptoms, and complications, many of which depend on the age of the infant/child and the size of the defect. Treatment may include management with medications, or open heart surgery to repair or resect, or to temporarily correct the defect until the child is older and growth takes place.

MEDICAL CARE

Diuretics: chlorothiazide (Diuril), spironolactone (Aldactone) PO, or furosemide (Lasrx) PO or IV, depending on acuity of condition and need to promote fluid excretion by decreasing reabsorption of water, potassium, and sodium by the kidneys .

Cardiac glycosides: digoxin (Lanoxin) tablets or elixir PO or IV-form; administered to prevent or treat congestive heart failure resulting from congenital heart defect by increasing the force of and decreasing the rate of cardiac contractions.

Antibiotics: penicillin G potassium (Pentids solution or tablets) PO, or erythromycin (Ilosone tablets, chewables, suspension) PO if patient is penicillin-sensitive as prophylaxis for bacterial endocarditis.

Prostaglandin synthesis inhibitors: indomethacin (Indocin) IV to close PDA.

Prostaglandin hormones: alprostadil (Prostin VR Pediatric) IV to maintain open PDA when needed for blood flow.

Electrolytes: potassium chloride tablet (Klorvess), elixir (Pan-Kloride) PO as potassium replacement with use of diuretic therapy.

Chest x-ray: reveals cardiomegaly involving left side of heart, no enlargement depending on defect or cardiomegaly involving right ventricle, increased pulmonary blood flow or congested lungs, egg-shaped heart and narrowed mediastinum.

Electrocardiography (ECG): reveals abnormal changes associated with right ventricular and/or atrial hypertrophy, possible abnormal changes associated with left ventricular hypertrophy in older children, may not reveal any abnormality depending on specific defect; identifies arrhythmias.

Echocardiography (contrast, two-dimensional or real time, M-mode): reveals cardiomegaly, atrial or ventricular changes and location and size, great vessel location and size, valve function and any abnormalities or obstructions of the valves, increase in left atrial to aortic ratio, location of shunting in heart.

Doppler: reveals circulation abnormalities and congested lung areas, done with or without echocardiography.

Cardiac catheterization: reveals abnormalities in communication between chambers, oxygen, and pressure levels in the chambers; location and number of septal defects.

Angiography: reveals cardiac defect by revealing detailed heart structure.

Electrolyte panel: reveals possible decreased potassium and increased sodium.

Complete blood count (CBC): increased WBC with infection, decreased Hgb and Hct with anemia, increased RBC, decreased platelet count.

Prothrombin or partial thromboplastin times (PT, APPT): reveals bleeding tendency and evaluates components of the blood-clotting mechanisms.

Blood urea nitrogen (BUN): reveals increase when heart is not able to perfuse kidneys.

Arterial blood gases (ABG): reveals decreased pH and PO_2 and increased PCO_2 resulting from changes in pulmonary blood flow.

Surgical shunt: increases blood flow to the lungs for severely hypoxic newborns creating an artificial connection between the right or left subclavian artery and the pulmonary artery on the same side (modified Blalock-Taussig shunt).

NURSING CARE PLANS

Essential nursing diagnoses and plans associated with these conditions:

Decreased cardiac output (3)

Related to: Structural factors of congenital heart defect
Defining characteristics: Variations in hemodynamic readings (hypertension, bounding, pulses, tachycardia), ECG changes, arrhythmias, fatigue, dyspnea, oliguria, cyanosis or absence of cyanosis, murmur, decreased peripheral pulses, widened pulse pressure, squatting or knee-chest position

Ineffective breathing pattern (45)

Related to: Decreased energy and fatigue, pulmonary complications
Defining characteristics: Dyspnea, hypoxia (blue baby), tachypnea, abnormal ABGs, cyanosis

Altered nutrition: less than body requirements (168)

Related to: Inability to ingest, digest, or absorb nutrients because of biological factors
Defining characteristics: Poor feeding, fatigue, slow growth, lack of interest in food, prolonged impaired cardiac function, decreasing perfusion to gastrointestinal organs

Altered growth and development (423)

Related to: Effects of acute or chronic illness or disability
Defining characteristics: Altered physical growth, delay or difficulty in performing motor or social skills typical of age, dependence and isolation

SPECIFIC DIAGNOSES AND CARE PLANS

Activity intolerance

Related to: Generalized weakness
Defining characteristics: Presence of circulatory/ respiratory problem, verbal complaint of fatigue or weakness, needs to rest after short period of play
Related to: Imbalance between oxygen supply and demand
Defining characteristics: Abnormal heart rate or blood pressure response to activity, exertional dyspnea

Outcome Criteria

Ability to maintain activity at an optimal level within limitations imposed by symptoms of the defect

Interventions	Rationales
Assess level of fatigue, ability to perform ADL and other activities in relation to severity of condition	Provides information about energy reserves and response to activity
Assess dyspnea on exertion, skin color changes during rest and when active	Indicates hypoxia and increased oxygen need during energy expenditure
Allow for rest periods between care, disturb only when necessary for care and procedures	Promotes rest and conserves energy
Avoid allowing infant to cry for long periods of time, use soft nipple for feeding; cross-cut nipple, requiring less energy for infant to feed; if unable for infant to ingest sufficient calories by mouth, gavage-feed infant	Conserves energy
Provide toys and games for quiet play and diversion appropriate for age of child, allow to limit own activities as much as possible	Promotes growth, diversion, and physical and mental development

Interventions	Rationales
Provide optimal environmental temperature; when bathing infant, expose only the area being bathed and keep the infant covered to prevent heat loss	Avoids hot or cold extremes which increase oxygen and energy needs

Information, Instruction, Demonstration

Interventions	Rationales
Explain need to conserve energy and encourage rest	Avoids fatigue
Inform of activity or exercise restrictions and to set own limits for exercise and activity	Prevents fatigue while engaging in activities as nearly normal as possible
Inform to request assistance when needed for daily activities	Prevents overtiring and fatigue
Assist to plan for care and rest schedule	Provides for rest and prevents overexertion, minimizes energy expenditure

Discharge or Maintenance Evaluation

- Controls activities that are fatiguing
- Maintains rest and activity schedule
- Engages in activities appropriate for age and energy level

Risk for infection

Related to: Chronic illness
Defining characteristics: Debilitated condition, IV-site contamination, susceptibility to bacterial endocarditis, immobility, change in VS

Outcome Criteria

Absence of infection

Interventions	Rationales
Assess temperature, IV site if present, increased WBC, increased pulse and respirations	Provides information indicating potential infection

Interventions	Rationales
Provide adequate rest and nutritional needs for age	Protects against potential infection by increasing body resistance and defenses
Wash hands before giving care	Prevents transmission of microorganisms to infant/child
Avoid allowing those with infections to have contact with infant/child	Prevents transmission of infectious agents to infant/child with compromised defense
Administer antibiotic therapy	Preventive measure administered as prophylaxis
Use sterile technique for IV maintenance if present	Prevents contamination, which causes infection

Information, Instruction, Demonstration

Interventions	Rationales
Inform to avoid contact with those in family or friends that have an infection	Infections are easily transmitted to a debilitated child
Instruct parent(s) and child in personal hygiene practices (rest, nutrition, activity, bathroom for elimination, bathing)	Prevents reduced defenses or exposure to possible contaminants

Discharge or Maintenance Evaluation

- Measures taken to prevent exposure to infection
- Medical asepsis, personal hygiene measures taken for daily care
- Correct administration of antibiotic administration when needed to prevent complication of bacterial endocarditis
- Reports changes in VS, temperature to physician

Risk for injury

Related to: Internal factor of cardiac function from congenital defects and medication administration
Defining characteristics: Digoxin toxicity (vomiting, dysrhythmia), hypokalemia (muscle weakness, hypotension, irritability, drowsiness), congestive heart

failure (tachycardia, dyspnea fatigue, restlessness, cough, cyanosis, orthopnea, edema, weight gain, neck vein distention, decreased BP, cardiomegaly), hypoxemia, possible cardiac surgery

Outcome Criteria

Recognition and reporting of signs and symptoms of complications associated with congenital heart defect

Interventions	Rationales
Assess for risk of drug toxicity, cardiac complication of heart failure	Early identification of signs and symptoms of complications allows preventive measures and adjustments to be made
Assess for possibility of open heart surgery, need for diagnostic tests and procedures	Allows for preparation and support of parent(s) and infant/child
Administer digoxin or indomethacin in correct dosages, check dosages, take apical pulse for a full minute before administering digoxin, assess for drug responses	Promotes safe administration of cardiotonic to decrease and strengthen heart rate (digoxin), or to promote closing of ductus (indomethacin)
Assist and support family's feelings and decision regarding surgery	Provides needed support to allay anxiety and promote caring attitude

Information, Instruction, Demonstration

Interventions	Rationales
Instruct in administration of cardiotonic, taking apical pulse, when to withhold (less than 70-80 in child and 90-100 in infant), to notify physician of low pulse or irregular pulse, signs of toxicity	Ensures safe and accurate administration of cardiac glycoside
Prepare parent(s) and child (use play doll) for diagnostic procedures and/or surgery; should be extensive, consistent, and comprehensive, including surgical procedure to be performed	Assists in allaying anxiety and understanding that diagnostic tests are usually done before surgery

Interventions	Rationales
and expected results, prognosis and whether corrective, palliative, temporary, or permanent	
Inform of actions to take if child becomes cyanotic (knee-chest or squatting position, elevating head and chest), when to call physician	Encourages calmness during attack and teaches actions that will relieve episode and associated fear

Discharge or Maintenance Evaluation

- Correctly administers prescribed medications with absence of side effects
- Verbalizes signs and symptoms of complications to report
- Takes apical pulse correctly
- Expresses feelings regarding possible need for surgery
- Intervenes to relieve cyanotic episodes
- Verbalizes understanding of procedures and tests to be done

Ineffective family coping: Compromised

Related to: Situational and developmental crises of family and child

Defining characteristics: Family expresses concern and fear about infant/child's disease and condition, displays protective behavior disproportionate to need to grow and develop, chronic anxiety and possible hospitalization and surgery

Outcome Criteria

Decreased anxiety and increased development of coping skills with infant/child's illness and changes in family processes

Interventions	Rationales
Assess anxiety level, erratic behaviors (anger, tension, disorganization), perception of crisis situation	Information affecting ability of family to cope with infant/child's cardiac condition
Assess coping methods used and effectiveness	Identifies need to develop new coping skills if existing methods are ineffective in changing behaviors exhibited

Interventions	Rationales
Assess level of anxiety need for information and support	Provides information about need for interventions to relieve anxiety and concern
Encourage expression of feelings and provide factual information about infant/child	Reduces anxiety and enhances family's understanding of condition
Assist in identifying and using techniques to cope with and solve problems and gain control over the situation	Provides support for problem solving and management of situation
Provide anticipatory guidance for crisis resolution and allow for grieving process	Assists family in adapting to situation and developing new coping mechanisms

Information, Instruction, Demonstration

Interventions	Rationales
Inform and reinforce appropriate coping behaviors, support family decisions	Promotes behavior change and adaptation to care of infant/child
Inform that overprotective behaviors may hinder growth and development during infancy/childhood	Knowledge will enhance family understanding of condition and of adverse effects of behaviors
Inform of need to maintain health of family members and social contacts	Chronic anxiety, fatigue, and isolation as result of infant care will affect health and care capabilities of family
Inform of disease process and behaviors, physical effects, and symptoms of condition	Relieves anxiety of parents when they know what to expect
Clarify any misinformation and answer questions regarding disease process	Prevents unnecessary anxiety resulting from inaccurate knowledge or beliefs
Inform parent(s) to include ill infant/child in family activities rather than family revolving around needs of infant/child	Promotes normal growth and development of family and infant/child

Interventions	Rationales
Inform to maintain consistent behavior limits and modification techniques	Prevents behavioral problems and child control over family, which interfere with child's growth and family relationships
Instruct parent(s) in nutritional and activity needs and/or limitations and approaches that will assist in establishing an effective pattern	Assists in coping with effects and special needs of infant/child with cardiac defect

Discharge or Maintenance Evaluation

- Optimal health of family members, caretaker maintained
- Statements that anxiety reduced and coping techniques utilized effectively
- Maintenance of social contacts of family
- Reduction of overprotective behaviors in infant/child care
- Statements of adjustment and progressive adaptation to special physical and behavioral needs
- Ability of family to adopt a positive view of infant/child's condition and need for normal growth and development
- Appropriate growth and development advances for age group
- Uses behavior modification techniques

Congenital Heart Diseases

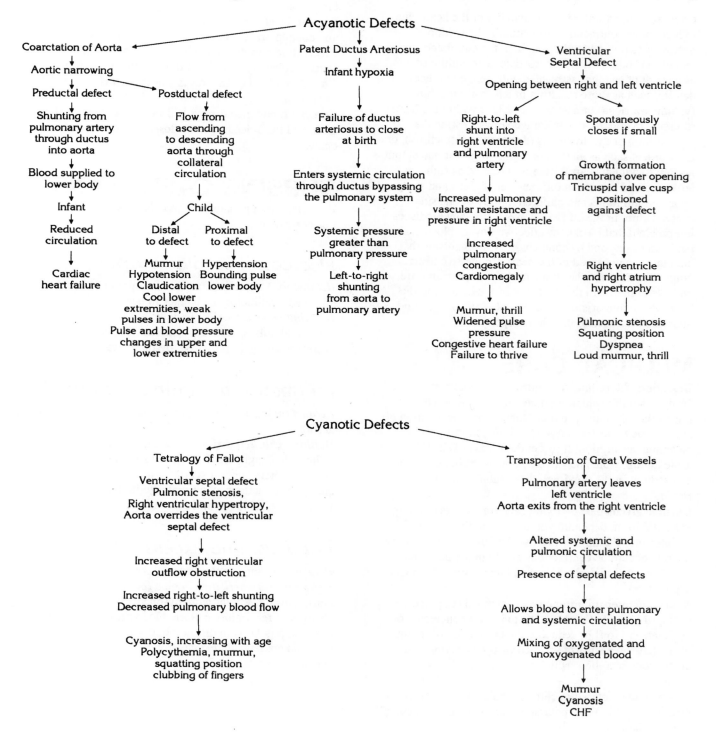

Acyanotic Defects

Coarctation of Aorta
↓
Aortic narrowing
↓
Preductal defect → Postductal defect
↓
Shunting from pulmonary artery through ductus into aorta
↓
Blood supplied to lower body
↓
Infant
↓
Reduced circulation
↓
Cardiac heart failure

Postductal defect
↓
Flow from ascending to descending aorta through collateral circulation
↓
Child
↓
Distal to defect / Proximal to defect
↓
Murmur / Hypertension
Hypotension / Bounding pulse
Claudication / lower body
Cool lower extremities, weak pulses in lower body
Pulse and blood pressure changes in upper and lower extremities

Patent Ductus Arteriosus
↓
Infant hypoxia
↓
Failure of ductus arteriosus to close at birth
↓
Enters systemic circulation through ductus bypassing the pulmonary system
↓
Systemic pressure greater than pulmonary pressure
↓
Left-to-right shunting from aorta to pulmonary artery

Ventricular Septal Defect
↓
Opening between right and left ventricle
↓
Right-to-left shunt into right ventricle and pulmonary artery
↓
Increased pulmonary vascular resistance and pressure in right ventricle
↓
Increased pulmonary congestion Cardiomegaly
↓
Murmur, thrill
Widened pulse pressure
Congestive heart failure
Failure to thrive

Spontaneously closes if small
↓
Growth formation of membrane over opening
Tricuspid valve cusp positioned against defect
↓
Right ventricle and right atrium hypertrophy
↓
Pulmonic stenosis
Squating position
Dyspnea
Loud murmur, thrill

Cyanotic Defects

Tetralogy of Fallot
↓
Ventricular septal defect
Pulmonic stenosis,
Right ventricular hypertropy,
Aorta overrides the ventricular septal defect
↓
Increased right ventricular outflow obstruction
↓
Increased right-to-left shunting
Decreased pulmonary blood flow
↓
Cyanosis, increasing with age
Polycythemia, murmur,
squatting position
clubbing of fingers

Transposition of Great Vessels
↓
Pulmonary artery leaves left ventricle
Aorta exits from the right ventricle
↓
Altered systemic and pulmonic circulation
↓
Presence of septal defects
↓
Allows blood to enter pulmonary and systemic circulation
↓
Mixing of oxygenated and unoxygenated blood
↓
Murmur
Cyanosis
CHF

Congestive Heart Failure

Congestive heart failure is the inability of the heart, due to ineffective contractions, to maintain the workload necessary to pump blood throughout the circulatory system of the body. In children, cardiac heart failure occurs as a result of changes associated with congenital heart defects, such as those resulting in left-to-right shunts (volume overload) or obstructive lesions within the heart (pressure overload), of cardiomyopathy affecting the myocardium or dysrhythmias (decreased contractility), or of disorders such as anemia or sepsis (high cardiac output needs). In adults, heart failure is classified as right- or left-sided and presents a different set of signs and symptoms, but in infants and children, failure of one side causes failure in the other side. Normally, any predisposing problem that blocks the effective flow of blood causes the heart to respond by compensatory mechanisms that maintain the workload of the heart. Congestive heart failure occurs when the compensatory mechanisms are not able to maintain the workload of the heart, and the body tissues and organs are deprived of the oxygen and nutrients they need to function properly.

MEDICAL CARE

Diuretics: chlorothiazide (Diuril), spironolactone (Aldactone) PO, which promotes fluid excretion by acting on the distal and proximal tubules or blocks action of aldosterone to decrease water, sodium chloride, and potassium absorption; furosemide (Lasix) PO or IV for acute failure, which acts to block reabsorption of water and sodium in the proximal, distal tubules and loop of Henle.

Cardiac glycosides: digoxin (Lanoxin) tablets or elixir PO or IV form, depending on treatment, for acute or maintenance therapy to increase the force of and decrease the rate of cardiac contractions and to dilate pulmonary blood vessels; relieves anxiety and restlessness from CNS depression.

Renin-angiotensin antagonists: captopril (Capoten), enalapril Maleate (Vasotec) PO to inhibit conversion of angiotensin I to II by reducing the production of renin; ultimately the result is to reduce vasoconstriction and aldosterone secretion, which reduce the work of the heart.

Electrolytes: potassium chloride tablet (Klorvess), elixir (Pan-Kloride) PO as a potassium replacement with use of diuretic therapy.

Analgesics/sedatives: morphine sulfate SC or IV to relax smooth muscle.

Chest x-ray: reveals cardiac dilatation and hypertrophy.

Electrocardiography: reveals ventricular hypertrophy and arrhythmias.

Echocardiography: reveals abnormal valve function via ultrasound.

Digoxin level: reveals therapeutic level of 0.8-2.0 mcg/L and done to prevent toxicity and regulate dosage.

Electrolyte panel: reveals hypokalemia, which will cause cardiac arrhythmias if diuretic therapy given.

Complete blood count: reveals decreased Hgb and Hct in anemia.

Arterial blood gases: reveals decreased PO_2 and pH and increased PCO_2 leading to acidosis with pulmonary. changes.

NURSING CARE PLANS

Essential nursing diagnoses and plans associated with this condition:

Decreased cardiac output (3)

Related to: Mechanical factors of alterations in preload, afterload, and inotropic changes in heart
Defining characteristics: Fatigue; oliguria; decreased peripheral pulses; pale, cool extremities; tachycardia; decreased BP; gallop rhythm, dyspnea, crackles

Ineffective breathing pattern (45)

Related to: Decreased lung expansion, pulmonary congestion
Defining characteristics: Dyspnea, tachypnea, orthopnea, cough, nasal flaring, respiratory depth changes, altered chest excursion, use of accessory muscles with retractions, abnormal arterial blood gases, wheezing, crackles, grunting, cyanosis

Fluid volume excess (5)

Related to: Compromised regulatory mechanisms
Defining characteristics: Edema (periorbital, peripheral), effusion, weight gain, dyspnea, orthognea, crackles, changes in respiratory pattern, blood pressure changes, oliguria, jugular vein distention, hepatomegaly, restlessness and anxiety, altered electrolytes, change in mental status

Altered nutrition: less than body requirements (168)

Related to: Internal factor of illness
Defining characteristics: Interrupted sleep, fatigue, lethargy, restlessness, irritability

Risk for fluid volume deficit (222)

Related to: Medication (diuretics)
Defining characteristics: Output greater than intake, weight loss, hypokalemia, hypernatremia

Altered tissue perfusion: cardiopulmonary, peripheral (6)

Related to: Hypervolemia, prolonged cardiac failure
Defining characteristics: Edema, dyspnea, change in color, temperature of extremities (mottled, cold), decreased peripheral pulses, effusion, changes in BP, tachypnea, orthopnea, tachycardia, cough

SPECIFIC DIAGNOSES AND CARE PLANS

Anxiety

Related to: Threat of death, threat of or change in health status, threat of change in environment (hospitalization)
Defining characteristics: Parent-increased apprehension that condition might worsen into life-threatening situation, increased concern and worry about possible hospitalization, increased tension and uncertainty, chronic worry. Child — unhappy and sad attitude; withdrawn or aggressive behavior; somatic and fatigue complaints; failure to thrive and participate in school, play, or social activities

Outcome Criteria

Reduced parental and child anxiety as adjustments to changes in life style and adaptation to underlying condition occur

Interventions	Rationales
Assess level and manifestations of anxiety in parent(s) and child	Provides information needed for interventions and clues to severity of anxiety

Interventions	Rationales
Allow expression of fears and concerns and time to ask questions about disorder and what to expect	Provides opportunity to vent feelings and secure information to reduce anxiety
Provide supportive, nonjudgmental environment and individualized, consistent care	Promotes trust and reduces anxiety
Hold and cuddle infant	Promotes comfort and security
Inform parent(s) and child of all procedures and treatments, anticipate needs	Relieves anxiety caused by fear of the unknown
Allow parent(s) to stay and open visitation and telephone communication; encourage to participate in care and to plan care similar to usual home patterns	Reduces anxiety by allowing presence and involvement in care and provides familiar persons and routine for child
Keep parent(s) informed of changes in condition, progress made	Promotes understanding and reduces anxiety about whether child is improving

Information, Instruction, Demonstration

Interventions	Rationales
Explain why hospitalization became necessary	Promotes understanding of disorder and underlying disease that causes this complication
Clarify any misinformation with simple, understandable language and honesty	Promotes knowledge and prevents anxiety caused by inaccurate information or beliefs
Instruct in signs and symptoms indicating possible heart failure (fatigue, tachycardia, anorexia, dyspnea, tachypnea) and measures to take	Provides information of what might be expected and what to report in order to allay anxiety

Discharge or Maintenance Evaluation

- Verbalizes that anxiety reduced by parent(s)
- Expresses increased comfort in caring for ill child/infant

- Symptoms of anxiety in the child decreasing or controlled

Activity intolerance

Related to: Imbalance between oxygen supply and demand
Defining characteristics: Abnormal heart rate or blood pressure response to activity, exertional dyspnea, fatigue, weakness, respiratory/circulatory problem

Outcome Criteria

Maintenance of activity within limitations imposed by condition

Interventions	Rationales
Assess level of fatigue, responses to activity	Provides information about change in vital signs and energy level
Allow for rest periods between care, disturb only when necessary and then perform care and treatments during one period of time	Promotes rest, conserves energy and reduces heart workload
Avoid allowing infant to cry for long periods of time; use soft nipple with large opening for feeding and feed frequently, slowly, and in small amounts	Conserves energy and prevents fatigue
Provide meals for child frequently and in smaller amounts	Conserves energy
Provide toys and quiet, age-appropriate play	Allows for play without depleting energy reserves
Provide optimal environmental temperature	Extremes of temperature increase oxygen and energy needs, which increase work of heart

Information, Instruction, Demonstration

Interventions	Rationales
Explain reason for need to conserve energy and encourage rest	Promotes compliance with activity restrictions
Inform of activities allowed, type of play recommended, and rationale	Prevents fatigue while still allowing activities as near normal as possible
Assist in planning for rest and activity schedule	Provides for rest, prevents overexertion and symptoms, minimizes energy expenditure
Inform of continued stimulation-type activities (visual, auditory, tactile, mental, and physical)	Promotes normal growth and development

Discharge or Maintenance Evaluation

- Controls activities that are fatiguing and cause symptoms
- Maintains rest and activity schedule
- Engages in stimulating activities appropriate for age and energy level

Knowledge deficit of parent(s), child

Related to: Lack of information about disorder and treatments/care
Defining characteristics: Verbalization of need for information about disease, medications, dietary restrictions

Outcome Criteria

Adequate knowledge for compliance of treatments to reduce workload of heart

Interventions	Rationales
Assess knowledge of disease, causes and methods to prevent or control condition, willingness and interest to implement care to reduce work of heart, ability and readiness to learn	Promotes plan of instruction that is realistic to ensure compliance of medical regimen, prevents repetition of information
Provide information about disorder causes and risk factors; use clear, understandable language, pictures, pamphlets, models, video tapes, anatomical doll in teaching	Ensures understanding and aids in reinforcement of learning

Interventions	Rationales
Instruct and assist in planning menus that include sodium restriction, fluids if prescribed, additional calories	Allows input, control over planning for sodium, and fluid restriction may be needed to prevent fluid retention, additional calories provided for higher metabolic needs
Instruct in administration of cardiac glycosides and diuretics, including dosage, frequency, route, side effects to report, expected results	Ensures correct administration of drugs to prevent heart failure and drug toxicity
Instruct in taking pulse for 1 minute and allow return demonstration	Apical pulse taken before administration of cardiac glycoside
Inform of effects of disorder on infant/child (growth and physical development)	Disorder slows growth and development for age
Inform of need to report infection or changes in breathing, pulse, irritability, restlessness, edema, temperature (increase), or weight	Reduction in body defenses predisposes to infectious process, signs and symptoms reported to prevent progressive heart failure

Discharge or Maintenance Evaluation

- Verbalizes knowledge of disease process, causes and risk factor
- Adapts and complies with dietary, fluid restrictions
- Caretaker and family support for medical regimen
- Correctly administers medications and verbalizes side effects and symptoms of digitalis toxicity, hypokalemia
- Verbalizes signs and symptoms of congestive heart failure and importance of reporting to physician

Congestive Heart Failure

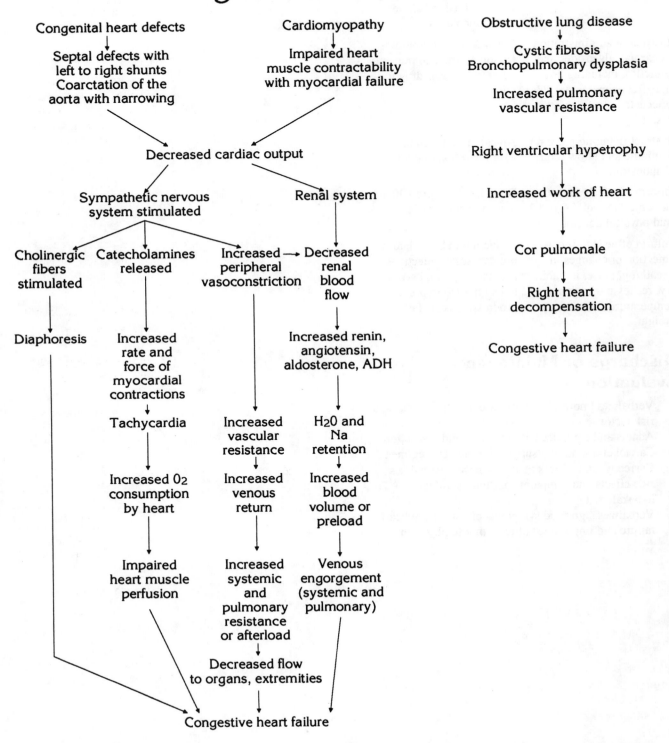

Congenital heart defects

Septal defects with
left to right shunts
Coarctation of the
aorta with narrowing

Cardiomyopathy

Impaired heart
muscle contractability
with myocardial failure

Obstructive lung disease

Cystic fibrosis
Bronchopulmonary dysplasia

Increased pulmonary
vascular resistance

Right ventricular hypetrophy

Increased work of heart

Cor pulmonale

Right heart
decompensation

Congestive heart failure

Decreased cardiac output

Sympathetic nervous
system stimulated

Renal system

Cholinergic
fibers
stimulated

Catecholamines
released

Increased → Decreased
peripheral   renal
vasoconstriction blood
flow

Diaphoresis

Increased
rate and
force of
myocardial
contractions

Tachycardia

Increased O_2
consumption
by heart

Impaired
heart muscle
perfusion

Increased
vascular
resistance

Increased
venous
return

Increased
systemic
and
pulmonary
resistance
or afterload

Decreased flow
to organs, extremities

Increased renin,
angiotensin,
aldosterone, ADH

H_2O and
Na
retention

Increased
blood
volume or
preload

Venous
engorgement
(systemic and
pulmonary)

Congestive heart failure

Dysrhythmias

Dysrhythmias is a term used to describe cardiac rate and rhythm abnormalities or irregularities. They may originate from any site in the heart, as any cell in the myocardium has the ability to discharge an impulse. In children, they may occur as the result of cardiac surgery or congenital heart defects and are less common than in adults. Treatment consists of medications, and in some cases, a permanent pacemaker to manage conduction disturbances in the heart.

MEDICAL CARE

Antiarrhythmics: verapamil hydrochloride (Isoptin) PO or IV, depending on acuteness of condition, to slow SA and AV node conduction in tachyarrhythmias.
Cardiac glycosides: digoxin (Lanoxin) PO to slow and strengthen heart beat.
Chest x-ray: reveals correct placement of pacemaker catheter.
Electrocardiography: reveals deviations suggesting arrhythmias that assist in diagnosis of cardiac conditions and provide rhythm strips to monitor pacer function; test to determine pharmacologic treatment of dysrhythmias; similar to cardiac catheterization, which artificially induces a dysrhythmia and administers different drugs IV to see which will terminate the dysrhythmia.
Transesophageal recording: stimulates heart to record any dysrhythmias.

NURSING CARE PLANS

Decreased cardiac output (3)

Related to: Electrical factors of alteration in rate, rhythm, and conduction
Defining characteristics: Arrhythmias, ECG changes, changes in apical and peripheral pulses, failing batteries or break in pacemaker catheter

SPECIFIC DIAGNOSES AND CARE PLANS

Risk for infection

Related to: Inadequate primary defenses (broken skin)
Defining characteristics: Redness, heat, pain, and swelling at site of pacemaker insertion, cardiac electrode site, or IV site if present

Outcome Criteria

Absence of infectious process at site of permanent generator electrodes or infusion

Interventions	Rationales
Assess site of generator insertion in subcutaneous pocket in chest for warmth, redness, pain, and drainage	Indicates infectious process at pacemaker site
Assess IV site for edema, infiltration, redness, and warmth if IV present	Indicates phlebitis or dislodgement of infusion catheter for administration of fluids and IV medications
Assess skin under electrodes for erythema, irritation, or rash if cardiac monitoring present	Infection can result from skin irritation and breakdown caused by electrode gel and adhesive pads
Maintain sterile technique for dressing changes, IV site changes, and care of any breaks in skin	Prevents contamination by pathogenic microorganisms
Change IV site and tubing every 24-72 hours according to protocol	Prevents bacterial growth and prolonged irritation to vein
Gently wash and dry electrode sites when removed and before reapplication	Prevents prolonged irritation to skin
Administer antibiotic therapy	Prevents irritation to vein and phlebitis

Information, Instruction, Demonstration

Interventions	Rationales
Observation of pacemaker site and reporting signs and symptoms of infection	Provides for prompt treatment if infection is present
Taking oral or axillary temperature	Monitors for infection
Technique for care of site during and after healing	Maintains sterility or cleanliness of site
Observation of pacemaker site and reporting signs and symptoms of infection	Provides for prompt treatment if infection is present

Discharge or Maintenance Evaluation

- Site(s) free of inflammation and infection, intact and healing
- Verbalization of signs and symptoms to report
- Daily assessment and care of site

Risk for injury

Related to: Internal regulatory function
Defining characteristics: Negative response to medications (digoxin toxicity), pacemaker or catheter malfunction, failure of pacemaker to capture or sense arrhythmias

Outcome Criteria

Proper functioning and maintenance of pacemaker system with pulse rate, rhythm, and duration occurring as programmed; digoxin level maintained at therapeutic level; electrolytes within normal ranges

Interventions	Rationales
Assess pulse, changes in cardiac output, changes in ECG	Decreases in pulse and cardiac output indicate battery depletion; ECG changes may indicate loss of capture, arrhythmias from malpositioning of pacing catheter
Assess digoxin, potassium and calcium levels	Electrolyte imbalance may result in arrhythmias, too much or too little dosages, or cardiotonic causes arrhythmias
Monitor effect of antiarrhythmics by taking pulse rate and rhythm; carefully administer correct dosage at correct rate	Ensures desired effect of medications
Troubleshoot for sensing of capture failure	Prevents pacemaker failure or corrects functional problems
Provide ROM to shoulder if appropriate and ordered	Prevents loss of function of shoulder on side of pacemaker insertion

Information, Instruction, Demonstration

Interventions	Rationales
Describe to parent(s) and child the device and its parts, how it functions, and type of lead used; use manufacturer's instruction pamphlet, drawing, and models	Provides understanding of type and function of pacemaker; parts include the generator with the battery and electronic circuitry, which produces the impulse to the heart, and a lead, which operates as a conductor of the impulse to the heart; lead may be epicardial or transvenous
Method of taking pulse (apical) for 1 minute	Monitors effect of medication and changes to report
Procedure for transmission of ECG by telephone	Transmits ECG strips by phone to monitor for dysrhythmias, pacemaker function, and battery depletion
Activity limitations, types of activities to avoid that might affect pacemaker function (contact sports)	Activity tolerance usually improved with pacemaker
Importance of wearing identification with pacemaker type, site of insertion, physician name and number	Provides information for emergency care
Inform to avoid electrical interferences, microwave ovens, and to request hand scanner at airports	Some pacemakers are still affected by electrical interference of current leakage
Inform of importance of follow-up visits to physician	Ensures monitoring of condition and pacemaker function
Instruct in administration of antiarrhythmics; cardiac glycosides; diuretics, including name, actions, dosage, frequency, side effects, how to take, expected results	Ensures proper dosage, frequency, and knowledge of when to report side effects
Instruct in cardiopulmonary resuscitation	May be needed as an emergency measure to maintain normal rhythm

Discharge or Maintenance Evaluation

- Reports to and visits physician as recommended
- Checks pulse daily, states acceptable variations in pulse
- Correct administration of medications and when to withhold dose
- Wears or carries identification information
- Properly grounds all electrical equipment; avoids exposure to electrical interferences if necessary
- Sends transtelephone rhythm strips periodically or as directed
- Reviews manufacturer's instruction guide, states symptoms to report
- Uses home cardiac monitor correctly; applies electrodes, settings, alarms
- Demonstrates cardiopulmonary resuscitation correctly
- Participates in activities within identified limitations

Dysrhythmias

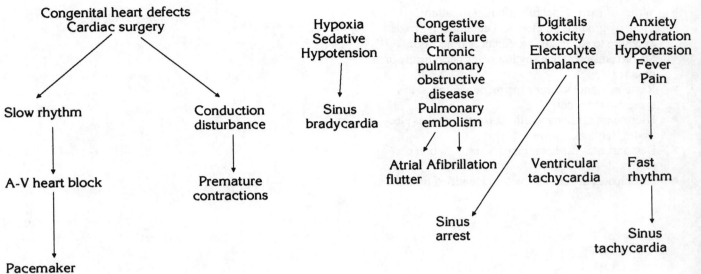

Congenital heart defects
Cardiac surgery

Slow rhythm → A-V heart block → Pacemaker implantation

Conduction disturbance → Premature contractions

Hypoxia
Sedative
Hypotension → Sinus bradycardia

Congestive heart failure
Chronic pulmonary obstructive disease
Pulmonary embolism → Atrial flutter / Afibrillation

Digitalis toxicity
Electrolyte imbalance → Ventricular tachycardia / Sinus arrest

Anxiety
Dehydration
Hypotension
Fever
Pain → Fast rhythm → Sinus tachycardia

Hypertension

Hypertension in children is reflected by the consistent readings of the systolic and/or diastolic blood pressure at the level of or above the ninety-fifth percentile for age and sex. It may be primary or secondary. Fifty to 80 percent of secondary hypertension is caused by renal parenchymal disease, therefore infants and children with hypertension and adolescents with severe hypertension need to be evaluated for renal pathology. Hypertension in children is of particular concern because of its close association to hypertension in those adults who were hypertensive as children. That children with an increased blood pressure usually do not display any overt symptoms has led to the inclusion of blood pressure determinations as part of routine examination in those 3 years and older. Children under 3 who have been diagnosed with a heart condition are also tested.

MEDICAL CARE

Diuretics: chlorothiazide (Diuril and Hydrochlorothiazide Chydrodiuril) PO promotes diuresis and elimination of sodium by preventing reabsorption; it also decreases cardiac output, which reduces peripheral vascular resistance.

Antihypertensives (beta-blockers): propranolol (Inderal), Atenolol PO to lower cardiac output, which decreases blood pressure; usually given with a diuretic.

Antihypertensives (angiotensin-converting enzyme inhibitor): captopril (Capoten), Lisinopril PO to lower total peripheral resistance by inhibiting angiotensin-converting enzyme.

Vasodilators: hydralazine (Apresoline), Minoxidil PO to relax smooth muscle of arterioles, resulting in reduced peripheral resistance.

Calcium channel blockers: Niphedipine (Procardia) PO lowers BP by decreasing vasoconstriction of the vessels.

Chest x-ray: reveals hypertrophy of left ventricle in sustained hypertension.

Electrocardiography: reveals cardiac abnormalities.

Urinalysis: reveals renal disease or infection.

Electrolytes: reveals hypokalemia, hypernatremia during diuretic therapy.

Lipid panel: reveals increases in lipoproteins, cholesterol, and triglyceride levels.

Blood urea nitrogen: reveals increases in impaired renal function in secondary hypertension.

Creatinine: reveals increases in impaired renal function in secondary hypertension.

Complete blood count: reveals increased WBC in presence of infection.

NURSING CARE PLANS

Essential nursing diagnoses and plans associated with this condition:

Fluid volume excess (5)

Related to: Compromised regulatory mechanisms, excessive sodium intake
Defining characteristics: Edema, weight gain, intake greater than output, blood pressure changes, altered electrolytes

Altered nutrition: More than body requirements

Related to: Excessive intake in relationship to metabolic need
Defining characteristics: Weight 10 percent over ideal for height and frame, dysfunctional eating pattern, hereditary predisposition

Altered tissue perfusion: Renal (6)

Related to: Interruption in renal, arterial, or venous flow
Defining characteristics: Edema, oliguria, hypertension

Risk for fluid volume deficit (222)

Related to: Medications (diuretic)
Defining characteristics: Increased urinary output, sudden weight loss, hypokalemia, dry skin and mucous membranes

SPECIFIC DIAGNOSES AND CARE PLANS

Risk for injury

Related to: Internal regulatory function
Defining characteristics: Uncontrolled hypertension; neurologic status (blurred vision, headache, irritability, dizziness, papilledema); future renal, heart, circulatory problems

Outcome Criteria

Maintenance of blood pressure within normal range for age, sex and height

Interventions	Rationales
Assess BP using a Doppler method on an infant and proper size cuff on child, noting proper application of cuff, position, and extremity used; use a cuff that covers 2/3 of the upper arm and inflatable bladder that encircles the child's arm circumference; take an infant's BP in a supine position; take a child's BP with the child seated and the arm supported at the level of the heart; obtain readings when infant/child is at rest q2h	Provides accurate systolic and diastolic readings to establish a pattern of elevations, although no definite readings are used to diagnose hypertension in children
Assess for headache, dizziness, nose-bleed, visual changes	Indicates increased BP, although symptoms in children are varied and some or none of the symptoms may be present
Provide quiet environment and reduce activities, stress and stimuli	May increase BP
Administer antihypertensives and diuretics as prescribed	Drug therapy is given diuretics as prescribed when BP does not respond to nonpharmacologic methods of reducing it; control is managed with the use of one drug and cautious addition of another drug, depending on side effects produced and achieved reduction of BP

Information, Instruction, Demonstration

Interventions	Rationales
Instruct in medication administration including action, dosage, frequency, side effects, importance of	Pharmacologic intervention to control hypertension

Interventions	Rationales
long-term therapy, physical and behavioral changes to report	
Demonstrate and have parent(s) return the demonstration of taking BP correctly and of maintaining a log of readings and what the BP indicates	Offers correct monitoring of BP for changes that might indicate need for initiation and/or changes in treatments for children with chronic hypertension
Inform to report any sustained elevation of BP, neurologic symptoms	Provides opportunity to prevent neurologic impairment or other complications
Inform that therapy is long term and of consequences of noncompliance	Provides realistic support and rationale to encourage compliance of drug therapy

Discharge or Maintenance Evaluation

- Blood pressure within normal ranges for age, sex and height
- Correct administration of prescribed medications Absence of signs and symptoms associated with elevated BP
- Continued monitoring of BP
- Verbalization of signs and symptoms, side effects to report

Knowledge deficit of parent(s), child

Related to: Lack of information or experience about disease and treatment
Defining characteristics: Verbalization of need for information about nonpharmacologic treatments

Outcome Criteria

Adequate knowledge for compliance of treatments to reduce BP

Interventions	Rationales
Assess knowledge of disease, causes and methods to control disease, willingness and interest to implement long-term care	Promotes plan of instruction that is realistic to ensure compliance of medical regimen, prevents repetition of information

Interventions	Rationales
Provide information and explanations in clear language; use pictures, pamphlets, video tapes, models in teaching about disorder, causes and risk factors	Ensures understanding based on readiness, aids reinforce learning
Instruct and assist in planning dietary menu that includes restrictions that help reduce BP	Weight reduction and restricted sodium, fat, and cholesterol intake may be part of the medical regimen
Instruct in an activity and exercise plan specific to child's needs and interests (swimming, cycling)	Assists in weight reduction and contributes to lowering BP
Instruct in relaxation techniques, such as breathing, biofeedback	Reduces stress that raises BP
Inform of importance of follow-up visits to physician	Provides early detection of complication and evaluation therapy
Inform of long-term nature of medical regimen and potential for cardiac, cerebral, and renal damage or complications that result from noncompliance	Provides rationale for acceptance of long-term care
Inform of availability of stress, weight reduction, or nutritional counseling	Provides specialized guidance if needed to ensure compliance and success

Discharge or Maintenance Evaluation

- Verbalization of knowledge of disease process, causes, and risk factors
- Adaptation and compliance with dietary restrictions, limit caffeine
- Daily participation in aerobic exercises, individualized activities
- Family participation in stress reduction and support for medical regimen
- Maintains schedule for physician visits
- Obtains additional information from American Heart Association
- Weight loss achieved until average for age, height, and frame reached
- Practices stress reduction techniques
- Seeks out counseling services if needed for weight loss

Hypertension

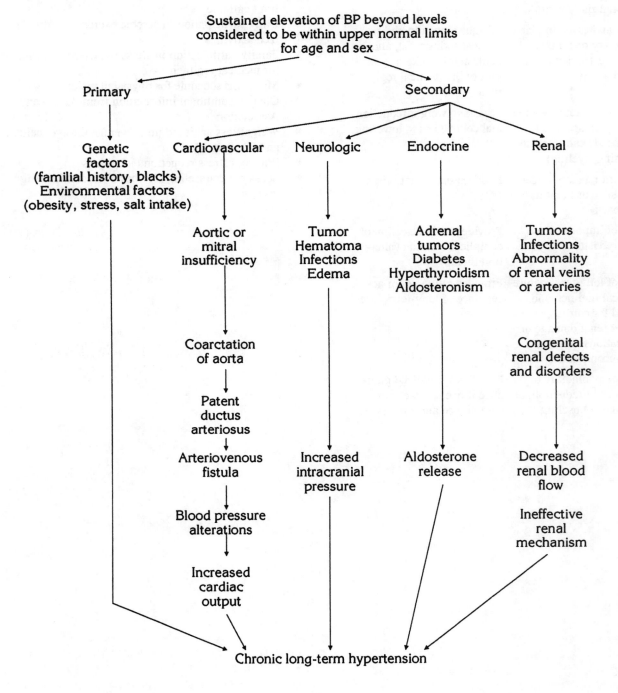

Sustained elevation of BP beyond levels
considered to be within upper normal limits
for age and sex

Primary

Secondary

Genetic
factors
(familial history, blacks)
Environmental factors
(obesity, stress, salt intake)

Cardiovascular

Neurologic

Endocrine

Renal

Aortic or
mitral
insufficiency

Tumor
Hematoma
Infections
Edema

Adrenal
tumors
Diabetes
Hyperthyroidism
Aldosteronism

Tumors
Infections
Abnormality
of renal veins
or arteries

Coarctation
of aorta

Congenital
renal defects
and disorders

Patent
ductus
arteriosus

Arteriovenous
fistula

Increased
intracranial
pressure

Aldosterone
release

Decreased
renal blood
flow

Blood pressure
alterations

Ineffective
renal
mechanism

Increased
cardiac
output

Chronic long-term hypertension

Kawasaki Disease (Mucocutaneous Lymph Node Syndrome)

Kawasaki Disease (KD) is an acute inflammation of systemic blood vessels of unknown cause. Most cases occur to children less than 5 years of age. The disease is self-limiting, but about 25% of those affected will develop cardiac sequelae (most commonly dilatation of the coronary arteries resulting in coronary aneurysms). The disease occurs in 3 phases: the acute phase is progressive inflammation of small blood vessels and is accompanied by high fever, inflammation of the pharynx, dry, reddened eyes, swollen hands and feet, rash, and cervical lymphadenopathy. In the subacute phase, the manifestations disappear, but there is inflammation of larger vessels and the child is at greatest risk for the development of coronary aneurysms. In the convalescent phase (6-8 weeks after onset), the clinical signs of KD are resolved, but lab values are not completely normal. There are no diagnostic tests for KD, so the diagnosis is made on the basis of the child exhibiting at least 5 of 6 criterion manifestations.

MEDICAL CARE

Hgb/Hct: the child with KD is often anemic at the time of diagnosis.
WBC: may show leukocytosis with a "shift to the left" (increased immature white blood cells during the acute phase).
Sedimentation rate: elevated, reflecting inflammation, and lasts 6-8 weeks.
Platelet count: thrombocytosis and hyper-coagulability occurs in the subacute phase and gradually returns to normal.
Liver enzymes: usually elevated during the acute phase.
EKG: monitors myocardial and coronary artery status.
Gamma globulin: IV gamma globulin is given during the first 10 days of the illness; usually given as a single dose of 2g/Kg over 8-12 hours.

Aspirin (ASA): used for its anti-inflammatory and anti-coagulant actions; given in large doses (80-100 mg/Kg/day) while the child is febrile, and then 3-5 mg/Kg/day until the platelet count returns to normal.

NURSING CARE PLANS

Essential nursing diagnoses and plans associated with this condition:

Hyperthermia (112)

Related to: Inflammatory disease process
Defining characteristics: High fever (103-105 degrees F), not responsive to antipyretics or antibiotics, lasting 5 or more days, and irritability

Risk for fluid volume deficit (222)

Related to: Decreased PO intake during uncomfortable acute phase, fluid losses through fever and increased metabolic rate
Defining characteristics: Refusal to take PO fluids, oliguria, poor skin turgor, dry mucous membranes, weight loss

SPECIFIC DIAGNOSES AND CARE PLANS

Pain

Related to: Inflammatory process (dry mucous membranes, conjunctivitis, pharyngitis), fever, joint pain, swollen hands and feet
Defining characteristics: Crying, extreme irritability, refusal to play, discomfort when being touched or moved

Outcome Criteria

Decrease in pain during the acute phase with complete resolution by the end of the phase

Interventions	Rationales
Assess level of pain by observation (crying, grimacing, vocal expressions of pain), having child rate pain using assessment scales, and by obtaining	Provides information upon which accurate assessments of pain and treatment effectiveness can be based

Interventions	Rationales
relevant pain information from parent(s) about child's expression of pain	
Use cool cloths on skin, lotion, and soft, loose clothing on child	Decreases skin discomfort
Use lubricating lip ointments and glycerin swabs on the oral mucosa; offer cool liquids and soft foods	Moistens dry oral mucosa to decrease discomfort and promote oral intake
Keep child's room quiet and semi-dark	Promotes rest; darkness decreases eye discomfort caused by conjunctivitis
Disturb child as little as possible; when necessary, handle gently and avoid unnecessary handling	Movement causes discomfort
Administer IV gamma globulin and high dose ASA therapy as directed	Decreases inflammatory process and helps decrease fever

Information, Instruction, Demonstration

Interventions	Rationales
Explain to parent(s) reason for child's discomfort/ irritability; ask parent(s) for information on child's expression of pain	Promotes understanding and cooperation; provides valuable assessment data
Explain to parent(s) that irritability may persist for up to 2 months; that peeling skin on hands and feet is normal and not painful	Promotes understanding and allows parent(s) to anticipate needs
If child has joint pain, explain to parent(s) that it may persist for several weeks; passive ROM exercises in a warm bath may help	Persistent joint pain is not uncommon; ROM with heat helps increase flexibility

Discharge or Maintenance Evaluation

- Child is afebrile
- Engages in age-appropriate, quiet play activity
- Reports decrease (or absence) of pain

- Parent(s) verbalize knowledge of continuing comfort needs

Anxiety

Related to: Acute, serious illness of unknown origin with possible cardiac sequelae
Defining characteristics: Verbalization of need for information about disease and medical treatment

Outcome Criteria

Adequate knowledge for compliance with treatment and follow-up care and decrease in anxiety

Interventions	Rationales
Assess knowledge of disease and treatments	Promotes plan of instruction appropriate to knowledge level of parent(s)
Provide information about the disease (the unknown etiology, the disease phases and manifestations, diagnostic tests and treatments)	Ensures understanding and promotes compliance; the unknown etiology helps allay any guilt parent(s) may have concerning the child contracting the disease
Support parent(s) in their efforts to comfort their irritable child; encourage them to "take a break" while the nurse cares for the child; reassure parent(s) that irritability is a manifestation of KD and that they should not feel embarrassed or guilty	Provides support to parent(s) during a stressful event
Monitor child closely during IV gamma globulin administration (temp, pulse, BP). Stop the infusion and report immediately any signs of reaction (chills, fever, dyspnea, nausea/vomiting)	Gamma globulin is a blood product and requires the same close observation for safe administration to prevent a reaction; this reassures parent(s) that their child is receiving appropriate care

Information, Instruction, Demonstration

Interventions	Rationales
Explain to parent(s) that touching the child may cause pain; demonstrate	Provides information parent(s) need to give comfort to their child

Interventions	Rationales
gentle handling of child as needed	
Explain to parent(s) that the child may have recurrent fever at home and demonstrate how to take the child's temperature and when to notify physician (temp. greater than 38.4° C/101° F)	Helps ensure child will receive needed care at home
Demonstrate ASA administration to parent(s) and instruct them to report any signs of toxicity (tinnitus, headache, dizziness, or confusion). Explain that ASA may cause easy bruising and that the ASA should be stopped and the physician notified if child exposed to chickenpox or influenza (risk of Reye's syndrome)	Helps ensure safe, proper administration of ASA at home
Explain to parent(s) that long-term physician follow-up is needed to assess child for possible sequelae	Ultimate cardiac sequelae is not usually known at discharge; knowledge helps parent(s) understand and comply with follow-up

Discharge or Maintenance Evaluation

- Parent(s) verbalize understanding of disease and treatment
- Parent(s) able to accurately assess their child's temperature and properly administer ASA
- Parent(s) verbalize knowledge of ASA toxicity and know what symptoms to report
- Parent(s) take child to physician for follow-up appointments

Kawasaki Disease

Abrupt onset of fever for 5 or more days
Bilateral conjunctival inflammation without exuclate
Dry, recloral mucosa
Peripheral edema, erythema of palms and soles
Polymorphous rash
Cervical lymphaden opathy

↓

Kawasaki Disease

↓

Leukocytosis
Elevated erythrocyte sedimentation
rate
Elevated liver enzymes
Thrombocytosis

↓

IV single large dose of gamma globulin
PO large doses of ASA
Baseline EKG

↓

↓   ↓

Complete resolution with no sequelae   Development of dilated coronary ar-
                                                                        teries
Low dose daily ASA until normal   Coronary aneurysms
platelet count
                                                              Low dose ASA therapy continued in-
                                                                        definitely
Follow-ups needed   Courmdin therapy may be given
                                                              On-going follow-up with cardiologist

Acute Rheumatic Fever (ARF)

Acute rheumatic fever is an autoimmune disease responsible for cardiac valve disease or rheumatic heart disease. It is associated with infections caused by the Group A Streptococcus and occurs about 2-6 weeks following a streptococcal upper respiratory infection. It is prevented by adequate treatment of the infection with appropriate antibiotic therapy within 9 days of onset of streptococcal infection before further complications can occur. Because rheumatic heart disease does not occur after only one attack of ARF and since children are susceptible to recurrent attacks of ARF, it is vital that an initial episode is diagnosed, treated, and that long-term prophylactic therapy (5 years or more) is given following the acute phase. There is no specific test for ARF; the diagnosis is based upon the manifestations using the revised Jones Criteria as a guideline. Jones Criteria consists of major manifestations (polyarthritis, carditis, chorea, subcutaneous nodules, and erythema marginatum) and minor manifestations (fever, arthralgia, EKG and laboratory changes). The presence of 2 major manifestations, or 1 major and 2 minor manifestations, supported by evidence of a preceding Group A streptococcal infection is indicative of ARF.

MEDICAL CARE

Antibiotics: benzathine penicillin G IM, penicillin G potassium (Pentids solution), ampicillin (Amcill tablets, suspension or pediatric drops) PO or erythromycin (Ilosone tablets, chewables, suspension PO if penicillin-sensitive).
Anti-inflammatory/antipyretic/analgesic: aspirin (Acetylsalicylic Acid tablets, suspension or liquid) PO to reduce temperature and reduce inflammatory process by inactivating the enzyme required for prostaglandin synthesis, which contributes to inflammatory process.
Antibiotics: penicillin G benzathine (Bicillin) IM monthly or penicillin G potassium (Pentids) PO daily as long-term therapy.
Electrocardiogram: reveals prolonged P-R interval.
Antistreptolysin-O titer: reveals increase 7 days after streptococcal infection with elevation above 330 Todd units, indicating recent infection.

Complete blood count: reveals increased WBC in presence of infectious process.
Erythrocyte sedimentation rate: reveals increase in presence of inflammatory process in rheumatoid disease.
C-reactive protein: reveals increase during inflammatory process and may be done in place of ESR.
Throat culture: reveals presence of streptococci, Group A.

NURSING CARE PLANS

Essential nursing diagnoses and plans associated with this condition:

Hyperthermia (112)

Related to: Illness or inflammatory disease
Defining characteristics: Low-grade increase in body temperature above normal range, temperature tends to spike in late afternoon

Altered nutrition: less than body requirements (168)

Related to: Inability to ingest food because of anorexia, increased metabolic rate and/or chores
Defining characteristics: Anorexia, fatigue, weight loss, abdominal pain

Impaired physical mobility (278)

Related to: Pain and discomfort
Defining characteristics: Joint pain of polyarthritis
Related to: Neuromuscular impairment from chorea
Defining characteristics: Decreased muscle control and strength, clumsiness, uncoordination, sudden and aimless movement of extremities, bedrest protocol

SPECIFIC DIAGNOSES AND CARE PLANS

Pain

Related to: Biological injuring agents, arthralgia
Defining characteristics: Verbal description of pain, guarding and protective behavior of painful joints, edema, redness, heat at affected joints

Outcome Criteria

Relief of acute pain and progressive absence of symptoms associated with arthralgia

Interventions	Rationales
Assess severity of pain, joints involved, level of joint movement	Provides information regarding pathologic changes in joints; joint involvement is reversible, usually affecting large joints, such as knees, hips, wrists, and elbows; an increase in numbers of affected joints occurs over a period of time
Assess behavior changes, such as crying, restlessness, refusal to move, irritability, aggressive or dependent behavior	Nonverbal responses to pain that are age-related as child or infant may be unable to describe pain; fear and anxiety associated with pain causes changes in behavioral responses
Administer analgesic and anti-inflammatory agent, and inform child that the medication will decrease the pain; administer a sustained-action analgesic before bedtime or 1 hour before anticipated movement	Relieves pain, edema in joints and promotes rest and comfort
Maintain bedrest during the acute stage of disease	Promotes comfort and reduces joint pain caused by movement
Elevate affected extremities above level of heart	Promotes circulation to the heart to relieve edema
Change position q2h while maintaining body alignment	Prevents contractures and promotes comfort
Move gently and support body parts; minimize handling of affected parts as much as possible	Prevents additional pain to affected parts
Apply bed cradle under outside covers over painful parts	Prevents pressure on painful joints
Provide toys, games for quiet, sedentary play	Provides diversionary activity to distract from pain

Interventions	Rationales
Use nonpharmacologic measures to decrease pain (distraction, cutaneous stimulation, imagery, relaxation, heat application)	Provides additional measures to decrease pain perception

Information, Instruction, Demonstration

Interventions	Rationales
Inform of limited activity or amount of joint movement allowed	Prevents increase or exacerbation of pain
Inform parent(s) and child of need for analgesia and that it will help him/her to feel better	Controls pain, and allows for uninterrupted sleep and activity within tolerance level
Inform parent(s) and child that joint involvement is temporary, that pain and edema will subside, and that joints will return to normal	Reduces anxiety associated with fear of permanent damage
Instruct in body positioning and handling of affected parts	Promotes comfort and prevents pain and contractures while on enforced bedrest

Discharge or Maintenance Evaluation

- Joint pain relieved and/or controlled
- Compliance with medication regimen for pain and inflammation
- Compliance with methods to protect joints from pain
- Limits movement and activity that cause discomfort; exacerbation of signs and symptoms of disease; risk of development of complication of valve damage

Risk for infection

Related to: Chronic recurrence of disease
Defining characteristics: Noncompliance with long-term medication regimen, evidence of exacerbation of signs and symptoms of disease, risk of development of complication of valve damage

Outcome Criteria

Absence of occurrence of reinfection

Interventions	Rationales
Assess compliance to prescribed antimicrobials; daily oral administration or monthly intramuscular injections	Long-term antibiotic therapy (as long as 5 years) as a preventive measure creates compliance difficulty, and need for IM injections may be necessary in order to ensure compliance
Assess for chest pain, dypsnea, cough, tachycardia during sleep, friction rub, gallop during acute stage of disease	Signs and symptoms of carditis, which may lead to endocarditis causing vegetation that becomes fibrous at the valve areas that is at increased risk with repeated infections
Administer antibiotic therapy during acute phase of disease	Inhibits cell wall synthesis of microorganisms, destroying causative agent

Information, Instruction, Demonstration

Interventions	Rationales
Instruct in long-term antibiotic regimen, need for protection before dental work or any invasive procedure, and inform of importance of compliance to prevent recurrence	Therapy starts after acute phase and medical supervision is needed for life as rheumatic fever may recur; a large percentage of children who have had the disease have heart disease later in life
Inform to report to physician any upper respiratory infections, elevated temperature, joint pain, inability to continue antibiotic therapy	May indicate recurrence of the disease or need to change or adjust medication

Discharge or Maintenance Evaluation

- Compliance with antibiotic regimen daily or monthly
- Notification of dentist regarding history of the disease and therapy
- Reporting of any symptoms to physician
- All preventative measures taken to avoid recurrence of disease

Rheumatic Fever

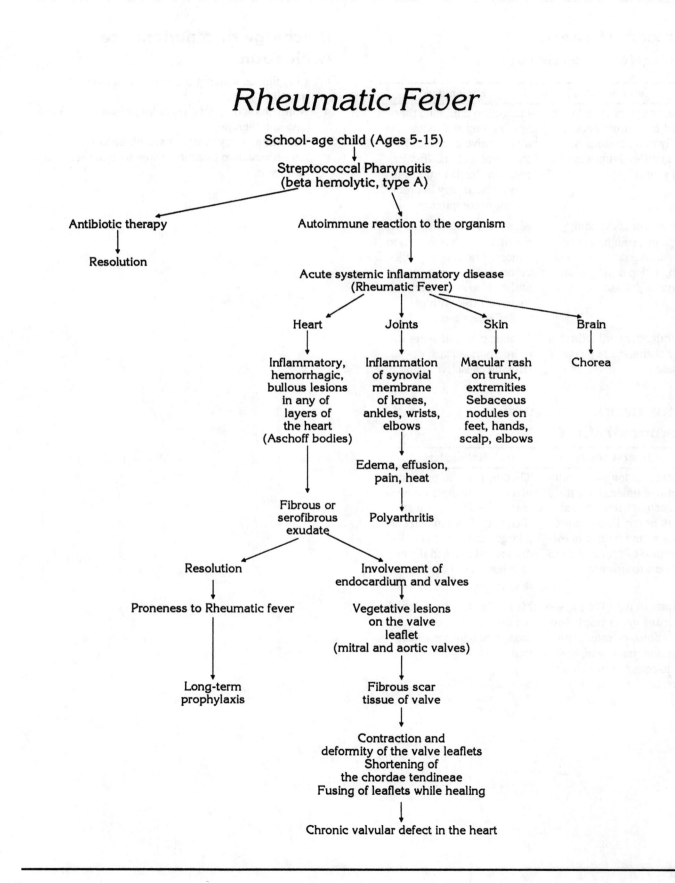

School-age child (Ages 5-15)

Streptococcal Pharyngitis
(beta hemolytic, type A)

Antibiotic therapy

Resolution

Autoimmune reaction to the organism

Acute systemic inflammatory disease
(Rheumatic Fever)

Heart

Joints

Skin

Brain

Inflammatory,
hemorrhagic,
bullous lesions
in any of
layers of
the heart
(Aschoff bodies)

Inflammation
of synovial
membrane
of knees,
ankles, wrists,
elbows

Macular rash
on trunk,
extremities
Sebaceous
nodules on
feet, hands,
scalp, elbows

Chorea

Edema, effusion,
pain, heat

Fibrous or
serofibrous
exudate

Polyarthritis

Resolution

Involvement of
endocardium and valves

Proneness to Rheumatic fever

Vegetative lesions
on the valve
leaflet
(mitral and aortic valves)

Long-term
prophylaxis

Fibrous scar
tissue of valve

Contraction and
deformity of the valve leaflets
Shortening of
the chordae tendineae
Fusing of leaflets while healing

Chronic valvular defect in the heart

Respiratory System

Respiratory System

The respiratory tract is a common site of major and minor disorders in infants and children, and any alteration in respiratory structure or function has a profound effect on the ability to supply the body with oxygen and remove carbon dioxide. A constant supply of oxygen is necessary to sustain organ function and survival, and any decrease in or cessation, obstruction, and infection, can compromise airway patency and pattern. This in turn changes the respiratory rate and efficiency. This tendency gradually decreases after the age of five. Each stage of life and its associated changes resulting from growth and developmental patterns establish different pulmonary parameters and susceptibility to diseases. Although the system generally functions the same as in an adult, anatomic changes that occur with growth influence the way that the infant or child responds to acute or chronic illnesses related to this system.

GENERAL RESPIRATORY CHANGES ASSOCIATED WITH PHYSICAL GROWTH AND DEVELOPMENT

Chest structure and bronchopulmonary movement

- Chest shape and anteroposterior diameter:
  Infant: rounded chest where diameter equals transverse diameter
  School age: changes gradually to lateral diameter ratio of 1:2 or 5:7 as chest assumes a more flattened anteroposterior diameter with growth
- Narrow, smaller lumen of airway system with increased airway resistance until age of five years
- Ability to respond to irritating stimuli by age 4-5 months as smooth muscle develops in airways, gradually reaching smooth muscle development of an adult by age of one year
- Glottis has more cephalad location in the infant than in the child; epiglottis is longer, and the narrowest part of the larynx located at the same level as the cricoid cartilage; larynx grows slowly during infancy and childhood, with a spurt of growth after childhood phase during preadolescence (voice change)
- Airways grow faster than cervical and thoracic spine, causing a descent of the larynx and trachea; the tracheal bifurcation gradually descends from opposite T3 in the infant to T4 by the end of the growth period, and the cricoid cartilage descends from C4 in the infant to C6 by the end of the growth period
- Diaphragm in the infant is attached higher in front and is longer, causing a decreased ability to contract with the same force of an older infant or child
- Lung growth changes from globular to lobular shape until twelve years of age
- Lung growth produces an increase in alveoli numbers and size as septa in the alveoli develop, divide, and increase their numbers at each terminal airway
- Branching of terminal bronchioles is increased as alveoli are increased as the child grows
- Collateral pathways develop between bronchioles and growth pores in alveolar walls during child's growth

Breathing pattern and ventilatory function

- Respiratory rate (ratio to pulse is 1:4)
Infant:	30-60/minute
Toddler:	25-40/minute
Preschool:	22-34/minute
Schoolage:	18-30/minute

  Rate decreases as metabolic needs decrease
- Respiratory depth (chest expansion)
Infant:	2-4 inches
Toddler:	4-6 inches
Preschool:	6-8 inches
Schoolage:	9-10 inches
- Respiratory pattern:
  Infant: obligate nasal and diaphragmatic breathing during first year of life
  Schoolage: changes gradually from infancy through childhood to a more thoracic breathing for girls and a more abdominal breathing for boys — volume of inspired air increases as lungs grow in size, resulting in a decreased amount of oxygen taken in and an increased amount of carbon dioxide expired
- Increased surface area available for gas exchange as alveoli increase in numbers and size
- Changes in compliance with age, from high compliance in the infant with a more pliant rib cage to gradually decreasing to normal compliance level; chest structure changes with growth

- Arterial blood gas values:
  PH: 7.35-7.45
  pO_2: 80-100 mm Hg (pressure of dissolved oxygen in the blood)
  pCO_2: 35-45 mm Hg (pressure of dissolved carbon dioxide in the blood)
  HCO_3: 22-28 mEq/L (bicarbonate level in the blood to reveal buffering effect on acid)

ESSENTIAL NURSING DIAGNOSES AND CARE PLANS

Ineffective airway clearance

Related to: Tracheobronchial infection, obstruction, secretions
Defining characteristics: Abnormal breath sounds (fine or coarse crackles, rhonchi, wheezes), changes in rate or depth of respirations, tachypnea, cyanosis, fever
Related to: Decreased energy and fatigue
Defining characteristics: Ineffective cough with or without sputum, labored respirations, inability to feed self, sleeplessness, lack of activity, limpness

Outcome Criteria

Return of respiratory status to baseline parameters for rate, depth and ease
Breath sounds clear with optimal air flow
Effective daily bronchoelimination, resulting in patent airways
Ability to cough up and remove secretions that are thin and clear
Absence of upper or lower respiratory infectious process

Interventions	Rationales
Assess respirations for rate (count for one full minute), depth and ease, presence of tachypnea (50-80/min), dyspnea and if it occurs during sleep or quiet time; note panting, nasal flaring, grunting, slowing, deep (hyperpnea) or shallow (hypopnea) breathing, stridor on inspiration, head bobbing during sleep	Reveals rate and type of respirations (baselines or deviations) that are related to age and size of the infant/child and presence of anxiety in the child, changes that indicate obstruction and consolidation of airways and lungs resulting in a decrease in lung surface are for gas diffusion, extreme changes in depth are abnormal, head bobbing indicates dyspnea in the infant and

Interventions	Rationales
	fatigue causing neck flexion, grunting indicates chest pain or impending respiratory failure
Assess breath sounds by auscultation, consolidation by percussion and fremitus	Provides indication of patent airways by auscultation, revealing crackles heard in the presence of secretions (fine and coarse), rhonchi (audible and palpable) in larger airway obstruction and wheezes in small bronchiolar narrowing (inspiration and expiration), diminished breath sounds in presence of decreased air flow and lung consolidation; indication of consolidation by presence of dullness on percussion and increased fremitus, decreased functional lung area by presence of tympany on percussion
Assess skin color changes, distribution and duration of cyanosis (nailbeds, skin, mucous membranes, circumoral) or pallor	Reveals presence and degree of cyanosis, indicating an uneven distribution of gas and blood in the lungs, and alveolar hypoventilation resulting from airway obstruction, the weakness of muscles used in respiration or respiratory center depression
Assess cough (moist, dry, hacking, paroxysmal, brassy, or croupy): onset, duration, frequency, if occurs at night, during day, or during activity; mucus production: when produced, amount, color (clear, yellow, green), consistency (thick, tenacious, frothy); ability to expectorate or if swallowing secretions, stuffy nose or nasal drainage	Reveals characteristics of cough as an indication of a respiratory condition that may be produced by infection or inflammation; small and narrow airways of an infant/child and the difficulty to cough up secretions cause obstruction from the stasis of secretions, which lead to infection and change in respiratory status

Interventions	Rationales	Interventions	Rationales
Elevate head of bed at least 30° for child and hold infant and young child in lap or in an upright position with head on shoulder; older child may sit up and rest head on a pillow on overbed table; check child's position frequently to ensure child does not slide down in bed	Facilitates chest expansion and respiratory efficiency by reducing pressure of abdominal organs on diaphragm	blowing up balloon, blowing bubbles, blowing a pinwheel or blowing cotton balls across the table in younger child	
Reposition on sides q2h; position child in proper body alignment	Prevents accumulation and pooling of secretions	Suction nasal and/or oropharyngeal, if needed and appropriate, using correct catheter and method, amount of negative pressure, and time limits; orotracheal with the administration of oxygen before and after suctioning if needed; use bulb syringe to suction mucus from infant's nose	Removes secretions when cough is nonproductive (older child if unable to regulate cough or breathe through mouth); if nose obstructed by mucus (infant or young child); type of suctioning dependent on amount, ability to drain or cough up, breath sounds in upper airways; catheter size is age dependent, maximum negative pressure of 60-90 cm H_2O with time limit of 5 seconds for infant, and 90-110 cm H_2O with 5 second time limit for child; prolonged suctioning causes vagal stimulation, oxygen desaturation, and bradycardia, and the use of high pressure damages the mucous membrane lining of airways
Provide cool steam vaporizer at bedside or mist tent	Promotes environmental air humidification that soothes dried mucous membranes and aids in liquefication of secretions for easier removal as inspiration of dry air reduces ciliary action and causes the retention of secretions		
Provide fluids at frequent intervals over 24 h time periods; encourage clear liquids, and avoid milk as much as possible	Maintains hydration status, and clear liquids liquefy and mobilize secretions; milk tends to thicken secretions		
Provide for periods of rest by organizing procedure and care and disturbing infant/child as little as possible in acute stages of illness	Prevents unnecessary energy expenditure resulting in fatigue	Administer pain medications as needed; assess level of pain using appropriate pain assessment tools, utilizing a preventative approach	Promotes compliance in deep breathing exercises and coughing to aid in the removal of secretions
Perform postural drainage between meals using gravity, percussion, and vibration unless contraindicated; hold infant on lap; support child with pillows	Promotes removal of secretions and sputum from airways; percussion and vibration loosen and dislodge secretions, and gravity drains the airways and lung segments through positioning	Provide mouth care qid and after suctioning	Prevents drying of oral mucous membranes
Assist to perform deep breathing and coughing exercises in child when in a relaxed position for postural drainage unless procedures are contraindicated; use incentive spirometer in older child,	Promotes deeper breathing by enlarging tracheobronchial tree and initiating cough reflex to remove secretions	Provide toys, games for quiet play, and a quiet environment	Prevents excessive energy expenditure and need for additional oxygen consumption, which changes respiratory status while still providing moderate activity and diversion of play

Interventions	Rationales
Place airway maintenance equipment and supplies at bedside (resuscitation bag, oxygen and suction equipment, endotracheal tube, tracheostomy tube, and supplies)	Provides immediate access to emergency equipment for interventions to treat airway obstruction if needed
Administer medications (mucolytics, bronchodilators, antibiotics, expectorants, decongestants, and/or antihistamines) orally, parenterally, via aerosol therapy with hand-held measured-dose inhaler, small volume nebulizer, IPPB according to physician order	Treats conditions affecting secretions, infection by liquefying secretions and enhancing outflow and removal of secretions (mucolytics, expectorants), relieving bronchospasms (bronchodilators), destroying infectious agents by interfering with cell way synthesis (antibiotics), reducing allergic responses and discomfort of nose stuffiness (decongestant, antihistamines), and by suppressing cough (cough suppressants) unless cough is desired to bring up secretions

Information, Instruction, Demonstration

Interventions	Rationales
Instruct parent(s)/child in handwashing techniques	Prevents transmission of microorganisms from touching or handling supplies, touching face of child by parent(s)/child without handwashing
Instruct parent(s)/child to avoid contact with those who have respiratory infections	Prevents transmission of microorganisms via airborne droplets
Inform parent(s) of need to maintain or increase fluids, type of fluids to include and avoid, to offer small amounts q1h to infant and 50-100 ml to child q2h during waking hours using small cup or straw	Liquefies secretions and maintains hydration

Interventions	Rationales
Instruct parent(s) in use of cool mist by vaporizer in room or placing child in bathroom of warm mist produced by running the shower with door closed; inform of safety measures to take when using vaporizer; type of mist (warm or cool) depends on the type of respiratory illness underlying; examples are: warm mist for acute spasmodic croup, cool mist for most other upper respiratory illnesses	Eases breathing by providing humidity to liquefy secretions
Demonstrate and instruct child in deep breathing and coughing exercises; allow to practice these exercises	Helps to raise and expectorate secretions by initiating cough reflex; raising secretions prevents accumulation of secretions in the lungs and airways which reduces surface area for gas exchange and predisposes to infection
Demonstrate and instruct parent(s) to perform postural drainage by gravity, percussion, vibration with hands, or use of automatic percussor/vibrator device	Promotes ventilation by dislodging and raising secretions, clears sputum and increases force of expirations
Teach the importance of physical exercise; activities with short burst of energy (baseball, sprinting, skiing) are recommended	Promotes better tolerance than endurance exercises
Recommend swimming as a form of physical exercise	Promotes saturation of inhaled air with moisture; exhaling underwater prolongs expiration and improves end expiratory pressures
Instruct parent(s) in use of bulb syringe to remove mucus from infant's nose, demonstrate and instruct in oropharyogeal suctioning if appropriate; allow return demonstration	Removes secretions in those too weak or unable to cough up secretions, removing mucus from nose of infant enhances breathing (obligate breather)

Interventions	Rationales
Instruct parent(s) and possibly older child in administration of medications via proper route with name and action of each drug: dosage; why given; frequency; time of day or night; side effects to report; how to administer in food — crushed, chewable, by measured dropper, or other recommended form; and method (nose drops, inhaler)	Ensures compliance with correct drug dosage and other considerations for administrations for desired results, and what to do if side effects occur
Instruct parent(s) and child to administer aerosols with use of hand-held inhaler, small volume nebulizer using oral or mask breathing apparatus; assembling of devices, cleaning and care of reusable supplies and equipment	Promotes proper administration and independence of child depending on age and ability

Discharge or Maintenance Evaluation

- Takes respirations for rate, depth, and ease and notes deviations from baseline parameters
- Maintains thin, clear secretions that can be coughed up or removed from airways by suctioning
- Performs deep breathing and coughing exercises, postural drainage, and vibration/percussion if appropriate
- Maintains proper care and disposal of supplies and prevention of transmission of infectious agents to child
- Complies with daily medication regimen via correct route and method, using correct dosage and form of drug(s)
- Maintains hydration status with increases in intake when needed

Ineffective breathing pattern

Related to: Inflammatory process
Defining characteristics: Shortness of breath, tachypnea, fremitus, temperature elevation, purulent sputum or yellowish-green color, cough, positive sputum/throat culture, throat pain and edema and redness
Related to: Decreased lung expansion

Defining characteristics: Dyspnea, respiratory depth changes, increased anteroposterior diameter (barrel chest), altered chest excursion
Related to: Tracheobronchial obstruction
Defining characteristics: Dyspnea, head bobbing in infant, drooling, tachypnea, abnormal arterial blood gases, cyanosis (skin, circumoral, mucous membranes), nasal flaring, respiratory depth changes, use of accessory muscles and retractions, altered chest excursion, prolonged expiratory phase, grunting, apnea during sleep, anxiety, air hunger, sitting up with mouth open to breathe, stridor on inspiration, persistent cough, throat edema
Related to: Anxiety
Defining characteristics: Dyspnea, tachypnea, fatigue, crying, hyperactivity

Outcome Criteria

Return of respiratory status to baseline parameters for rate, depth, and ease; optimal breathing pattern and ventilation
Breath sounds clear with optimal airflow
Effective breathing effort and improved chest expansion
Anxiety reduced or minimized
Control of respirations and factors that affect them
Absence of upper or lower respiratory infectious process

Interventions	Rationales
Assess respirations for rate (count for one full minute), depth and ease, presence of tachypnea (50-80/minute), dyspnea and use of accessory muscles and retractions (intercostal, subcostal, substernal, suprasternal), respiratory rhythm, nasal flaring; note expiratory phase, chest expansion, periods of apnea, head bobbing in infant during sleep	Reveals rate and type of respirations (baselines or deviations) that are related to age and size of the infant/child and presence of anxiety and disease processes, changes in patterns indicate the acuteness of a condition and the respiratory function that result from infection and obstruction; retractions that become severe are responses to a decrease in intrathoracic pressure that may extend to suprasternal area if lung consolidation is severe, nasal flaring occurs as the work of breathing increases, head bobbing occurs with dyspnea in infants

Interventions	Rationales
Assess configuration of chest by palpation; auscultate for breath sounds that indicate a movement restriction (absent or diminished, crackles or rhonchi)	Reveals an increased anteroposterior ratio common in children with chronic respiratory disease that results from hyperexpansion of the airways
Assess skin for pallor or cyanosis, distribution and duration of cyanosis (nailbeds, skin, mucous membranes, circumoral)	Reveals presence of hypoxemia causing cyanosis from an uneven distribution of gases and blood in the lungs, and alveolar hypoventilation caused by airway obstruction, weakness of muscles used in respirations
Assess for cough, pain when coughing, characteristics of cough and sputum, ability to mobilize and bring up secretions when amounts increase	Cough is an indication of a respiratory condition and if excessive may cause chest pain and interfere with respirations, accumulation of mucus in airways affects respiration if obstruction is present
Position with head elevated at least 30° or seated upright with head on pillows; position on side if more comfortable; tripod position for the child with epiglottitis; avoid tight clothing or bedding; for child with low muscle tone, use pillows and/or padding to maintain positioning	Facilitates chest expansion and respiratory efficiency by reducing pressure of abdominal organs on diaphragm; position of comfort is age related and dependent on degree of dyspnea
Perform deep breathing exercises and upper body exercises (isometric)	Strengthens intercostal and abdominal muscles, and diaphragm, which enhances breathing and prolongs expiratory phase
Assess child's pain and administer analgesics as prescribed; use a pain assessment tool appropriate to the child's age and developmental level; assess and record child's response to pain control measures; provide age-appropriate diversional activities as tolerated	Promotes improved oxygenation

Interventions	Rationales
Pace activities and exercises, and allow for rest periods and energy conservation	Prevents changes in respiratory pattern brought about from exertion and fatigue
Monitor blood gas levels and provide supplemental oxygen via hood, tent, cannula, or face mask as needed if hypoxia results from inadequate breathing pattern and ventilation; if an infant is apneic, provide access at bedside at all times	Maintains oxygen level in blood to maintain tissue and organ function, amount and type of oxygen administration dependent on hypoxia and changes in mentation
Administer bronchodilators via oral, subcutaneous, or aerosol therapy; antibiotics, or sedatives (cautiously) via oral therapy if respiratory efficiency is not reduced; antiasthmatics and steroids via oral or aerosol therapy	Relieves bronchospasms that affect respirations (tachypnea, rhonchi), prevents or treats infection, promotes rest and reduces anxiety to enhance breathing; prevents asthmatic attack and reinforces body defenses against allergic reactions
Provide a balanced diet according to child's preferences and ability to eat/drink	Promotes and supports the body's own natural defenses
Assess family's responses to child's illness and/or hospitalization; utilize the principles of family-centered caregiving, encouraging the parents to participate in their child's illness within their comfort level	Parents know their child's behaviors, temperament and reactions to previous illnesses and treatments better than the health care professionals; utilizing the parent's knowledge will promote understanding and improved caregiving

Information, Instruction, Demonstration

Interventions	Rationales
Inform and instruct parent(s) and child in handwashing and when to perform, disposal of tissues, covering mouth and nose when coughing to avoid those with respiratory infections	Prevents transmission of microorganisms to child from inanimate objects of airborne droplets

Interventions	Rationales
Demonstrate and instruct to parent(s) and child in possible positions for comfort and ventilation during activities and sleep	Facilitates ease of breathing
Inform parent(s) and child of activity restrictions and to avoid any activities beyond tolerance and energy level	Reduces potential dyspnea and fatigue
Instruct child in relaxation exercises, quiet play, and controlled breathing	Reduces anxiety in older child which increases respiratory rate
Inform parent(s) and child to avoid allergens, changes in environmental temperatures, humidity and pollutants, effect of pets, dust, dirty filters, plant odors, and other irritants in the home	Prevents responses that change respiratory pattern
Instruct and demonstrate oxygen administration (correct rate and method) and safety measures (fire prevention) to parent(s)	Supplies oxygen when needed in a correct and safe manner
Instruct and demonstrate medication regimen to parent(s) and older child and include route, dosage, action, what to expect, and how to administer according to form prescribed	Ensures accurate and safe administration for medications for optimal effect
Inform parent(s) to avoid giving child over-the-counter medications unless advised by physician	Prevents any undesirable interactions with prescribed drugs
Instruct parent(s) in disinfection, care of reusable supplies, and care of equipment used to administer medications	Reduces potential for infection and preserves equipment and supplies for long-term use
Instruct and demonstrate use of apnea monitor to parent(s) (application, setting, alarms, electric source) and how to perform cardiopulmonary resuscitation on infant if needed	Provides alert system for parent(s) to monitor changes in respirations and heart rate of infant with apnea episodes

Interventions	Rationales
Teach parents of the importance of good nutrition for themselves and their children	Enhances the child's own natural body defenses

Discharge or Maintenance Evaluation

- Takes respirations for rate, depth, and ease and notes deviations from baseline parameters
- Performs breathing and upper body exercises with improved chest expansion daily
- Complies with daily medication regimen via correct route and method, using correct dosage and drug forms
- Monitors infant during sleep for apneic episodes with apnea monitor
- Carries out measures to prevent transmission of infectious agents
- Maintains proper cleansing and care of equipment and supplies and disposal of contaminated articles
- Maintains an environment that prevents exposure to allergens or changes that affect breathing
- Paces activities with rest periods, controls or relieves breathing, difficult exercises or if pattern changes

Impaired gas exchange

Related to: Ventilation perfusion imbalance
Defining characteristics: Hypercapnia, hypoxia, inability to move secretions, confusion, restlessness, irritability

Outcome Criteria

Return of respiratory rate, depth, and ease to baseline parameters
Arterial blood gases within normal ranges for age
Absence of hypoxemia and changes in mentation and organ function

Interventions	Rationales
Assess respiratory status for rate, depth, and ease, (count for one minute), presence of dyspnea, tachypnea, chest movement, periods of apnea	Reveals respiratory effort, rate and depth (baselines or deviations), symmetry of movements, and use of accessory muscles, which affect the amount of air that reaches the alveoli for ventilation process and diffusion of oxygen (external respiration)

Interventions	Rationales
Assess for presence of cyanosis (skin, nailbeds, circumoral, and mucous membranes), ABGs for decreased pH and pO_2 and increased pCO_2 level trans-monitoring for $tcPO_2$ an $tcPCO_2$, pulse oximeter sensor for O_2 saturation level	Reveals status of hypoxemia and hypercapnia and potential for respiratory failure: cyanosis in children results from hypoventilation or an uneven distribution of gas and circulation through the lungs, usually caused by disease and breathing ab-normalities; gas levels pro-vide the basis for oxygen administration adjustment, need for position change; continuous monitoring by oximetry or transcutaneous electrode reduces need for arterial punctures to deter-mine hypoxemia and hypercapnia
Assess changes in con-sciousness and activity, presence of irritability and restlessness	Reveals hypoxic state as oxygen level in blood re-duces, causing decrease of oxygen to brain
Place child in semi or high Fowler's position, orthopenic position for older child unless contrain-dicated	Promotes chest expansion and ease of breathing, gas distribution, and pulmo-nary blood flow, all of which enhance gas ex-change
Administer oxygen via hood (infant), tent (young child), cannula, or face mask (older child) at rate prescribed, and adjust ac-cording to blood gas levels	Ensures adequate oxygen intake to maintain desired level; a PO_2 of less than 60 mm Hg and PCO_2 of more than 50-55 mm Hg may indicate need for reposi-tioning, stimulation, suctioning, or ventilator support
Provide sedation for rest-lessness, irritability as or-dered unless respirations are depressed	Promotes rest and ease of respiratory effort to sup-port ventilation, especially if anxiety present
Determine effect of disease process on gas exchange	Reveals any condition that may interfere with ventila-tion and the diffusion pro-cess, which will affect gas exchange

Interventions	Rationales
Note early stages of hypoxemia and effects on nervous system (mood changes, anxiety, confu-sion), circulatory system (tachycardia, hyperten-sion), respiratory system (altered depth and pattern, dyspnea, retractions, grunting, prolonged expi-ration), gastrointestinal system (anorexia)	Promotes careful evalua-tion of early signs and symptoms of insufficient alveolar ventilation and prevention of respiratory failure or arrest

Information, Instruction, Demonstration

Interventions	Rationales
Inform and discuss disease process, causes, signs and symptoms to parent(s) and child appropriate to age	Provides information about reason for how to control symptoms and promote general health
Explain all procedures and use of equipment to par-ent(s) and child appropri-ate to age	Reduces anxiety, which reduces oxygen require-ments in the child
Instruct and demonstrate oxygen administration	Maintains oxygen levels with amounts given
Instruct and demonstrate oxygen administration showing correct device to deliver O_2, amount to de-liver, frequency, type of oxygen system, safety fac-tors to parent(s); allow for return demonstration	Maintains oxygen levels with amounts given, pre-venting hypoxia as well as oxygen, toxicity methods and amounts vary with age and condition of in-fant/child
Instruct and demonstrate use of apnea monitor to parent(s); allow for return demonstration of applica-tion, setting, alarms, power source, inform of when and how to respond to changes in respiration and heart rate	Alerts parent(s) to pres-ence of prolonged periods of apnea in infant in order to prevent hypoxia and possible death
Inform parent(s) of respi-ratory signs and symptoms that must be reported indi-cating blood gas imbalance (fatigue, mental confusion, increasing dyspnea and tachypnea)	Assessing and reporting prevents potential for hypoxemia, hypercapnia, and more serious compli-cations of respiratory fail-ure

Discharge or Maintenance Evaluation

- Takes respiratory rate, depth, and ease, and notes deviations from baseline parameters
- Maintains position of comfort and optimal chest expansion and ventilation
- Complies with safe oxygen administration via correct method, device, and amount as needed whether continuous or intermittent
- Reports signs and symptoms of respiratory changes, skin color changes, mentation changes
- Monitors infant during sleep for apneic periods by correct use of apnea monitor
- Calls upon assistance from respiratory therapist available from durable medical equipment resource for oxygen administration
- Maintains proper cleansing and care of equipment and supplies and disposal of contaminated articles used in oxygen administration

Apnea/Sudden Infant Death Syndrome

Apnea in the infant is the periodic absence of breathing for more than 15 seconds in the full-term or more than 20 seconds in the preterm infant. It may be associated with gastroesophageal reflux, seizures, sepsis or the impairment of breathing during sleep in the infant, although it is not uncommon to find no apparent causative factor. Apnea occurs during infancy and is usually resolved by one year of age without resulting in the death of the infant. The apparent life-threatening event (ALTE) that is indicative of apnea may place the infant at risk of sudden infant death syndrome (SIDS) but is not considered a cause, as only a very small percentage of SIDS cases have experienced ALTE. SIDS is most common between three and eighteen weeks of age and results in the death of the infant. Both apnea and high-risk SIDS infants may be monitored by an apnea-monitoring device as a preventative measure. SIDS presents a crisis for the parents and family, which becomes the focus for nursing interventions that reflect care and support to assist them in coping with the sudden, unexplained, unpreventable loss.

MEDICAL CARE

Apnea monitor: a device that is attached to the infant by electrodes placed on a belt that is wrapped around the infant's chest; alarms sound when respiratory or heart rate changes occur that are more or less than the rates set revealing apneic episodes.

Oxygen therapy: treats hypoxia during apneic periods.

Chest x-ray: reveals respiratory infection if present.

Electrocardiogram: reveals presence of arrhythmias caused by bradycardia associated with apnea.

Electroencephalogram: reveals changes associated with seizures.

Pneumocardiogram: reveals cardiorespiratory patterns of heart and breathing rates, nasal airflow, and oxygen saturation.

Upper gastrointestinal x-ray: reveals reflux associated with apnea.

Arterial blood gases: monitors respiratory function for pO_2 and pCO_2 changes resulting from abnormal ventilatory drive.

Methylxanthines: a drug used to stimulate respiration; Theophyline PO and Aminophyline IV.

NURSING CARE PLANS

Essential nursing diagnoses and plans associated with these conditions:

Ineffective breathing pattern (45)

Related to: Tracheobronchial obstruction
Defining characteristics: Respiratory depth changes, apnea during sleep, cyanosis, abnormal arterial blood gases

Impaired gas exchange (47)

Related to: Ventilation perfusion imbalance
Defining characteristics: Preterm birth, hypoxia, apnea, bradycardia, hypercapnia, pallor

Altered nutrition: Less than body requirements (168)

Related to: Inability to ingest food because of biological factors
Defining characteristics: Choking and gasping during feeding, apneic or cyanotic episodes

SPECIFIC DIAGNOSES AND CARE PLANS

Risk for altered parenting

Related to: Lack of knowledge
Defining characteristics: Verbalization of role inadequacy, inappropriate caretaking behaviors (use of apnea monitoring device, cardiopulmonary resuscitation), request for information about care of infant and parenting skills
Related to: Unmet social and emotional maturation needs of parent(s)
Defining characteristics: Reluctance to leave infant with another caretaker, isolation from social activities, fear and anxiety about possible death of infant

Outcome Criteria

Verbalized readiness to deal with apneic episodes of infant
Demonstrates correct application and operation of apnea monitor
Performance of cardiopulmonary resuscitation (CPR)

Interventions	Rationales
Assess history of apnea, life-threatening event of infant, SIDS of siblings or cousins	Reveals risk factors associated with condition as basis for further evaluation
Assess for presence of apneic or cyanotic episodes, bradycardia, upper respiratory infection, poor feeding with choking during feedings	Identifies apneic episodes of more than 15 seconds in preterm or more than 20 seconds in full-term infant, associated factors, or potential for SIDS and need for monitoring
Anxiety level of parent(s), ability to participate in apnea monitoring and/or CPR as an intervention in event of episode	Fear and anxiety common to parents of apneic infant; feelings of guilt and inadequacy, fear of death of child presents obstacle to learning and interventions necessary for child's survival
Encourage and allow parent(s) to express feelings about unmet needs and ability to meet and develop self-expectations	Identifies potential for isolation and social deprivation of mother, strategies to achieve realistic expectations
Encourage touching and play activities between parent(s) and infant	Enhances bonding process and positive parental behaviors
Provide calm, supportive, and positive environment; encourage and praise positive parental behaviors	Reduces anxiety for enhanced learning of infant care procedures

Information, Instruction, Demonstration

Interventions	Rationales
Prepare written instructions for parent(s) of step-by-step procedures for monitoring or resuscitation	Provides reference as reinforcement of learning
Demonstrate for parent(s and allow for return demonstration of attaching electrodes to belt and monitor, applying belt to infant's chest, setting monitor, testing monitor alarms,	Apnea monitor may be prescribed by physician for use in home for apneic and "near-miss" infants, although use is controversial; monitors cardiac and respiratory activity with an
turning monitor ON, removal and care of monitor after use	alarm system that wakes parents when rates are not within prescribed boundaries; electrodes, lead wires, and cable pick up on breathing and heart activity signals and limit apnea time by sounding alarm
Instruct parents on safety issues of home apnea monitoring, as applicable: remove leads from infant when not attached to monitor; unplug power cord when cord is not plugged into monitor; use safety covers on electrical outlets to discourage siblings from inserting other objects	Prevent electrical accidents related to home monitor
Demonstrate for parent(s) and allow for return demonstration of CPR on infant model; instruct both parents or a parent and family member in assessment of infant and need for CPR, correct mouth-to-mouth and cardiac compression techniques; supply written instructions or booklet for review	CPR done to resuscitate infant with cessation of breathing and presence of cyanosis
Instruct parent(s) to notify electric company and nearest 911 unit that monitor is being used; provide telephone numbers for emergency services and instruct to keep near phone	Provides for emergency services if and when needed, including alternate electric sources
Instruct other significant family members (grandparents) and support persons as to care for the child with a home monitor, including CPR	Promotes positive copying as parents can lesson continuous responsibility of home apnea monitoring
Inform of parental tasks required for development of parenting skills, especially those for infant care	Parent(s) may not be aware that these tasks must be learned in relation to child's developmental needs

Interventions	Rationales
Explain the difference between apnea and SIDS, and discuss information available about controversy	Parental perception of the relationship between these conditions is often the basis for their fear of child's possible survival
Suggest referral to home care agency, contact with family members and friends, other support services	Provides range of support and assistance, which helps to reduce anxiety and promote social activities
Instruct parents to place healthy infants on their sides or back during sleep; avoid soft surfaces and gas-trapping objects (pillows) in the sleep environment	Decreases the risk of SIDS, according to some recent research; in 1994, the American Academy of Pediatrics and the Federal government made these recommendations, although they are somewhat controversial; education of parents so they can make their own informed decision.

Discharge or Maintenance Evaluation

- Applies, operates, and removes apnea monitor
- Cleanses and cares for monitor and supplies used in procedures
- Correctly performs CPR on infant model
- Verbalizes decreased anxiety and fear in caring for infant
- Can assess infant and intervene when needed
- Performs parental role activities
- Develops realistic expectations for infant and self
- Participates in social and other role activities
- Utilizes support services and follow-up care, physician services when needed
- Parents utilize safety precautions when home monitor is in use

Ineffective family coping: Compromised

Related to: Situational crisis the family may be facing
Defining characteristics: Family expresses concern and fear about infant's apnea episodes, displays protective behavior disproportionate to infant's need to grow and develop, describes a preoccupation with monitoring of infant apnea, chronic anxiety

Outcome Criteria

Increased development of coping skills, and comfort with infant apnea monitoring and changes in family processes brought about by infant condition

Interventions	Rationales
Assess anxiety level, erratic behaviors (anger, tension, disorganization) perception of crisis situation	Identifies information affecting ability of family to cope with infant apnea and monitoring
Assess coping methods used and effectiveness	Identifies need to develop new coping skills if existing methods are ineffective in changing exhibited behaviors
Encourage expression of feelings and provide factual information about infant apnea	Reduces anxiety and enhances family's understanding of condition
Assist to identify and use techniques to cope with and solve problems and gain control over the situation	Provides support for problem solving and management of situation
Provide anticipatory guidance for crisis resolution	Assists family to adapt to situation and develop new coping mechanisms

Information, Instruction, Demonstration

Interventions	Rationales
Inform parent(s) and reinforce appropriate coping behaviors	Promote behavior change and adaptation to care of infant during apnea
Inform parent(s) that overprotective behaviors may hinder growth and development during infancy	Enhances family understanding of condition and adverse effects of behaviors
Inform of need to maintain health of family members and social contacts	Provides information about chronic anxiety, fatigue, and isolation a result of infant care and about their effects on health and care capabilities of family

Discharge or Maintenance Evaluation

- Maintains optimal health of family members, caretaker
- Verbalizes that anxiety is reduced and coping techniques are utilized effectively
- Maintains social contacts
- Reduces overprotective behaviors in infant care
- Verbalizes adjustment and progressive adaptation to apnea episodes and monitoring
- Family adopts a positive view of infant's condition and realizes need for normal growth and development

Dysfunctional grieving

Related to: Loss of child as result of SIDS; absence of anticipatory grieving

Defining characteristics: Expressed distress; anger; guilt over loss; difficulty in expressing loss; sadness; crying; sudden, unexplained and unexpected death of infant; shock; grief; denial; social isolation

Outcome Criteria

Progressive grief resolution over period of time needed

Interventions	Rationales
Assess feelings of parent(s) and what they perceive happened to infant; listen to any feelings expressed	Allows feelings of anger, guilt, and sorrow to be expressed following death of infant
Provide privacy and remain with parents; avoid conversation and questions that may place any blame or cause guilt; reinforce parents that the cause of SIDS is unknown, with no absolute means to prevent or predict it	Provides support without adding to grief and feelings of guilt
Prepare infant for parent to view and hold; stay with parents during this experience	Allows parents to say goodbye to their child
Prepare parents adequately before they hold/see the infant; explain to parents the necessity of leaving in tube such as endotracheal	Promotes positive grief resolution if parents hold/see the infant and spend time saying goodbye on their own terms

Interventions	Rationales
tube, intravenous catheter due to autopsy; allow parent to determine the length of time they hold their infant; this varies by culture and individual parent needs	
Notify clergy or other support if requested; offer baptism/prayer to parents; arrange for clergy to be present, if applicable	Provides support and comfort
Provide parents the opportunity to call significant others; if unable, staff member should call	Presence of other family members and significant others often serves as support for grieving family
Answer any questions about SIDS and explain need for autopsy to verify diagnosis	Reinforces physician's explanation of disorder
Take pictures of infant and offer to parents; saving clothing infant was wearing, ID bracelets, hats, as part of a "momento packet" to be given to parents; if parents refuse packet, save for future retrieval	Promotes positive grief resolution
Assist parents to inform and help siblings understand loss; answer children's questions honestly and appropriately for age level	Children's concept of death develops with age, and help is needed to avoid feelings of blame and guilt by siblings
Assist to identify and use effective coping mechanisms applicable to situation	Promotes movement through grieving process by utilizing defense mechanisms that have worked in the past
Reassure parents that they are not responsible for the death of their child	Reinforces that SIDS is an unpreventable, unexplainable sudden death of an infant and that no one can be blamed
Obtain thorough history from parents, including parental resuscitation efforts and illness history	Provides optimal level of accurate information for medical examiner

Interventions	Rationales
(experienced or trained member of staff recommended due to sensitive nature of information)	
Contact the infant's primary care provider	Enhances the parental support system and enhances communication
Inform parents of autopsy process and how results will be obtained	Promotes improved understanding of SIDS; may lessen feelings of guilt

Information, Instruction, Demonstration

Interventions	Rationales
Coping skills and approaches that may be used	Promotes coping ability with consequences of loss
Inform of stages and importance of grieving and of behavior that is acceptable in resolving grief	Allows, in a nonjudgmental environment, for the initial shock and disbelief that are expected behaviors of grief
Refer family to counseling services, local SIDS chapter, community health nursing agency	Provides support and assistance during bereavement or chronic grief which may affect family relationships, presence of infertility or other problems
Correct any misinformation or misconceptions regarding the disorder	Assists with resolution of guilt and grieving

Discharge or Maintenance Evaluation

- Seeks out assistance when needed from community resources, local SIDS Foundation
- Verbalizes better understanding of SIDS
- Shares feelings with professionals and other members of family
- Participates in advocacy movements for legislation and community support for SIDS research and resources

Apena/Sudden Infant Death Syndrome

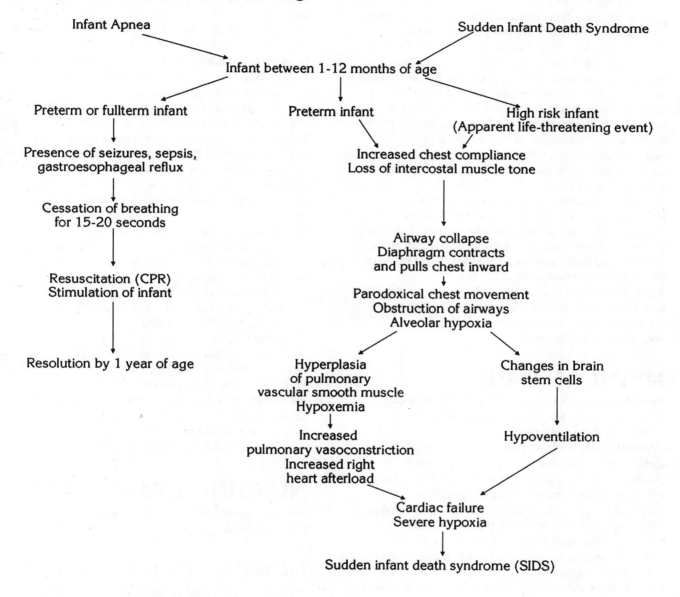

Asthma

Asthma in children is a reversible airway-reactive disease characterized by bronchospasm, increased mucus production, and edema of the mucosa of the bronchioles. The result is obstruction, air trapping, respiratory distress, and changes in ventilation. Asthma is the leading chronic disorder in children. Most children experience their first attacks between two and seven years of age with the onset of the most severe cases occurring after the age of seven. The onset of an attack may be gradual or immediate; continuous, with wheezing present at all times; or spasmodic, with intermittent attacks separated by intervals without symptoms.

As an attack progresses, alveoli that are hyperinflated and poorly ventilated may lead to impaired gas exchange, hypoxemia, hypercapnia, and eventual respiratory acidosis and failure. The two types of asthma are extrinsic (immune mechanisms) and intrinsic (imbalance in the autonomic nervous system), both of which affect the bronchial tissue and mast cell function that produces the characteristic symptoms of the disease.

Status asthmaticus is an acute condition characterized by an asthma attack that fails to respond to treatment and continues and increases in severity. It requires hospitalization of the child.

MEDICAL CARE

Bronchodilators/Xanthine: theophylline (Bronkodyl elixir, Theolair liquid, Theo-lV); produces bronchodilation by relaxing bronchial smooth muscle.

Bronchodilators/Adrenergic agonists: epinephrine hydrochloride (Sus-Phrine) given SC, epinephrine bitartrate (Bronkaid Mist Suspension) given via hand-held metered dose inhaler, racemic epinephrine (Vaponefrin) given via small volume nebulizer inhalant (SVN), isoproterenol hydrochloride or albuterol (Ventolin, Proventil) given via SVN or hand-held metered dose inhaler; produces bronchial dilatation to reduce bronchospasms.

Bronchodilators/Anticholinergics: ipratropium bromide (Atrovent) given via hand-held metered dose inhaler; acts on large airways to produce bronchodilatation.

Anti-inflammatory: prednisone (Deltasone) given PO, methylprednisolone sodium succinate (Solu-Medrol) given IV, beclomethasone dipropionate (Vancenase, Benconase) given via hand-held metered dose inhaler if child is over six years of age; reduces the inflammation and the airway obstruction that result.

Expectorants: potassium iodide (SSKI), guaifenesin (Robitussin) given PO in liquid form; reduces surface tension of secretions for easier removal.

Antiasthmatics: cromolyn sodium (Intel) given PO in solution or capsules or via hand-held metered dose inhaler in children over six years of age as a prophylactic agent in prevention of attacks; inhibits release of broncho-constrictors from mast cells (histamine and the slow acting substance of anaphylaxis).

Sedatives: phenobarbital (Luminal) given PO or rectally, hydroxyzine (Vistaril) given PO in tablet or liquid form; reduces anxiety and promotes rest.

Antibiotics: given PO or IV specific to organism identified in culture and in sensitivity test of sputum.

Oxygen therapy: treats hypoxemia as indicated by ABGs and is administered by tent, cannula, or face mask; use is usually reserved for status asthmaticus.

Chest x-ray: may reveal hyperinflation, infiltrates, or other pulmonary conditions such as atelectasis or pneumonia.

Pulmonary function: reveals decreased vital capacity and tidal volume, usually done on an older child.

Sputum culture: reveals large numbers of eosinophils and crystalloid fragments.

Arterial blood gases: reveals decreased pH, decreased pO_2, and increased pCO_2 as attack continues and ventilation perfusion imbalance occurs.

Complete blood count: reveals increased WBC if infection present, increased eosinophils in differential count of more than 5%, increased Hgb and Hct.

Skin tests: done by scratch or intradermal to identify specific allergens for hypersensitization injection therapy for an older child.

Inhalation tests: a bronchial challenge test to reveal specific allergens that precipitate symptoms.

NURSING CARE PLANS

Essential nursing diagnoses and plans associated with this condition:

Ineffective airway clearance (42)

Related to: Tracheobronchial infection, obstruction, secretion

Defining characteristics: Dyspnea; tachypnea; cough with or without sputum; uncontrollable cough that is hacking and paroxysmal, becomes rattling, and produces a clear, frothy sputum; abnormal breath sounds (wheezing on expiration and inspiration, fine and coarse crackles); circumoral and nailbed cyanosis; fever; assuming orthopneic position

Ineffective breathing pattern (45)

Related to: Inflammatory process, tracheobronchial obstruction, anxiety

Defining characteristics: Dyspnea, tachypnea, cough, nasal flaring, prolonged expiratory phase, intercostal and suprasternal retractions in infant, hyperresonance on percussion, shallow and irregular respirations, barrel chest configuration, abnormal ABGs, cyanosis, anxiety, restlessness, apprehension, speaks in short, broken phrases or unable to speak

Impaired gas exchange (47)

Related to: Ventilation perfusion imbalance

Defining characteristics: Restlessness, irritability, hypoxemia, hypercapnia, confusion, somnolence

Risk for fluid volume deficit (222)

Related to: Loss of fluid through normal routes, altered intake

Defining characteristics: Difficulty in drinking during panting, tachypnea, and dyspnea; thirst; dry skin and mucous membranes; diaphoresis; insensible loss

Sleep pattern disturbance (114)

Related to: Internal factors of chronic illness

Defining characteristics: Interrupted sleep from dyspnea, tachypnea, irritability, restlessness, inability to remain in prone or supine positions

Altered nutrition: Less than body requirements (168)

Related to: Inability to ingest food because of biological factors

Defining characteristics: Anorexia, nausea, vomiting, weight loss, dyspnea and tachypnea preventing intake of food

SPECIFIC DIAGNOSES AND CARE PLANS

Anxiety

Related to: Threat of or change in health status

Defining characteristics: Increased apprehension, fear with asthma attack, change in respiratory status, exposure to known or unknown allergens, tension and uncertainty about possible hospitalization for acute attack

Outcome Criteria

Reduced parental and child anxiety verbalized as asthma attacks minimized or controlled

Utilizes anxiety controlling measures of breathing exercises, quiet play, staying with child during respiratory changes

Interventions	Rationales
Assess level of parental and child anxiety before, during, and after attack	Provides information about anxiety level of child and parent(s) as respirations become more difficult and fear of suffocation is present, and about fear of subsequent attacks
Provide calm, supportive, and nonjudgmental environment, especially during an attack	Reduces anxiety and calming effect slows and eases respirations for improved ventilation
Allow parent(s) and child to express fears and concerns and to ask questions about disease and what to expect	Provides opportunity to vent feelings and secure information to reduce anxiety, especially if they know how to prevent or reduce frequency of attacks
Prepare parent(s) and child before all procedures and treatments	Relieves anxiety caused by fear of unknown
Stay with child during acute attack	Provides comfort and support to the child
Encourage quiet play and avoid any disciplinary actions	Provides distractions from changes in breathing pattern and prevents emotional upsets, which increase respiratory difficulty or may initiate an acute attack
If hospitalized, allow open visitation, and telephoning; encourage parent(s) to stay with child if possible, to bring toy or blanket from home, and to maintain home schedules for sleep, feeding, play as appropriate	Relieves anxiety for parent(s) and child when familiar people and routines are available

Information, Instruction, Demonstration

Interventions	Rationales
Explain to parent(s) and child the reason for and what to expect before and/or during attack; use drawings, pictures, models, and video tapes for child	Promotes understanding of what is happening during attack and the possible causes in order to allay anxiety
Inform parent(s) and child of the reversibility of the disease, how the medications and treatment resolve the attack	Reduces anxiety caused by fear of suffocation
Clarify any misinformation and answer all questions honestly in simple understandable language for the parent(s) and child	Prevents unnecessary anxiety that results from inaccurate information or beliefs
Instruct parent(s) and child in environmental control and exercise limitations	Provides anticipatory teaching that assists parent(s) and child in preventing attacks

Discharge or Maintenance Evaluation

- Expresses reduction in anxiety about possible attack
- Resolves misconceptions about the disease by verbalizing what causes the disease, what to expect, and how to prevent attack
- Supports and comforts child during an attack with calmness and understanding
- Participates in anxiety controlling measures like breathing exercises, quiet play

Risk for activity intolerance

Related to: Respiratory problem, fatigue
Defining characteristics: Prolonged dyspnea from asthma attack; lethargy; exhausted appearance, inability to eat, speak, play

Outcome Criteria

Return to activity within disease limitations after attack
Fatigue kept at a minimum during attack
Fatigue prevented or controlled by providing medical regimen to control attack

Interventions	Rationales
Assess presence of weakness and fatigue caused by respiratory changes	Provides information about energy reserves as dyspnea and work of breathing over period of time exhausts these reserves
Schedule and provide rest periods in a quiet environment	Promotes adequate rest and reduces stimuli
Disturb only when necessary, perform all care at one time instead of spreading over a long period of time, avoid performing any care or procedures during an attack	Conserves energy and prevents interruption in rest
Provide for quiet play, reading, TV, games while at rest	Prevents alteration in respiratory status and energy depletion caused by excessive activity

Information, Instruction, Demonstration

Interventions	Rationales
Explain reason for need to conserve energy and avoid fatigue to parent(s) and child	Promotes understanding of effect of activity on breathing and need for rest to prevent fatigue
Instruct in planning a schedule for bathing, feeding, rest that will conserve energy and prevent attack or promote resolution of an attack	Provides care while promoting activities of daily care
Inform of activity or exercise restrictions if these trigger attack; suggest medically approved activities (swimming, bicycling)	Provides preventative measures to offset possible attack

Discharge or Maintenance Evaluation

- Controls activities that cause fatigue or precipitate attack
- Provides rest and activity periods scheduled daily
- Fatigue minimized or absent

Health-seeking behaviors: Prevention of asthma attack and secondary infections of respiratory tract

Related to: Lack of understanding of preventative measures and need for behavior changes

Defining characteristics: Expressed desire for increased control of health practices and effect of current environmental conditions and behaviors on health status, increased frequency of attacks

Outcome Criteria

Absence of reduction of respiratory infections
Symptoms of impending or actual asthma attack controlled
Optimal health status maintained

Interventions	Rationales
Assess for knowledge of factors related to attacks, past history of respiratory infections and measures taken to maintain health of child	Provides basis for information needed for health maintenance, as respiratory changes or infection can trigger an asthma attack
Assess for use of over-the-counter medications, type used and effects	Identifies whether products available for treatment of respiratory diseases should or should not be used, as they may interact with prescribed medications, causing attack to become more severe
Assess health history of allergies in family members, what does or doesn't precipitate attack, and what behaviors result from the attack	Identifies familial tendency to airway reactive disease or history of allergic rhinitis, eczema, urticaria
Assess for knowledge of long-term effects of disease, which may eventually lead to obstructive disease of the lungs	Provides information related to prognosis, which depends on severity and frequency of attacks, and possible relationship to future health

Information, Instruction, Demonstration

Interventions	Rationales
Instruct parent(s)/child in handwashing technique, allow for demonstration	Prevents transmission of microorganisms from touching or handling supplies, touching face of child by parent(s) or child without handwash
Instruct child to avoid contact with those who have respiratory infections, how to cover mouth and nose when coughing or sneezing, and to dispose of tissues	Prevents transmission of microorganisms by airborne droplets
Inform parent(s) and child of physiology and signs and symptoms of the disease and possible precipitating factors influencing an attack	Provides information that will enhance performance of preventative measures and compliance to medical regimen
Inform parent(s) and child in signs and symptoms indicating the onset of an attack (change in respirations, wheezing, dyspnea)	Teach actions to be taken to prevent a severe attack and when to notify physician
Inform child to avoid excessive activity, stressful situations	Provides information on how to avoid situations that may provoke an attack
Inform parent(s) of effect of allergens and how to avoid exposure to offending environmental factors (cold air, humidity, air pollution, sprays, plants)	Reduces exposure to factors that precipitate an attack
Inform parent(s) of actions to change home environment to reduce dust, exposure to pets and indoor plants, changing of filters, avoidance of foods (yellow dye), drugs (aspirin)	Reduces exposure to factors that precipitate an attack
Instruct child in breathing exercises and controlled breathing	Prevents attack before it begins and increases ventilation

Interventions	Rationales
Inform and instruct parent(s) and child in medication administration (bronchodilators, antiasthmatics, anti-inflammatory agents) and how to manage method of administration; advise to avoid over-the-counter drugs without physician advice	Promotes compliance in order to prevent attack and maintain wellness
Inform parent(s) of skin testing for sensitivities to allergens	Identifies allergies for hyper-sensitization regimen
Suggest community agencies to contact for information and support	Offers support to families with child suffering from asthma

Discharge or Maintenance Evaluation

- Demonstrates age-related measures to take to prevent transmission of infectious agents
- Avoids exposure to known allergens
- Complies with medication regimen and correctly administers medications via tablet, liquid, metered dose, or small volume nebulizer inhaler, subcutaneous injections as prescribed
- Verbalization of understanding of disease and importance of control of precipitating factors and symptoms of an attack
- Verbalized understanding of daily requirements to prevent attack
- Maintains infection-free health status
- Contacts local agency for American Lung Association and Asthma and Allergy Foundation of America for programs, manuals, video tapes for parent(s), child, and family to assist in management of disease
- Maintains school schedule within limitations imposed by disease, with notification of condition to school nurse, teacher, coach and other appropriate staff

Altered family processes

Related to: Child within the family diagnosed with asthma, a chronic illness
Defining characteristics: Parental stress, which may result in parental dysfunction; stress may be manifested by excessive worry, withdrawal, denial, difficulty in making child-rearing decisions, overprotectiveness; alterations in the parent-child relationship which may hinder adjustment and decrease parent's ability to maximize child's growth and development potential

Outcome Criteria

Parents verbalize feelings and concerns related to the implications of the disease on the entire family
Family demonstrates acceptance, adjustment, and coping behaviors related to the symptoms and effects of asthma
Family provides an environment which fosters optimal growth and development of the child

Interventions	Rationales
Provide an opportunity for the family to adjust to the diagnosis; anticipate the normal grief reaction of "loss of the perfect child"	Reaction may occur in the early adjustment phase, after the diagnosis of a chronic disease, depending on the severity
Explore the family's feelings regarding the child and the diagnosis	Indicators of family-related psychologic stress often are obtained during open discussions as part of a history-taking; family stressors, if found early, can be the focus of preventative services to promote adaptation
Explore the family's specific feelings regarding: guilt, anger, disappointment, irritation, and fear; discuss with parents their fears: dealing with the child's anxiety, fear of complications, fear of death, fear of tests and procedures, fear of treatments, and the child's potential inability to feel "normal" as compared to peers; help family to identify realistic and unrealistic fears	Validates the normalcy of their feelings which promotes stress reduction and positive coping skills
Assess the family's coping skills and resources; help the family gain confidence	Promotes reinforcement of positive coping skills
Foster positive family relationships; serve as a role model regarding attitudes and behaviors towards the child	Promotes the family's ability to cope in a positive manner

Interventions	Rationales
Assess interpersonal relationships within the family and support systems, with emphasis on the family's relationship with the child diagnosed with asthma; intervene appropriately with evidence of maladaptation; refer to counseling if appropriate	Promotes early identification of interpersonal problems, especially within the parent-child relationship
Provide support to the family; assess family's own support systems and encourage their appropriate use; refer to community agencies and support groups, as applicable	Promotes positive adaptation within the family
Assess siblings and peers at intervals, as appropriate, providing time for questions and feelings	Promotes positive relationships within siblings and peers, which can be altered by chronic illness which requires increased parental attention, etc.

Information, Instruction, Demonstration

Interventions	Rationales
Instruct the family regarding the disorder, treatments, and implications; reinforce all information given; provide accurate information, paced at a rate appropriate for the family	Promotes a sense of control and alleviates stress; reinforcement and individualizing the approach promotes better understanding
Instruct family in methods to promote the child's physical, psychological, and cognitive development, based on child's current developmental level	Provides parents accurate information on growth and development
Assist family in the development and implementation of a home plan of care, utilizing age-appropriate goals consistent with activity tolerance	Provides for an optimal level of care at home; parental input into that plan of care may serve to increase compliance and foster positive adaptation

Interventions	Rationales
Explain to child/family the possible benefits of hyposensitization therapy where allergies cannot be avoided, as applicable	Prevents potential asthma exacerbation when allergen induced
Teach child and family correct use of metered dose inhaler, nebulizer, and peak flow meter; emphasize understanding of equipment usage, cleaning, and strategies for compliance	Prevents and/or minimizes asthma exacerbation by early identification
Instruct child and family on preventative treatment when applicable (i.e., prevention of exercise-induced asthma can be accomplished by use of certain medications prophylactically)	Prevents and/or minimizes asthma exacerbations
Instruct child and family on good health practices, such as balanced nutritional diet, adequate rest, good hygiene, and follow-up care	Promotes the body's own natural defenses
Instruct child and parents on methods to prevent infections: good hand washing, cleaning and care of equipment used, and avoidance of exposures	Prevention of infection may minimize asthma exacerbations
Instruct parents as to the signs of depression, especially in the adolescent; make appropriate referrals as needed	Promotes timely communication between parent and healthcare provider if concerns arise

Discharge or Maintenance Evaluation

- Family has open discussions and identifies problem areas
- Family develops and uses appropriate problem solving techniques to resolve differences
- Family verbalizes feelings and fears
- Child with asthma is incorporated into the family, with appropriate caregiving becoming part of the routine

- Family maintains supportive relationships with each other, utilizing positive coping skills
- Family relationships are maintained and stress/anxiety minimized
- Parents/child demonstrate correct use of equipment utilized, including cleaning
- Parents/child verbalize and practice sound health practices, such as nutrition, rest, prevention of infections, and exercise
- Parents recognize signs of depression and seek appropriate medical attention, as applicable

Asthma

Increased airway reactivity

Left branch:

Extrinsic factors
Allergens (antigen)

↓

Immunologic response

↓

Antigen deposited on mucosa;
coating destroyed by lysozymes

↓

Release of foreign protein
initiating immune response

↓

IgE and IgA attach to mast cells and
basophils; then react to the antigen
(hypersensitivity reaction)

↓

Release of granules in mast
cells containing histamine,
anaphylaxis, prostaglandins and
eosinophil and platelets factors

↓

Contraction of bronchial muscle
Capillary dilatation
Increased permeability of vessels
Stimulation of mucous gland secretions

↓

Theophylline
Sympathomimetic

↓

Inhibition of mediator
production by mast cells

↓

Reduced bronchospasms

↓

Bronchial relaxation

Right branch:

Intrinsic factors of
exercise, food, drugs
respiratory infection
physical or emotional stress

↓

environmental changes

↓

Autonomic nervous system response
Vagal stimulation
Reduced beta-adrenergic response

↓

Release of mediator substances

↓

Muscle contraction of bronchi

↓

Bronchospasms
Edema
Muscosal secretions
Inflammation

↓

Increased resistance in airway

↓

Increased air trapping in lungs
Hyperinflation of alveoli

↓

Increased work of breathing (fatigue)
Increased oxygen consumption

↓

Increasing dyspnea, tachypnea
Gas exchange compromised
Increased cardiac output

↓

Theophylline, corticosteroid,
sympathomimetic, atropine

↓

Respiratory failure

↓

Resolution   Death

Bronchiolitis

Bronchiolitis is an acute viral inflammation of the lower respiratory tract involving the bronchioles and alveoli. Accumulated thick mucus, exudate, and cellular debris and the mucosal edema from the inflammatory process obstruct the smaller airways (bronchioles). This causes a reduction in expiration, air trapping, and hyperinflation of the alveoli. The obstruction interferes with gas exchange, in severe cases causing hypoxemia and hypercapnia, which could lead to respiratory acidosis. Children in a debilitated state experiencing this disorder with other serious diseases are hospitalized.

MEDICAL CARE

Bronchodilators: theophylline (Bronkodyl elixir, Theolair liquid) PO to treat bronchial mucosal edema by relaxation of the bronchi and bronchiole smooth muscle; favorable response may indicate asthma if episodes of bronchiolitis are frequent.

Antipyretics: acetaminophen (Tylenol tablets, Pedric wafers or elixir, Liquiprin drops) PO to reduce fever. Ibuprofen (nonsteroidal anti-inflammatory) for children 6 months-12 years; Motrin or Advil liquid suspension or tablets PO to reduce fever and inflammation.

Antivirals: ribavirin (Vilena, Viramid) via aerosol inhalation (hood, tent, or mask) during first 3 days of illness to prevent replication of the syncytial virus; usually reserved for use in those with or at risk for severe illnesses or complications.

Chest x-ray: reveals hyperinflation, atelectasis and areas of collapse, flattened diaphragm indicating air trapping; areas of consolidation may need differentiation from pneumonia.

Nasal/Nasopharyngeal culture: reveals respiratory synctial virus by enzyme-linked immunosorbent assay method.

Arterial blood gases: reveals decreased pH, pO_2 under 60 mm Hg, pCO_2 over 45 mm Hg, indicating respiratory compromise and potential failure.

Complete blood count: reveals increased WBC, indicating infectious process.

NURSING CARE PLANS

Essential nursing diagnoses and plans associated with this condition:

Ineffective airway clearance (42)

Related to: Tracheobronchial infection, obstruction, secretion

Defining characteristics: Abnormal breath sounds (diminished or absent, crackles, wheezes); audible and palpable rhonchi; hyperresonance; change in rate and depth of respirations; tachypnea (50-80/min); paroxysmal, non-productive, and harsh, hacking cough; dyspnea and shallow respiratory excursion; fever; increased mucus and nasal discharge

Ineffective breathing pattern (45)

Related to: Inflammatory process, tracheobronchial obstruction

Defining characteristics: Dyspnea, tachypnea, cough, nasal flaring, shallow respiratory excursion, suprasternal and subcostal retractions, abnormal ABGs

Impaired gas exchange (47)

Related to: Ventilation perfusion imbalance

Defining characteristics: Hypoxia, hypercapnia, irritability, restlessness, fatigue, inability to move secretions

Altered nutrition: Less than body requirements (168)

Related to: inability to ingest food because of biological factors

Defining characteristics: dyspnea, fatigue, and weakness, causing difficulty in feeding, anorexia

Risk for fluid volume deficit (222)

Related to: Excessive losses through normal routes, altered fluid intake

Defining characteristics: Tachypnea, fatigue, increased temperature, dry skin and mucous membranes, increased pulse rate, weight loss

Hyperthermia (112)

Related to: Illness of lower respiratory infection

Defining characteristics: Low-grade, moderate fever; malaise

SPECIFIC DIAGNOSES AND CARE PLANS

Anxiety

Related to: Change in health status of infant or small child, threat of or actual hospitalization of infant/small child

Defining characteristics: Increased apprehension that condition might worsen; expressed concern and worry about impending hospitalization, need for treatment such as mist tent, IV therapy while hospitalized

Outcome Criteria

Reduced parental and child anxiety verbalized as illness is resolved

Verbalized understanding of causes of fear and anxiety, and positive effect of treatment regimen

Interventions	Rationales
Assess source and level of anxiety, how anxiety is manifested, and need for information that will relieve anxiety	Provides information about anxiety level and the need for interventions to relieve it; sources of anxiety may include fear and uncertainty about treatment and recovery, guilt for presence of illness, possible loss of parental role, and loss of responsibility if hospitalized
Allow expression of concerns and opportunity to ask questions about condition and recovery of ill infant/small child	Provides opportunity to vent feelings, and to secure information needed to reduce anxiety
Communicate with parent(s) and answer questions calmly and honestly	Promotes calm and supportive environment
Encourage parent(s) to remain calm and involved in care and decision-making regarding infant/small child noting any improvement that results	Promotes constant monitoring of infant/small child for improvement or worsening of symptoms
Allow parent(s) to stay with infant/small child or allow open visitation and telephoning, have parents assist in care (holding, feeding, diapering) and suggest routines and methods of treatment	Allows parent(s) to care for and support infant/small child; absence and wondering about condition of infant/small child may increase anxiety

Information, Instruction, Demonstration

Interventions	Rationales
Inform parent(s) of disease process and behaviors, physical effects and symptoms of disease	Provides information to relieve anxiety by informing parent(s) of what to expect
Explain reason for each procedure or type of therapy, effects of any diagnostic tests to parent(s) and child as appropriate for age	Prevents anxiety by reducing fear of unknown
Inform parent(s) that the most acute phase of disease is the first 24-72 hours followed by rapid and complete recovery, and that antibiotics are ineffective against this viral causation agent	Prevents anxiety by providing information about usual course of the most distressing time of illness
Clarify any misinformation and answer questions in lay terms when parent(s) are able to listen, give same explanation other staff and/or physician gave regarding disease process and transmission	Prevents unnecessary anxiety resulting from inaccurate knowledge or beliefs, or inconsistencies in information

Discharge or Maintenance Evaluation

- Expresses reduction in anxiety about disease process, therapy and prognosis
- Participates in care and decision-making regarding infant/small child
- Verbalizes positive effect of caring for and supporting ill infant/small child
- Visits and/or telephones the hospital if unable to stay

Fatigue

Related to: States of respiratory discomfort and effort

Defining characteristics: Lethargy or listlessness, emotional liability or irritability, exhausted appearance, inability to eat, limpness

Outcome Criteria

Return of energy level and increased endurance function
Improved respiratory function and return to baseline parameters for rate, depth and ease
Ability to eat, drink, and play within limits imposed by illness

Interventions	Rationales
Assess for extreme weakness and fatigue; ability to rest, sleep, and amount; movement in bed	Provides information to determine effects of dyspnea and work of breathing over period of time, which becomes exhaustive and depletes infant/small child energy reserves and ability to rest, eat, drink
Disturb infant/small child only when necessary, perform all care at one time instead of spreading over a long period of time	Conserves energy and prevents interruptions in rest
Schedule and provide rest periods in a quiet, comfortable environment (temperature and humidity)	Promotes adequate rest and reduces stimuli to order to decrease risk for fatigue
Allow quiet play with familiar toy while maintaining bedrest	Rest decreases fatigue and respiratory distress; quiet play prevents excessive activity, which depletes energy and increases respirations

Information, Instruction, Demonstration

Interventions	Rationales
Explain reason for need for infant/small child to conserve energy and avoid fatigue	Promotes understanding of response to respiratory distress and importance of rest and support to prevent fatigue
Inform parent(s) of measures to take to prevent fatigue in infant/small child (holding and/or rocking, feeding in small amounts, playing with child, offering diversions such as TV, toys)	Provides support to infant/small child and conserves energy
Inform parent(s) to pick up infant/small child if crying longer than 1-2 minutes	Prevents fatigue, as prolonged crying is exhaustive
Instruct parent(s) to develop a plan to provide feeding, bathing, changing diaper around rest periods	Prevents interruption in rest and sleep

Discharge or Maintenance Evaluation

- Decreased respiratory rate and excursion
- Provides rest and sleep periods imposed by illness
- Reduces and/or minimizes fatigue
- Participates in activities that do not compromise energy and breathing pattern
- Maintains ability to eat, drink, and play within limits imposed by illness

Knowledge deficit of parent(s), caretaker

Related to: Lack of information on how to prevent transmission of respiratory syncytial virus
Defining characteristics: Promotion of health-seeking behaviors within the hospital and home to prevent complications and speedy recovery
Related to: The use of the drug Ribavirin, when applicable (anti-viral drug used to treat RSV infection)
Defining characteristics: Direct or indirect contact with the virus, cross-infection of family members, parent(s) request for information about preventative measures

Outcome Criteria

Absence of cross-infection to others and secondary infection in infant/small child
Respiratory rate, depth, and ease remains within baseline parameters

Interventions	Rationales
Assess existing knowledge of disease prevention and transmission	Provides baseline for type of information needed to prevent infection transmission to child
Inform that the virus is transmitted by direct and indirect contact via the nose and eyes, and that hands should be kept away from these areas	Explains that kissing and cuddling infant/small child, and fomites that are on hard, smooth surfaces are sources of contact with the virus

Interventions	Rationales
Instruction in handwashing technique for child, family members and staff	Prevents transmission by the hands, which are the main sources of contamination and carriers of organisms to the face area
Advise that plastic goggles may be worn when caring for infant/small child	Prevents risk of contact with virus via the eyes
Inform of potential for spread of virus to other family members and need for segregation of infant/small child from others	Explains that virus is easily transmitted, with an incidence as high as half of family members acquiring viral infections
If hospitalized, isolate and use gloves, gown precautions; confine care assignments to patients with respiratory conditions	Protects from exposure to secretions and transmission of virus to other patients

Information, Instruction, Demonstration

Interventions	Rationales
Instruct parents and child if applicable, on the administration of medications prescribed	Improves consistency of medication administration and the recognition of adverse side effects
Instruct parents on the signs and symptoms of respiratory distress and infection, including fever, dyspnea, tachypnea, and expectoration of yellow/green sputum	Encourages parents to seek prompt medical attention, as needed
Instruct parents on the importance of good nutrition and hydration, emphasizing a high color balanced diet and increased fluids	Promotes liquification of secretions and replaces calories used to fight infection, thereby boosting the child's own natural body defenses
Instruct parents on the importance of providing cool mist humidity and instructions on the proper use	Promotes liquification of secretions
Instruct parents in the use of cover gowns over their clothes when they are in	Prevents the potential spread of the virus to others

Interventions	Rationales
direct contact with the child, when applicable	
Encourage and teach parents to provide care for the hospitalized child at a level they are comfortable with and within the constraints of necessary treatments	Promotes parental identity and control; may lessen anxiety and stress
Instruct parents regarding the drug Ribavirin used during hospitalization: • Side effects • Type and purposes of isolation, including use of masks, gloves, and/or gowns as applicable • Precautions utilized for parents, staff, and visitors, including information regarding potential risks of environmental exposure; advise pregnant women not to directly care for child; decrease potential exposure by temporarily stopping the aerosols when tent/hood is opened and administer drug in well-ventilated rooms (at least 6 air exchanges per hour) • Strict handwashing before and after leaving the child's room	Promotes understanding which may lessen anxiety; prevents accidental exposures to the drug
Instruct child, as applicable, and family members on the appropriate disposal of soiled tissues, etc.	Prevent the transmission of the disease
Instruct parents on the importance of limiting the number of visitors and screening them for recent illness	Prevent transmission of the disease to others; prevent further complications in the child with RSV

Discharge or Maintenance Evaluation

- Protects self, family members, and child from exposure to the virus
- Verbalizes methods of preventing small child from touching face and other areas with hands and handwashing procedure for child
- Verbalizes how virus is transmitted and precautions necessary to take to prevent spread of disease and/or secondary infection
- Demonstrates handwashing technique and verbalizes when to perform during care of infant/small child
- Parents accurately administer prescribed medications and report adverse effects
- Parents provide rest and good nutrition for the child
- Parents use humidity, as applicable, and understand delivery methods
- Parents remain active in caretaking at a level with which they are comfortable
- Parents understand the use of the drug Ribavirin, potential side effects and precautions utilized during administration

Bronchiolitis

Upper Respiratory Infection

↓

Respiratory syncytial virus (RSV)
Adenovirus, rhinovirus, parainfluenza virus

↓

Inflammation/edema of bronchiolar mucosa

↓

Sloughing of cells in lining of bronchioles
Increased mucus production

↓

Obstruction of small and medium airways

↙   ↘

Air Trapping in alveoli   Narrowed lumina of airways

↓   ↓

Hyperinflation   Increased airway resistance
Hypoxia

↓   ↓

Collapse of walls of alveoli   Dyspnea, tachypnea,
Atelectasis   nasal flaring
                                         Chest retractions of
                                         sternum and
                                  lower ribs on inspiration
                              Crackles, rhonchi, wheezes
                           Cough that is paroxysmal and dry

↓   ↓

Treatment regimen ⟵————————   Hypoxemia/respiratory acidosis
                                   Diminished or absent breath sound
                                       Cyanosis

↓   ↓

Recovery   Respiratory or cardiac
Repeated attacks of   failure in severe cases
wheezing/asthma

Bronchopulmonary Dysplasia

Bronchopulmonary dysplasia (BPD) is a chronic lung condition most common in infants that were preterm or of small gestational age (SGA) at birth. It is characterized by degrees of lung damage past the age of 1 month, caused by the use of assistive ventilation with the administration of high concentrations of oxygen to treat Idiopathic Respiratory Distress Syndrome (IRDS) or other serious disorders of the neonate. The lung and airway damage affects pulmonary function which leads to oxygen dependence, abnormal ABGs, and chest findings on x-ray examination, as well as susceptibility to pulmonary infections resulting in frequent and/or lengthy hospitalizations. BPD may resolve by the time the child is 3-4 years of age.

MEDICAL CARE

Bronchodilators: theophylline (Bronckodyl elixir, Theolar liquid) given PO or aminophylline (theophylline ethylendediamine) given IV to produce bronchodilation by relaxing bronchial smooth muscle if dyspnea present.

Antimicrobials: cefaclor (Ceclor suspension), amoxicillin (Amcill pediatric drops) given PO or ampicillin sodium (Omnipen-N), carbenicillin disodium (Geopen) given IV, vancomycin (IV), third generation cephalosporins (IV) or other antibiotics to treat infection based on culture results and severity of infection.

Diuretics: furosemide (Lasix) given IV, spironolactone (PO) to promote fluid removal and excretion which will reduce edema if heart failure present.

Cardiac glycosides: digitalis (Digoxin) given IV to increase force and strength of heart contractions if heart failure or pulmonary hypertension present.

Corticosteroids: dexamethasone (IV, PO) given to decrease the inflammation of the lung tissue.

Oxygen therapy: treats hypoxemia as indicated by ABGs or transcutaneous O_2 monitoring or ear oximetry; oxygen level delivered varies according to severity of disease, per nasal cannula or endotracheal tube.

Chest x-ray: reveals bilateral infiltration, with areas of hyperaeration and cystic areas at base of lungs as disease progresses; "whiteout" and consolidation visible if condition worsens or increases in healing tissue visible if improving.

Electrocardiogram: reveals right ventricular hypertrophy and possible failure.

Pulmonary function: reveals prolonged ratio between inspiratory and expiratory phases.

Throat/tracheal cultures: reveals and identifies infectious agent and sensitivity to specific antimicrobial treatment if infection present.

Arterial blood gases: reveals hypoxemic state by decreases in pO_2 of less than 55-60 mm Hg and increases in pCO_2 of more than 45-65 mm Hg which determine oxygen administration adjustments based on chronic hypoxemia associated with this condition; increased HCO_3 in presence of respiratory failure (chronic or acute).

Electrolyte panel: reveals hypokalemia if diuretics given, calcium and phosphorus deficits if nutrition inadequate.

Complete blood count: reveals increased WBC if infection is present.

NURSING CARE PLANS

Ineffective breathing pattern (45)

Related to: Inflammatory process
Defining characteristics: Dyspnea, tachypnea, use of accessory muscles, increased anteroposterior diameter, abnormal ABGs, cyanosis, recurrent wheezing, crackles and presence of respiratory infections (bronchitis, bronchiolitis, pneumonia)

Impaired gas exchange (47)

Related to: Ventilation perfusion imbalance
Defining characteristics: Hypoxemia, hypercapnia, restlessness, confusion, irritability, somnolence

Altered nutrition: Less than body requirements (168)

Related to: Inability to ingest food
Defining characteristics: Hypoxia during feeding, poor feeder, decreased weight gain, increased energy/metabolic need for work of breathing, altered physical growth

Fluid volume excess (5)

Related to: Compromised regulatory mechanisms (presence of right heart failure)
Defining characteristics: Edema, pulmonary effusion, weight gain, dyspnea, crackles, change in respiratory pattern, pulmonary congestion

Altered growth and development (419)

Related to: Separation from significant others
Defining characteristics: Frequent or prolonged hospitalizations
Related to: Environmental and stimulation deficiencies
Defining characteristics: Isolation, listlessness, decreased responses
Related to: Effects of physical disability/chronic illness
Defining characteristics: Inability to perform self-care or self-control of activities appropriate for age; delay or difficulty in performing motor, mental, social skills typical of age group

SPECIFIC DIAGNOSES AND CARE PLANS

Risk for infection

Related to: Chronic respiratory disease
Defining characteristics: Reduced ciliary activity, lung damage, decreased lung capacity and accessory muscles' inability to move secretions, increased temperature, yellow or green sputum in increased amounts, diminished breath sounds; presence of respiratory and suction of family membranes

Outcome Criteria

Absence or reduction in frequency of respiratory infections
Respiratory status at baseline parameters maintained
Airway patency with effective removal of secretions and absence of stasis of secretions

Interventions	Rationales
Assess for change in breathing pattern, color of mucus, rise in temperature, diminished breath sounds; presence of respiratory infection of family members	Indicates presence or potential for infection, which may be life threatening in infants with this disease
Avoid exposure to persons with respiratory infections; isolate from infectious patients	Infants have a low respiratory reserve and are prone to infection transmission from others
Utilize handwashing technique before giving care to infant	Prevents transmission of microorganisms to infant

Interventions	Rationales
Remove secretions by physiotherapy or suctioning via sterile technique	Stasis of secretions provide medium for infection
Obtain sputum for culture	Identifies presence of pathogenic organisms

Information, Instruction, Demonstration

Interventions	Rationales
Demonstrate handwashing techniques and allow for return demonstration before caring for infant/child	Prevents cross-contamination by hands
Inform of infant/child susceptibility to infection and for infant/child to avoid contact with anyone with a respiratory infection	Any illness, even a minor one will compromise the infant/child's respiratory status
Inform to maintain an environment free of smoke, sprays, or other irritating substances	Avoids irritation of airways that might affect ease of respirations
Inform to provide adequate fluid and nutritional intake	Maintains fluid and nutritional requirements of infant
Instruct in cardiopulmonary resuscitation (CPR)	Provides anticipatory knowledge to perform life-saving measure if needed
Inform of need to have periodic x-rays and laboratory tests	Assist physician in monitoring progress of disease
Inform to report any changes in mucus or respiratory distress to physician	Provides for immediate interventions, if needed, to control infection

Discharge or Maintenance Evaluation

- Takes measures to avoid exposure to respiratory infections
- Maintains respiratory status within baseline parameters
- Effectively removes mucus of thin consistency and clear color
- Performs handwashing technique

- Adheres to diagnostic test schedule and interaction with physician when needed
- Provides appropriate fluid and nutritional requirements

Ineffective family coping: Compromised

Related to: Prolonged disease that exhausts supportive capacity of significant people

Defining characteristics: Preoccupation of significant persons with anxiety, guilt, fear regardless of infant/child illness; display of protective behaviors by significant persons that are disproportionate to infant/child needs (too much or too little), frequent hospitalizations, prolonged hospitalization

Related to: Inadequate or incorrect information or understanding by a primary person and/or significant persons

Defining characteristics: Verbalization by significant persons of inadequate knowledge base that interferes with care and support of infant/child

Outcome Criteria

Development of family coping skills in dealing with infant/child illness, hospitalization or potential for hospitalization, and care of infant/child with prolonged illness

Interventions	Rationales
Assess anxiety, fear, erratic behavior, perception of crisis situation by family members	Provides information affecting family ability to cope with infant/child prolonged illness
Assess coping methods used and effectiveness	Identifies coping methods that work and need to develop new coping skills
Encourage expression of feelings and questions in accepting, nonjudgmental environment	Reduces anxiety and enhances family's understanding of infant's condition
Encourage family involvement in care during and after hospitalization	Provides for reduction of anxiety and fear of equipment used in care
Allow for open visitation, encourage telephone calls to hospital by family members	Encourages bonding and assists in coping with infant/child hospitalization if family unable to stay
Provide place for family members to rest, freshen up	Promotes comfort of family

Interventions	Rationales
Suggest social worker referral if needed	Provides support and resources for financial or infant/child care relief
Give positive feedback and praise family efforts in developing coping and problem-solving techniques and caring for infant	Encourages parent(s) and family to participate in care and gain some control over the situation

Information, Instruction, Demonstration

Interventions	Rationales
Inform and reinforce appropriate coping behaviors	Promotes behavior change and adaption to care of infant with oxygen dependence
Inform that overprotective behaviors may hinder growth and development during infancy and that, with lung growth, pulmonary function may become normal and adverse effects of behavior	Knowledge will enhance family understanding of condition
Inform of need to maintain health of family members, emotional status of parent(s)	Chronic anxiety, fatigue will affect health and care capabilities of family
Provide information regarding infant's condition and progress, oxygen dependence needs, and reason for care and medications	Reduces anxiety of parent(s) and family and anticipates need for knowledge about disease and care
Inform that assistance may be secured by telephoning hospital after discharge	Provides family with resource in crisis situation
Instruct and demonstrate cardiopulmonary resuscitation (CPR), oxygen administration, and safety measures to eliminate fire hazards	Enables family to manage emergency situation and maintain safe oxygen administration

Discharge or Maintenance Evaluation

- Returns demonstration of CPR
- Verbalizes that improved coping skills will be practiced by family
- Family involved in support and care of infant/ child
- Verbalizes understanding of infant/child long-term care needs
- Administers oxygen and medication regimen correctly and safely
- Verbalizes reduced anxiety and fear of repeated hospitalizations after receiving information about family expectations during hospitalizations

ADDITIONAL NURSING DIAGNOSIS

Sleep pattern disturbance

Related to: Exposure to the Neonatal Intensive Care Unit (NICU) environment
Defining characteristics: Maladaptive behaviors such as alterations in heart rate, respirations, color changes, erratic body movements, difficulty with feedings or prolonged periods of wakefulness

Outcome Criteria

Limited changes in heart rate and respiratory rate with caregiving or when exposed to environmental demands
Limited color changes with caregiving, handling during technical procedures, or during social interactions
Better tolerance of feedings as evidenced by a decrease in residual volume after feedings and less regurgitation
Smoother and better organized body movements during and between caregiving
Smoother transitions between sleep states and wake states
Improved use of self-consoling behaviors, such as hand to mouth or hand to face movements, sucking (fingers, tubing, pacifier), hand or feet clasping, foot bracing, and maintaining flexion of extremities
Improved ability to block out repetitive stimuli (habituation) with decreased body movements during sleep or during transition from awake to sleep states
Improved ability to be consoled from outside sources; i.e., being held, talked to, rocked

Interventions	Rationales
Introduce one caregiving intervention at a time, observing responses; allow	Prevents overstimulation and further maladaptation to the environment.
for "time out" if infant displays stress signals, such as finger splaying, grimacing, tongue extension, worried alertness, spitting up, back arching, gaze aversion, yawning, hiccuping, color changes, or changes in cardiac or respiratory functioning	
Cluster caregiving, while not over-stimulating infant; continuously monitor infant for signs of stress during caregiving, providing rest periods as needed	Promotes longer periods of alert and/or deep sleep which will enhance the body's own natural defenses; providing rest periods will allow infant to recover prior to initiation of additional caregiving; prevents sudden disruptions in sleep; promotes stability and adaptive behaviors
Remain at bedside after procedures/caregiving to assess infant's response; if maladaptive responses occur, use "time-out" to allow infant to adapt	Prevents or minimizes maladaptive responses which often occurs up to 20 minutes after caregiving is completed
Alter physical environment by decreasing light and sound	Prevents or decreases maladaptive behaviors; both light and sound levels in the NICU have been implicated in interfering with sleep and stable physiological functioning
Facilitate handling by providing containment: holding infant's arms and legs in a flexed position, close to their midline using the caregiver's hands and/or positioning aids such as rolled blankets; premature or ill infants should be positioned prone or sidelying, maintaining soft flexion	Promotes flexion and stabilizes infant's motor and physiologic systems
Place the infant in a flexed position with hands to midline, or swaddled with hands free; providing paci-	Promotes self-consoling/ soothing behaviors which facilitate organization and adaptive behaviors

Interventions	Rationales
fier and/or fingers to suck on; providing objects to encourage hand grasping such as blankets, tubing, and fingers during caregiving	
Consistency of caregiving: a primary team identified to work collaboratively with the parents in developing an individualized plan of care reviewed daily and discussed at intervals with the parents	Promotes element of trust for both the infant and family, improving parent--infant relationships; allows caregivers to identify infant's behavioral cues
Provide individualized feeding support determined by the infant's own needs and strengths; feeding focus should be positive and pleasurable, with attention to infant's cues or signals	Promotes positive feeding experiences, which facilitates weight gain and feeding competency
Provide optimal level of family support through utilization of family centered care giving principles: enhanced parental involvement in all aspects of care giving and decision-making; promote family comfort with home-like environment	Promotes feelings of belonging and control which enhances parent-infant relationship

Information, Instruction, and Demonstration

Interventions	Rationales
Assist parents in learning their infant's signals or cues and interpreting them appropriately	Promotes positive parenting role and minimizes infant's maladaptive behaviors, promoting improved long-term growth and development
Instruct and encourage parents in caregiving activities throughout the NICU stay, at a level parents are comfortable with	Promotes improved parental confidence, enhances parenting skills, and improves parent-infant relationship/interactions

Interventions	Rationales
Assist parents in promoting infant adaptive behaviors through use of containment, swaddling, promotion and maintenance of flexion, non-nutritive sucking, and finger grasping	Promotes positive adaptive behaviors in the infant and increases parental participation and feelings of control
Assist and encourage parents to personalize infant bed space by bringing in clothes, blankets to be used over isolettes/cribs, and pictures from home	Promotes positive parental identity and feelings of control
Assist, instruct, and encourage parental participation in Kangaroo care or skin-to-skin holding when infant is medically stable; this method is accomplished by placing infant on parent's chest under their clothing	Promotes stable physiologic functioning, maintains thermoregulation, improves quiet/alert sleep periods, improves weight gain, promotes positive parent/infant relationship and improves parental confidence
Assist parents in making the difficult transition from hospital to home; allow ample time for teaching and communication of needs and feelings; validate feelings of anxiety as normal; give brief and accurate information, with time for clarification and provide supplemental written materials; allow parents permission to be in control of decisions and maintain structure in their own lives; discuss feelings of anger and guilt openly; adapt teaching and communication techniques to different family styles, customs, and cultures	Promotes feelings of control and mastery through education and open communication; this will enhance the parent-infant relationship and foster the child's growth and development

Discharge or Maintenance Evaluation

- Infant displays adaptive behaviors, such as physiologic stability evidenced by stable heart rate, respiratory rate, color changes, improved sleep states, ability to interact with others, and utilization of self-consoling behaviors

- Infant maintained in flexed position (prone or side-lying) with utilization of containment, swaddling, and nesting to maintain desired position
- Light and sound levels in the environment modified and monitored to facilitate infant sleep states and organization
- Parents verbalize understanding of and demonstrate mastery of caregiving techniques necessary for home care
- Parents verbalize and demonstrate understanding of infant's individual cues and can facilitate infant's adaptive responses

Bronchopulmonary Dysplasia

Hyaline membrane disease (IRDS)

Severe disorders during
neonatal period

Congenital heart disorder
Necrotizing enterocolitis
Meconium aspiration
Cerebral hemorrhage

Endotracheal intubation
Mechanical ventilation (positive pressure)
Prolonged high concentrations of oxygen

Epithelial damage

Thickened and fibrotic alveoli walls
Metaplasia of bronchiolar epithelium
Inhibited ciliary activity

Atelectasis
Hyperinflation of alveoli (cystlike)
Respiratory distress

Resolution in 6-12 months
with treatment

Normal pulmonary function
by 3-7 years of age

Some obstructive and restrictive
pulmonary effects
Activity intolerance

Increased oxygen requirement
Interstitial emphysema
Pneumonia

Fluid retention
Pulmonary hypertension
Respiratory failure
Right heart failure

Cystic Fibrosis

Cystic fibrosis (mucoviscidosis) is the most common hereditary disease of children. It is an autosomal-recessive trait disorder affecting the exocrine glands. The increased activity of the mucus mechanical obstruction forms accumulation in ducts and glands. Organs affected are the pancreas, small intestine, liver, lungs, and reproductive organs. Severity of the disease varies. Although an increased survival rate has been evident in recent years, death is the final result as progressive pulmonary complications occur and create a serious threat to the child's life. Children with cystic fibrosis and their families are continuously faced with the daily implementation of a medical regimen that may deplete their physical, emotional, and financial resources. Since the disease is chronic, hospitalization may be frequent.

MEDICAL CARE

Bronchodilators/Adrenergic agonists: isoetharine hydrochloride (Bronkosol) given via small volume nebulizer, isoetharine mesylate (Bronkometer) given via hand-held inhalator to relieve bronchospasms and facilitate removal of pulmonary secretions by bronchial dilatation and smooth muscle relaxation.

Mucolytics: acetylcysteine (Mucomyst) used in the nebulizing solution for mist tent, face mask to liquefy mucus, propylene glycerol and distilled water solution, normal saline used in mist therapy to stabilize the droplet and prevent vaporization; recombinant human deoxyribonuclease (Dnase) used as an aerosolized medication to decrease the viscosity of mucus.

Vitamins: if liver involved, vitamin A, D, E and K given as replacement in water-miscible preparations.

Expectorants: potassium iodide (SSKI), iodinated glycerol (Organidin), hydriodic acid syrup given PO to thin mucus secretions and facilitate expectoration.

Enzyme/Digestants: pancrelipase (Viokase) given PO to replace enzyme deficiency in powder, granules, packet, or tablet form to assist in digestion and bowel elimination.

Antibiotics: selection dependent on identification and sensitivity to organism revealed by culture, whether therapy is prophylactic, and term of treatment; penicillin G (Pentids solution) given PO, penicillin G potassium (Pfizerpen) given IM or IV, methicillin (Staphcillin) given IV for treatment of staphylococcal infections; vancomycin IV, Third generation Cephalosporins PO, IV.

Oxygen therapy: continuous, low-volume oxygen administered with caution in presence of respiratory distress.

Chest x-ray: reveals patchy areas of atelectasis and generalized obstructive emphysema, with later infiltratives and disemination of bronchopneumonia evident.

Pulmonary function: reveals severity of lung involvement and general condition.

Iontophoresis of pilocarpine sweat test: reveals sweat chloride content greater than 60 mEq/L, obtained by electrode stimulation of the sweat glands and measurement of the chloride content in the laboratory, is the most definitive test for cystic fibrosis.

Stool test: reveals fecal fat in a 5-day stool collection specimen and calculated to determine impaired fat absorption.

Alanine aminotransferase (ALT)/Aspartate aminotransferase (AST): reveals elevation of these enzymes in liver damage.

NURSING CARE PLANS

Essential nursing diagnoses and plans associated with this condition:

Ineffective airway clearance (42)

Related to: Tracheobronchial secretions and obstruction; decreased energy and fatigue
Defining characteristics: Dyspnea; tachypnea; increasing amount of thick, tenacious sputum; nonproductive cough; wheezy respirations with expiratory obstruction

Ineffective breathing pattern (45)

Related to: Tracheobronchial obstruction; decreased energy and fatigue
Defining characteristics: Dyspnea, tachypnea, cough, increased anteroposterior diameter (barrel chest), cyanosis, prolonged expiratory phase, finger and toe clubbing with continued ventilatory impairment

Altered nutrition: Less than body requirements (168)

Related to: Inability to digest food or absorb nutrients because of biological factors
Defining characteristics: Reduced weight gain; failure to thrive; weight loss with adequate food intake and increased appetite; vomiting; thin and wasted appearance of extremities and buttocks; absence of pancreatic enzymes, causing increased amount of stool; foul smelling loosely formed bulky stools; steatorrhea, prolapse of the rectum

Risk for fluid volume deficit (222)

Related to: Excessive losses through normal routes
Defining characteristics: Tachypnea, vomiting, diarrhea, profuse sweating, loss of sodium and chloride

Decreased cardiac output (3)

Related to: Electrical factors of rate and rhythm
Defining characteristics: Arrhythmias; ECG changes; variations in hemodynamic readings (VS and BP); dyspnea; pale, cold, clammy skin; cyanosis; edema; complication of heart failure

Sleep pattern disturbance (114)

Related to: Internal factor of illness effects
Defining characteristics: Interrupted sleep, cough, dyspnea, fatigue, increasing irritability, restlessness, lethargy, listlessness

Risk for impaired skin integrity (397)

Related to: External mechanical factor of pressure
Defining characteristics: Disruption of skin surface, redness or rash on genitalia and buttocks, redness and irritation at bony prominences, use of bedpan

Altered growth and development (419)

Related to: Effects of physical illness and disability
Defining characteristics: Altered physical growth, delay or difficulty in performing motor, social skills typical of age group
Related to: Separation from significant others
Defining characteristics: Frequent hospitalizations

SPECIFIC DIAGNOSES AND CARE PLANS

Risk for activity intolerance

Related to: Deconditioned status
Defining characteristics: Weakness, fatigue, inability to participate in self-care, physical and social activities
Related to: Respiratory problems
Defining characteristics: Dyspnea, tachypnea, exertional discomfort

Outcome Criteria

Return of activity within disease limitations
Weakness and fatigue kept at a minimum or controlled

Interventions	Rationales
Assess level of fatigue and activity in relation to respiratory status	Provides information about energy reserves as dyspnea and work of breathing over period of time exhausts these reserves
Schedule and provide rest periods in a quiet environment	Promotes adequate rest and reduces stimuli
Disturb only when necessary for care and procedures; provide quiet play appropriate for age (TV, games, reading), interests, and energy level	Conserves energy and prevents interruption in rest; prevents alteration in respiratory status and energy depletion caused by excessive activity
Perform respiratory physiotherapy; avoid treatment before or after meals	Reduces work while promoting effectiveness of breathing
Perform breathing exercises	Improves ventilation and strengthens chest muscles

Information, Instruction, Demonstration

Interventions	Rationales
Explain to parent(s) and child the reasons for need to conserve energy and to rest to avoid fatigue	Promotes understanding of effect of activity on breathing and importance of rest to prevent fatigue
Inform parent(s) and child of activity or exercise restrictions, how to engage in activities without tiring or affecting respiratory status; discuss types of activities child enjoys	Measures to prevent fatigue while engaging in as near normal participation as possible
Instruct child to ask for assistance if needed for daily activities; assist to plan a schedule for ADL that will conserve energy	Prevents overtiring and fatigue

Discharge or Maintenance Evaluation

- Controls activities that are fatiguing
- Prevents fatigue with rest periods provided when needed
- Work of breathing minimized and anxiety and apprehension controlled during activities

Risk for infection

Related to: Chronic pulmonary disease
Defining characteristics: Presence of and stasis of mucous in respiratory tract, increased environmental exposure, change in respiratory pattern and mucus color, temperature

Outcome Criteria

Absence of infection with implementation of preventative measures

Interventions	Rationales
Assess for change in breathing pattern, color of mucus, diminished breath sounds, ability to cough and raise secretions	Indicates presence of respiratory infection
Avoid exposure to persons with respiratory infections; isolate from infectious patients and carry out respiratory precautions	Prevents transmission of microorganisms as disease increases susceptibility to infection
Utilize handwashing technique before giving care	Prevents transmission of microorganisms to child
Assist to cough or remove secretions by suctioning	Stasis of secretions provide medium for infection
Use medical asepsis techniques or sterile techniques when administering respiratory care	Prevents exposure to infectious agents
Administer antibiotics	Provides prophylactic antibiotics, which are often prescribed as a preventative measure

Information, Instruction, Demonstration

Interventions	Rationales
Demonstrate handwashing technique to parent(s) and child and allow for return demonstration	Prevents cross-contamination by hands
Inform parent(s) of child's high susceptibility to infection and to avoid contact of child with persons or family members with respiratory infections	Prevents any infection that will compromise respiratory status and that could be life threatening
Instruct parent(s) in antibiotic regimen and inform of need to have influenza immunization and to avoid cough suppressants	Promotes use of preventative measures to control possible infection, cough suppressants prevent cough needed to bring up secretions
Inform parent(s) to report any changes in mucus or respiratory status to physician	Provides for immediate interventions to control infection

Discharge or Maintenance Evaluation

- Maintains respiratory status within baseline parameters
- Takes measures to avoid exposure to respiratory infections
- Utilizes medical asepsis
- Clears airway of mucus effectively
- Complies with antibiotic regimen, avoids medications not recommended by physician
- Secures yearly influenza immunization

Anticipatory grieving

Related to: Perceived potential loss of significant other by parent(s), perceived potential loss of physiopsychosocial well-being by child
Defining characteristics: Expression of distress at potential loss, poor prognosis for child (premature death), anger, guilt, sadness, fear, long-term chronic illness of child

Outcome Criteria

Progressive grief resolution and relinquishing of emotional attachment to the child over prolonged period of time of illness by parent(s)

Management of stages of grieving by parent(s) and child

Interventions	Rationales
Assess stage of grief process, problems encountered, feelings regarding potential loss	Allows for information regarding stage of grieving, as time to work through grieving varies with individuals and the longer the illness, the better able the parent(s) and family will be able to move through the stages towards acceptance
Provide emotional and spiritual comfort in an accepting environment	Provides for emotional needs of parent(s); assists them in coping with ill child
Avoid conversation that will cause guilt or anger	Provides support without adding stressors that are difficult to resolve
Answer all questions honestly, clarify any misconceptions	Promotes trust and reduces parental anxiety
Accept parental responses and allow for their expression of feelings	Allows for reactions necessary to work through grieving
Assist in identifying and using effective coping mechanisms and in understanding situations over which they have no control	Promotes use of defense mechanisms to progress through grief
Encourage parent(s) to assist child with normal development and discipline	Promotes sense of normalcy and well-being for child
Allow child to talk about any concerns regarding death and respond to questions honestly	Promotes expression of feelings and concerns for understanding grieving process and behaviors

Information, Instruction, Demonstration

Interventions	Rationales
Inform parent(s) and child of stages of growing and of behaviors that are acceptable in resolving grief	Promotes understanding of feelings and behaviors that are manifested by grief
Instruct parent(s) in coping skills and approaches that may be used	Promotes coping ability over prolonged period of illness
Refer to counseling services, clergy, local support agencies for cystic fibrosis, Cystic Fibrosis Foundation	Provides support and assistance in adapting to chronic illness and potential early death of child
Inform parent(s) and child of disease process and what can be expected from chronic nature and systems involved with the illness	Provides a realistic view of the child's illness
Depending on child's age and development, provide information on a need-to-know basis with honesty and in small amounts during each interaction	Promotes trust and understanding to allow for work of grieving

Discharge or Maintenance Evaluation

- Verbalizes understanding of grief process and responses
- Shares feelings with professionals and other members of family
- Secures assistance from support persons and/or groups
- Identifies and uses coping skills that assist in adaption to the chronic illness
- Performs normal parental tasks/interactions with child

Anxiety

Related to: Threat of or change in health status; threat of or change in environment (hospitalization), threat of death, threat of illness occurring in healthy children or future children

Defining characteristics: Parent — increased apprehension that condition might worsen or infection develop, expressed concern and worry about possible hospitaliza-

tion, fear of consequences of disease, increased tension and uncertainty;
child — unhappy and sad attitude, withdrawal or aggressive behavior, somatic and fatigue complaints, poor school attendance and performance

Outcome Criteria

Reduced parental and child anxiety as adjustments to changes in life-style and adaption to disease occur

Interventions	Rationales
Assess source and level of anxiety, how anxiety is manifested, and need for information that will relieve anxiety of child	Provides information about anxiety level and the need for interventions to relieve it, sources may include fear and uncertainty about treatment and recovery, guilt for presence of illness, possible loss of parental role, and loss of responsibility if hospitalized
Allow parent(s) and child to express fears and concerns and to ask questions about disease and what to expect	Provides opportunity to vent feelings and secure information to reduce anxiety
Communicate with parent(s) and answer questions calmly and honestly	Promotes calm and supportive environment
Provide supportive and nonjudgmental environment	Promotes trust and reduces anxiety
Inform parent(s) and child of all procedures and treatments	Relieves anxiety caused by fear of the unknown
Allow parent(s) to stay with child, allow open visitation and telephone communications; encourage to participate in care that is planned around usual home routines	Reduces anxiety for child by allowing presence and involvement in care, and familiar routines and persons
If hospitalization frequent, assign same personnel to care for child if appropriate	Promotes trust and comfort and reduces anxiety when cared for by familiar persons

Information, Instruction, Demonstration

Interventions	Rationales
Explain reasons for change in condition and need for hospitalization	Promotes understanding of disease complications and nature of chronic disease
Explain to parent(s) and child as appropriate for age, reason for each procedure or type of therapy, effects of any diagnostic tests	Prevents anxiety by reducing fear of unknown
Clarify any misinformation with honesty and in simple, understandable language	Prevents unnecessary anxiety resulting from inaccurate information or beliefs
Refer to counseling, community groups for cystic fibrosis	Provides support to parent(s) and child, and information from those with similar problems, which reduces anxiety

Discharge or Maintenance Evaluation

- Verbalizes that anxiety reduced by parent(s) and child
- Secures information and support from community agencies
- Expresses increased comfort when participating in care and support of child
- Symptoms of anxiety in the child decreasing or controlled
- Child participates in school and social activities
- Verbalizes understanding of causes of fear and anxiety, and of positive effect for treatment or regimen

Altered family processes

Related to: Situational transition of long-term illness
Defining characteristics: Family system unable to meet physical, emotional needs of its members; inability to express or accept wide range of feelings; family unable to deal with or adapt to chronic illness of child in a constructive manner; excessive involvement with ill child by parent(s)/siblings; evidence of marital and social discord exhibited by parent(s); guilt expressed by parent(s)/siblings; irritability as a response to the ill child; lack of support from family/friends

Outcome Criteria

Progressive adaptation and acceptance by family members of care for child with long-term illness, while retaining individual and family functions

Interventions	Rationales
Assess family ability to cope with ill child, strain on family relationships, developmental level of family, response of siblings, knowledge of health practices, family rule behavior and attitude toward long-term care, economic pressures and resources to care for long-term illness	Provides information about family attitudes and coping abilities, which directly affect the child's health and feeling of well-being; chronic illness of a child in a family may strengthen a family or strain family relationships; members may develop emotional problems when family is under stress
Assist individual family members to identify stressors and behaviors and to define them in positive terms (bad, indifferent, rebellious)	Individual problems that are defined and explored have meaning for the entire family
Assist family members in expressing problems and exploring solutions, responsibilities	Provides opportunity to express feelings, problems, and problem-solving strategies by whole family
Assist in establishing short- and long-term goals in maintaining child care and family integration of child into home routine	Promotes inclusion of ill child in family routines and activities
Support and encourage parental caretaking efforts	Reinforces roles and reduces stress in family members

Information, Instruction, Demonstration

Interventions	Rationales
Inform of and discuss family dynamics and need to tolerate conflict and individual behaviors	Provides knowledge and assists in understanding family behaviors leading to problem resolution
Discuss needs of all family members and inform of methods to provide care and attention to all members	Allows for ongoing responsibility for care of all family members

Interventions	Rationales
Inform parent(s) of local agencies, respite care, support groups for family assistance, Cystic Fibrosis Foundation	Provides information, economic and emotional support for family as a group or individual
Inform family of methods to maintain child's independence and role in the family and that discipline of child and well children should be the same	Ensures acceptance of child into family routines
Inform that family health must be maintained and social contacts encouraged	Health and attitude of family promotes ill child's coping ability
Provide information to parent(s) about where health care may be secured (dentist, physical therapy, pulmonary physiotherapy)	Ensures ongoing health care for child with chronic illness

Discharge or Maintenance Evaluation

- Family has open discussions and identifies problem areas
- Family develops and uses problem solving techniques to resolve differences
- Family health and social responsibilities met
- Family demonstrates constructive responses to problem
- Ill child integrated into family life, with care becoming a part of family's daily routines
- Parent(s) secure genetic counseling if appropriate
- Family secures assistance from community agencies
- Family displays supportive behaviors for each other
- Family relationships preserved and stressors minimized

Home maintenance management, impaired

Related to: Complexity of home care management of cystic fibrosis patient; lifelong chronicity of the disease
Defining characteristics: Frequent exacerbations of respiratory infections; inadequate understanding of illness and home care components; child not functioning up to full potential in terms of growth and development, independence issues; stressors within family relationships

Outcome Criteria

Absence or decrease in respiratory infections
Symptoms of cystic fibrosis controlled within confines of severity of illness; optimal health status maintained
Family relationships assessed and maintained

Information, Instruction, Demonstration

Interventions	Rationales
Develop a flexible home plan of care, with input from all family members, as applicable	Promotes less disruption to family routines
Assist parents in locating the appropriate equipment and supplies necessary for home care; provide opportunities to learn and practice use prior to discharge; anticipate problems	Promotes feelings of control; may decrease anxiety and stressors
Instruct parents in all aspects of home care; reinforce teaching with written materials; return demonstrations encouraged, as applicable: oral hygiene chest physiotherapy (CPT) — parents adjust frequency based on individual child's needs; use of games and childhood activities can be incorporated into the therapy which will increase the likelihood of success (somersaults, wheelbarrow); antibiotic therapy (oral or IV) for respiratory exacerbations; facilitate arrangements with home health nursing as applicable; nutrition management including pancreatic enzyme replacement, health practices — adequate rest, good hygiene, importance of follow-up care, exercise, prevention of illness	Promotes understanding of care needed for child at home to provide optimal health and promote normal growth and development; promotes body's own natural defenses

Interventions	Rationales
Instruct parents on the signs of depression, especially in adolescents; make appropriate referral as needed	Promotes good communication between parent and health professional if a concern arises
Organize and coordinate services from various health professionals involved in the home care of the child, including home health nursing, respiratory therapy, physicians, social services, as applicable	Promotes family support which is crucial for a positive adaptation to care at home; may lessen anxiety and stressors
Discuss impact of caregiving at home with family members to assess potential problems; include siblings	Promotes improved communication between family members and health professionals; promotes positive relationships between parent-child and child-sibling

Discharge or Maintenance Evaluation

- Family provides health care for child at home, maintaining physiologic functioning at an optimal level
- Family demonstrates constructive responses to problems encountered
- Ill child integrated into family life, with care becoming a part of the family's daily routine
- Family's access and receive adequate support from health care services involved in home care management
- Recombinant human deoxyribonuclease (DNase) used as an aerosolized medication to decrease the viscosity of mucus

Cystic Fibrosis

Genetic factor (Autosomal recessive trait)

Potential for alteration in secretory process of exocrine glands

Risks to Respiratory System	Risks to Gastrointestinal System	Risks to Reproductive System	Sweat Glands
Collection and stasis of thick, tenacious secretions (mucus) Bronchial obstruction	Secretions carried to intestines, pancreas, liver, and salivary glands through wide or narrow ducts	Absence or obstruction of vas deferens Undeveloped epididymis Decreased spermatogenesis; absence of sperm Plugged cervix with viscid mucus	Reduced resorption of Na and Cl
Atelectasis Pneumonia Infection Invasion of bronchial epithelium and tissues	Duct obstruction		Increased Na and Cl in sweat
	Biliary fibrosis and dysfunction Fibrosis and degeneration of pancreas tissue and secretory cells Lack of enzymes in duodenum to digest protein, fats and carbohydrates		Electrolyte imbalance Dehydration
Mucopurulent exudate in respiratory tract			
Chronic respiratory disease		Sterility	
Right ventricular hypertrophy Cor pulmonale	Intestinal obstruction Fibrocystic disease of pancreas Malabsorption of nutrients Portal hypertension Liver failure		

Epiglottitis

Epiglottitis is the acute inflammation of the epiglottis and surrounding laryngeal area with the associated edema that constitutes an emergency situation as the supraglottic area becomes obstructed. It results in respiratory distress that must be relieved by endotracheal intubation or tracheostomy in severe cases. Onset is rapid (over 4-12 hours) and breathing pattern usually re-established within 72 hours following intubation and antimicrobial therapy. Children most commonly affected are between 3 and 7 years of age.

MEDICAL CARE

Antipyretics/Analgesics: acetaminophen (Tylenol tablets, Pedric wafers or elixir, Liquiprin drops) given PO to reduce fever and relieve throat pain and pain from swallowing. Ibuprofen (nonsteroidal anti-inflammatory) for children 6 months-12 years; Motrin or Advil liquid suspension or tablets PO to reduce fever and inflammation.

Antibiotics: ampicillin (Amcill suspension) given PO, or ampicillin sodium (Omnipen-N) given IV; chloramphenicol (Chloromycetin Palmitate suspension) given PO; cefuroxime sodium (Zinacefl given IV to treat infection by inhibiting cell wall synthesis of microorganisms; preferred treatment route is via IV.

Immunization: hemophilus, type B vaccination, to protect against the Hemophilus influenza, type B, the most common cause of epiglottitis.

Oxygen therapy: treats potential hypoxia administered by tent, mask, or cannula or via endotrachial tube; assists in preventing obstruction of airway by thick secretions by providing humidity with oxygen.

Neck x-ray: may be done to view lateral neck to diagnose condition.

Throat culture: reveals and identifies causative agent and sensitivity to specific antimicrobial therapy. Done only under direct supervision of a physician, emergency equipment for intubation should be readily available.

Blood culture: reveals and identifies causative agent or presence of other infectious agent.

Arterial blood gases: reveals decreased pH, pO_2; increased pCO_2 as respiratory distress becomes more acute and ventilation perfusion disturbance occurs.

Corticosteroids: reduces inflammation of the epiglottitis, improving oxygenation. Dexamethasone Sodium Phosphate (Decadron) IV.

NURSING CARE PLANS

Essential nursing diagnoses and plans associated with this condition:

Ineffective airway clearance (42)

Related to: Epiglottic infection, obstruction, secretion
Defining characteristics: Sudden increase in temperature, dyspnea, tachypnea, drooling, difficulty in swallowing, bright red epiglottis with edema, decreased breath sounds, muffled voice, sore throat, presence of tracheostomy or endotracheal tube

Ineffective breathing pattern (45)

Related to: Inflammatory process, obstruction
Defining characteristics: Air hunger, dyspnea, tachypnea, use of accessory muscles (intercostal, sub or suprasternal retractions), cough, assumption of three-point position, sitting up with mouth open and chin forward, stridor or croaking sound on inspiration

Risk for fluid volume deficit (222)

Related to: Loss of fluid through normal routes (respirations and temperature), altered intake
Defining characteristics: Increased body temperature, dry skin and mucous membranes, decreased skin turgor, increased pulse and respirations, sore throat and difficulty in swallowing, refusal to drink fluids

Hyperthermia (112)

Related to: Illness of inflammation/infection of epiglottal area
Defining characteristics: Sudden increase in body temperature above normal range, as high as 101 degrees F, warm to touch, increased pulse and respirations, positive culture

SPECIFIC DIAGNOSES AND CARE PLANS

Anxiety

Related to: Change in health status of child; change in environment (hospitalization); change in role functioning (parenting)

Defining characteristics: Verbalization of extreme fear and apprehension by parent(s); agitation, crying, irritability, air hunger and extreme expression of fear (child)

Outcome Criteria

Reduced parental and child anxiety and calmer appearance as child returns to respiratory baselines

Interventions	Rationales
Assess severity of fear and anxiety of parent(s) and child	Provides information about presence of extreme anxiety as symptoms of disease become more acute and breathing more difficult
Provide calm and supportive environment and inform parent(s) that best care is being given to child	Provides reassurance and reduces anxiety of parent(s)
Allow child to assume position of comfort, provide familiar object (toy, blanket); tripod position may offer the most comfort	Promotes comfort and security for child
Remain with child at all times during acute stages	Provides constant assessment for emergency interventions and reassurance for parent(s)
Allow parent(s) to stay with child, provide a place for rest	Promotes security needs for child and assists in reducing parental anxiety
Inform of all procedures, care, and changes in the child's condition	Reduces anxiety caused by fear of the unknown
Avoid any care or procedures that are not necessary during acute stage	Prevents increase of anxiety which increases respiratory distress
Allow for expression of fears and feelings of parent(s) and child and for behaviors caused by severe anxiety	Reduces anxiety and embarrassment

Information, Instruction, Demonstration

Interventions	Rationales
Orient parent(s) and child to room, equipment, supplies and policies	Familiarizes them to hospital environment
Provide succinct, simply stated information about disease and treatment regimen to parent(s)	Reduces anxiety by knowing what to expect and reason for therapy
Inform parent(s) that swelling subsides 24 hours after antibiotic therapy initiated and epiglottis usually returned to normal in about 3 days	Provides confirmation of positive outcome and reduces anxiety

Discharge or Maintenance Evaluation

- Express a reduction in anxiety as acute stage of disease is relieved
- Parent(s) stays and supports child while hospitalized
- Child's fear and air hunger relieved, and progressive calmness of child is established

Risk for suffocation

Related to: Disease process
Defining characteristics: Supraglottic edema; obstruction; dysphasia; hypoxia; cyanosis; extreme anxiety, with struggle to breathe

Outcome Criteria

Preventative measures taken to ensure patent airway

Interventions	Rationales
Assess for changes in skin color from pallor to cyanosis, severe dyspnea and sternal and intercostal retractions, lethargy, increased pulse	Provides information about increasing airway obstruction
Allow to sit up and avoid forcing child to lie down	Lying down may cause epiglottis to fall backward, causing airway obstruction

Interventions	Rationales
Avoid inspecting throat with tongue blade or obtaining throat culture unless immediate emergency equipment and personnel at hand	Leads to airway spasms and obstruction
Administer O₂ and monitor via pulse oximeter	Promotes oxygenation of tissues and prevents hypoxemia
Have emergency intubation equipment at hand and assist with endotracheal intubation or tracheostomy if necessary, or prepare for procedure in surgery	Establishes airway if obstruction present and respiratory failure and asphyxia imminent

Information, Instruction, Demonstration

Interventions	Rationales
Provide parent(s) with explanation of care and all procedures and reason and procedure for emergency intubation or tracheostomy if needed while hospitalized	Explanations provide information and support for parent(s) who are not familiar with procedures
Inform parent(s) of reason for restraints if emergency procedure done, that swelling is reduced after 24 hours of therapy and tube will probably be removed after 3 days	Prepares parent(s) with information of what to expect
Instruct parent(s) in symptoms to report if child not hospitalized	Early reporting of possible airway obstruction allows for measures to be taken to prevent asphyxia

Discharge or Maintenance Evaluation

- Prevents airway obstruction and maintains airway patency
- Prevents suffocation as a result of endotracheal intubation or tracheostomy procedure
- Respiratory/ventilatory status within normal parameters established

Knowledge deficit (potential or actual)

Related to: The promotion of health-seeking behaviors within the hospital and/or home to prevent complications and speed recovery
Defining characteristics: Parent(s) request information about caregiving and preventative measures; child readmitted to hospital with complications

Information, Instruction, Demonstration

Interventions	Rationales
Instruct parent(s) and child (if applicable) on the administration of prescribed medications	Promotes understanding which may improve consistency of medication administration and recognition of adverse effects
Instruct parent(s) as to the signs and symptoms of respiratory distress	Encourages parent(s) to seek prompt medical treatment as necessary
Instruct parent(s) on the importance of rest and good nutrition, as applicable	Prevents secondary infections; promotes body's own natural defenses
Encourage and teach parent(s) to provide care for the hospitalized child at a level they are comfortable with and within the constraints of necessary treatments	Promotes parental identity and control; may lessen anxiety and stress
Instruct child and family members, as applicable, on good handwashing techniques and the proper disposal of soiled tissues, etc.	Prevents transmission of illness

Discharge or Maintenance Evaluation

- Parent(s) administer medications appropriately and recognize side effects
- Parent(s) recognize the signs of impending respiratory distress and seek medical attention, as needed
- Parent(s) provide adequate rest and nutrition
- Parent(s) use good hand washing and waste disposal techniques
- Parent(s) participate in the care of their child while hospitalized, as appropriate

Epiglottitis

Upper respiratory infection
Haemophilus influenzae, Type B (most common)
Group A Streptococcus

↓

Inflammation/edema of epiglottis and surrounding area

↓

Severe, rapid progression of infection and symptoms of obstruction
Airway obstruction with severe respiratory distress

Endotracheal intubation
Tracheostomy

Asphyxia

↓

↓

Resolution

Death

Laryngotracheo-bronchitis

Laryngotracheobronchitis is the most common form of croup. It is characterized by an acute viral infection of the larynx, trachea, and bronchi which causes obstruction below the level of the vocal cords. Spasmodic croup is croup of sudden onset, occurring mainly at night and characterized by laryngeal obstruction at the level of the vocal cords caused by viral infections or allergens. Both occur as a result of upper respiratory infection, edema, and spasms that cause respiratory distress in varying degrees depending on the amount of obstruction. The disease most commonly affects infants and small children between 3 months and 3 years of age and occurs in the winter months. Hospitalization is reserved for those with severe symptoms and compromised respiratory function caused by the obstruction.

MEDICAL CARE

Antipyretics: acetaminophen (Tylenol tablets, Pedric wafers or elixir, Liquiprin solution drops) given PO to reduce fever; Ibuprofen (nonsteroidal anti-inflammatory) for children 6 months-12 years; Motrin or Advil liquid suspension or tablets PO to decrease fever and inflammation.

Bronchodilators: racemic epinephrine (Vaponefrin) inhalant given by nebulizer or intermittent positive pressure breathing device (IPPB) to relax respiratory smooth muscle and relieve stridor respirations.

Sedatives: phenobarbital (Luminal) given PO to promote restin spasmodic croup if respirations not depressed by its use.

Anti-inflammatory: dexamethason (Decadron) given PO; dexamethasone sodium phosphate (Decardron Phosphate) given IV to increase body defenses against infection, although its effectiveness in reducing edema in this condition is questionable.

Antibiotics: ampicillin (Amcill suspension) given PO or ampicillin sodium (Omnipen-N) IV to treat infection by inhibiting cell wall synthesis of microorganisms; antibiotic selection dependent on culture sensitivity results; chloramphenicol (Chloromycetin Palmitate suspension) given PO if identified bacteria resistant to ampicillin.

Oxygen therapy: treats hypoxemia based on reduced pO_2 levels of ABGs, administered by tent or hood.

Chest/Neck x-rays: differentiates between croup disorders and epiglottitis.

Throat culture: reveals and identifies infectious agent and sensitivity to specific antimicrobial therapy.

Arterial blood gases: reveals hypoxemic states that require oxygen therapy; decreased pH and changes in oxygen and carbon dioxide levels, indicating respiratory acidosis or failure in severe cases.

Complete Blood Count: reveals increased WBC if infection present.

NURSING CARE PLANS

Essential nursing diagnoses and plans associated with this condition:

Ineffective airway clearance (42)

Related to: Tracheobronchial obstruction, secretions
Defining characteristics: Dyspnea; thick secretions; tachypnea; hoarseness; persistent barking cough; diminished breath sounds, with scattered crackles and rhonchi; cyanosis; restlessness; tachycardia; hypoxemia; hypercapnia

Ineffective breathing pattern (45)

Related to: Inflammatory process, laryngotracheo-bronchial constriction and obstruction
Defining characteristics: Dyspnea, tachypnea, abnormal ABGs, barking, metallic sounding cough, nasal flaring, inspiratory stridor, subclavicular and substernal retractions, cyanosis or pallor, restlessness, irritability

Risk for fluid volume deficit (222)

Related to: Loss of fluid through normal routes (respirations and temperature), altered intake
Defining characteristics: Low grade temperature, dry skin and mucous membranes, increased pulse and respirations, difficult swallowing, poor skin turgor, sunken fontanels, and absence of tears

Sleep pattern disturbance (114)

Related to: Internal factor of illness (difficulty breathing)
Defining characteristics: Interrupted sleep caused by cough, restlessness, irritability

SPECIFIC DIAGNOSES AND CARE PLANS

Anxiety

Related to: Change in health status of infant/small child; threat to or change in environment (hospitalization)
Defining characteristics: Increased apprehension that condition might worsen and hospitalization might be necessary (parental); crying and clinging behaviors, refusal to eat or play (infant or small child); persistent cough and breathing difficulty (infant/small child)

Outcome Criteria

Reduced parental and child anxiety, with appropriate explanations of disease and care as illness is resolved

Interventions	Rationales
Assess level and sources of anxiety of parent(s) and child and identify behaviors caused by anxiety	Provides information about need for interventions to relieve anxiety and concern
Allow parents to express concerns and to ask questions about course of disease and what to expect	Provides opportunity to vent feelings, secure information needed to reduce anxiety
Encourage parent(s) and child to remain calm and provide a quiet environment	Anxiety affects respirations and calm environment reduces anxiety
Inform parent(s) and child of all procedures, especially use of croup tent, care and any changes in condition	Relieves anxiety resulting from fear of the unknown
Allow parent(s) to stay with infant/small child if hospitalized, bring toy, blanket from home; allow visits from siblings	Allows parent(s) to care for and support child and provide familiar objects and people to reduce child's anxiety
If hospitalized, carry out home routines for feeding, sleep	Prevents anxiety associated with changes in daily rituals

Information, Instruction, Demonstration

Interventions	Rationales
Explain reason for and what to expect for each procedure or type of therapy; use drawings and pictures, video tapes for child	Reduces fear caused by anxiety
Explain course of disease to parent(s) and child, that recovery is fairly prompt with proper therapy, and that cough may persist for a week or more after recovery	Reduces anxiety caused by the sound of the breathing and appearance of the infant/small child
Clarify any misinformation and answer all questions regarding the disease process and manifestations	Prevents unnecessary anxiety resulting from inaccurate information or beliefs
If tent is used, instruct and assist parent(s) in interacting with child	Promotes support to child and relieves anxiety
Inform and discuss signs and symptoms indicating increasing severity of disease and actions to take	Reduces anxiety caused by increasing acuteness of condition by knowledge of what to do and when to report to physician

Discharge or Maintenance Evaluation

- Expresses a reduction in anxiety with explanations of disease and therapy
- Verbalizes the positive effect of caring for and supporting their sick infant/small child
- Visits, calls hospital when unable to stay with child

Fatigue

Related to: States of discomfort (dyspnea)
Defining characteristics: Lethargy or listlessness, emotional lability or irritability, exhausted appearance, inability to eat

Outcome Criteria

Return of energy level and increased endurance with improved respiratory function (decreased cough and stridor)

Interventions	Rationales
Assess for extreme weakness and fatigue, ability to rest and sleep	Dyspnea and work of breathing over period of time exhausts the infant/child's energy reserves affecting ability to rest, eat, drink
Disturb only when necessary, perform all care at one time instead of spreading over a long period of time	Conserves energy and prevents interruptions in rest
Schedule and provide rest periods in a quiet, comfortable environment (temperature and humidity)	Promotes adequate rest and reduces stimuli to decrease fatigue
Allow quiet play while maintaining bedrest	Rest decreases fatigue and respiratory distress; quiet play prevents excessive activity, which depletes energy and increases respirations
Explain reason for need to conserve energy and avoid fatigue to parent(s) and child	Promotes understanding of infant/young child's response to respiratory distress and importance of rest and support to prevent fatigue
Inform of measures to take to prevent fatigue (holding and/or rocking infant/young child, feeding slowly in small amounts, playing with child, offer TV and other diversions)	Provides support to infant/small child and conserves energy
Inform parent(s) of method to decrease crying and importance of not allowing an infant to cry longer than 1-2 minutes	Prevents fatigue, as prolonged crying exhausts infant
Instruct to make a plan for providing bathing, feeding, changing diaper around rest periods	Prevents interruption in rest or sleep

Discharge or Maintenance Evaluation

- Minimized fatigue with rest and sleep periods provided

- Infant/small child eats and drinks within limits and methods imposed by illness
- Participates in activities that do not compromise energy and breathing pattern
- Maintains respiratory status at baseline parameters

Knowledge deficit of parent(s), caretaker

Related to: Promotion of health-seeking behaviors within the hospital and home to prevent complications and speed recovery

Defining characteristics: Parents request information about the home care of the child and/or preventative measures; child is rehospitalized and/or develops complications

Outcome Criteria

Parent(s) provide optimal health care for the child at home
Parent(s) participate in caregiving
Absence of cross-infection to others and/or secondary infection in child

Interventions	Rationales
Instruct parent(s) and child as applicable, on the administration of prescribed medications	Improves consistency of medication administration and recognition of adverse side effects
Instruct parent(s) on the importance of rest	Prevents secondary infections and/or relapses
Instruct parent(s) on the importance of good nutrition and hydration, emphasizing a high calorie balanced diet and increased fluids	Promotes liquification of secretions, and replaces calories used to fight infections, boosting the child's own natural defenses
Instruct parent(s) on the importance of providing humidity (warm mist for spasmotic croup) and the appropriate methods of delivering humidity	Promotes liquification of secretions, decreases bronchial spasms
Encourage and teach parent(s) to provide care for the hospitalized child at a level they are comfortable with, and within the constraints of necessary treatments	Promotes parental identity and control; may lessen anxiety and stress

Interventions	Rationales
Instruct parent(s) on good handwashing techniques, and the appropriate disposal of soiled tissues, etc.	Prevents transmission of illness
Instruct parent(s) on the importance of limiting visitors and screening them for recent illness	Prevents transmission of illness; prevents or minimizes risk of complications for the infected child

Discharge or Maintenance Evaluation

- Parent(s) accurately administer prescribed medications and report adverse effects
- Parent(s) provide rest and good nutrition, fluids for the child
- Parent(s) utilize humidity, as applicable, and understand delivery methods
- Parent(s) remain active in caretaking at a level with which they are comfortable
- Parent(s) use good hand washing techniques and soiled tissue disposal
- Parent(s) verbalize an understanding of the signs of respiratory distress and seek prompt medical attention, as needed

Laryngotracheobronchitis

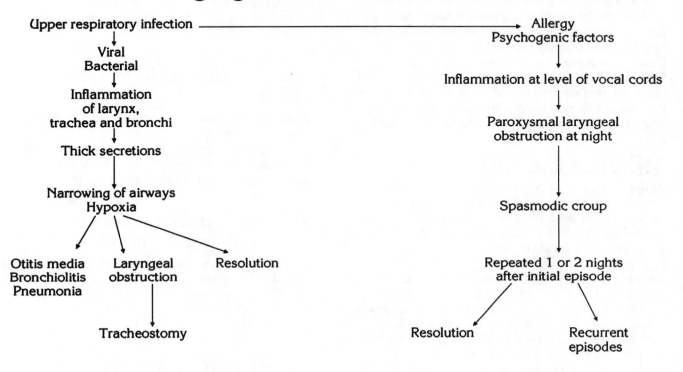

Upper respiratory infection ⟶ Allergy
Psychogenic factors

↓

Viral
Bacterial

↓

Inflammation
of larynx,
trachea and bronchi

↓

Thick secretions

↓

Narrowing of airways
Hypoxia

Otitis media
Bronchiolitis
Pneumonia

Laryngeal
obstruction

Resolution

Tracheostomy

Inflammation at level of vocal cords

↓

Paroxysmal laryngeal
obstruction at night

↓

Spasmodic croup

↓

Repeated 1 or 2 nights
after initial episode

Resolution

Recurrent
episodes

Pneumonia

Pneumonia is a lower respiratory condition characterized by the inflammation or infection of the pulmonary parenchyma. It is caused by bacteria, viruses, or fungi, or by the aspiration of a foreign substance. It may occur as a primary infection or secondary to another illness or infection. Pneumonia is most common in infants and small children, but it can occur throughout childhood. Signs and symptoms of the disease depend on the age, causative agent, extent of the disease, and the degree of obstruction it causes and the systemic reaction to the infection. The treatment and care is similar for all types of pneumonia.

MEDICAL CARE

Antipyretics: acetaminophen (Tylenol tablets, Pedric wafers or elixir, Liquiprin solution drops) given PO to reduce fever; Ibuprofen (nonsteroidal anti-inflammatory) for children 6 months-12 years; Motrin or Advil liquid suspension or tablets PO to reduce fever and inflammation.

Antibiotics: penicillin G (Pentids solution) given PO; penicillin G benzathine (Bicillin) given IM; penicillin G potassium (Pfizerpen) given IM or IV to treat pneumococcal, streptococcal, or staphylococcal pneumonia; methicillin (Staphcillin or oxacillin sodium (Bactocill) given IM or IV to treat staphylococcal pneumonia; Erythromycin, Trimethoprimsulfamethoxazole, Climadycin, Chloramphenicol, or cephalosporins for penicillin-allergic children.

Oxygen therapy: treats hypoxemia, administered by oxygen tent or hood.

Chest x-ray: reveals patchy areas of consolidation in one lobe or throughout lung, varying sizes of pneumatoceles or disseminated infiltration dependent on causative agent.

Sputum culture: reveals and identifies infectious agent and sensitivity to specific antimicrobial therapy.

Blood culture: reveals positive reaction for causative agent.

Complete blood count: increased WBC of 15,000 or over 20,000/cu mm.

Antistreptolysin-O titer: elevation indicates recent streptococcal infection if above 333 Todd units.

NURSING CARE PLANS

Essential nursing diagnoses and plans associated with this condition:

Ineffective breathing pattern (45)

Related to: Inflammatory process
Defining characteristics: Dyspnea, tachypnea, grunting and nonproductive cough in small child, nasal flaring, decreased dull breath sounds, crackles, productive cough in older child, use of accessory muscles with retractions, circumoral cyanosis, shallow respirations, increased fremitus

Risk for fluid volume deficit (222)

Related to: Excessive losses through normal routes, altered fluid intake
Defining characteristics: Increased temperature and pulse rate tachypnea, vomiting and diarrhea in young child, reduced fluids in proportion to output

Altered nutrition: Less than body requirements (168)

Related to: Inability to ingest food or digest food because of biological factors
Defining characteristics: Lack of interest in food, anorexia, cough, abdominal pain, vomiting and diarrhea in younger child

SPECIFIC DIAGNOSES AND CARE PLANS

Hyperthermia

Related to: Illness of lower respiratory tract infection
Defining characteristics: Abrupt onset of high body temperature (102°-105°F in infants and 104°-105°F in older child), tachycardia, tachypnea, chills, myalgia, warm to touch, flushed cheeks, convulsions in infant/young child

Outcome Criteria

Reduced parental anxiety with understanding of disease and what can be expected until illness is resolved

Interventions	Rationales
Assess sources and level of anxiety, how anxiety is manifested, and need for information and support	Provides information about the need for interventions to relieve anxiety and concern

Interventions	Rationales
Allow to express concerns and ask questions regarding condition of ill child	Provides opportunity to vent feelings, secure information needed to reduce anxiety
Encourage to remain calm and involved in care and decision-making regarding child's needs and to note any improvements that result	Promotes constant monitoring of child's condition for improvement or worsening of symptoms
Allow parent to stay with child or visit when able and to call when concerned if hospitalized; assist in care (hold, feed, bathe, clothe, and diaper) and provide information about child's daily routines	Allows parent to care for and support child instead of increasing anxiety if not with child

Information, Instruction, Demonstration

Interventions	Rationales
Inform of disease process, behaviors, physical effects, and symptoms of condition	Relieves anxiety by knowing what to expect
Explain to parent(s) and child in age-related fashion reason for each procedure or therapy, effects of any diagnostic tests, and how procedures are performed	Prevents anxiety by reducing fear of unknown

Discharge or Maintenance Evaluation

- Expresses a reduction in anxiety following explanations of disease process and therapy
- Verbalizes the positive effect and understanding of caring for and supporting their sick child
- Participates in care of child, visits and/or calls hospital if unable to stay

Risk for injury

Related to: Internal factor of pulmonary complications in infant/child
Defining characteristics: Fluid accumulation in the pleural cavity, dyspnea, pneumothorax, empyema, de-

creased breath sounds with crackles, seizure activity with high temperature, staphylococcal-type pneumonia in infant, pneumococcal-type pneumonia in child

Outcome Criteria

Absence or resolution of pulmonary complications

Interventions	Rationales
Assess vital signs and breath sounds, cough and ability to cough up secretions	Changes revealed in early stages of complications and reveals airway patency and dyspnea caused by fluid accumulation in pleural cavity and secretion accumulation in airways
Prepare infant/child for procedure and assist with thoracentesis; use therapeutic play to prepare child	Performed to drain fluid to be cultured or to instill antibiotics if infection present
Monitor temperature for sudden rise	Reveals a sudden, rapid rise in temperature which may trigger a febrile seizure
Report detection of possible respiratory complications early (chest pain, dyspnea, cyansois, abdominal distention)	Allows for immediate preventative measures to be taken during course of disease

Information, Instruction, Demonstration

Interventions	Rationales
Inform parent(s) that complications are uncommon because of effectiveness of antibiotic therapy	Promotes a positive feeling in parent(s) for recovery of child
Inform parent(s) that recovery from the disease is usually rapid and uneventful if symptoms are reported early for proper treatment	Promotes awareness and compliance of parent(s) to note respiratory changes and report them immediately to prevent complications
Inform parent(s) and child to report changes in respirations, sputum, temperature elevation	Indicates possible pulmonary infection

Discharge or Maintenance Evaluation

- Respirations within baseline parameters according to age for rate, depth and ease, absence of crackles, dyspnea
- Temperature within normal range for 24-48 hours
- Absence of signs and symptoms of pulmonary complication
- Culture of chest fluid negative for infectious organisms

Knowledge deficit of parent(s), caretaker

Related to: Unfamiliarity with disease and complications, measures to control and prevent transmission of respiratory disease

Defining characteristics: Verbalization of need for information about medications, activity and rest, nutritional and fluid requirements and medical asepsis techniques to prevent spread of infection

Outcome Criteria

Adequate knowledge for safe and compliant administration of antibiotic regimen and requirements for basic needs

Interventions	Rationales
Assess knowledge of disease and methods to control and resolve disease; willingness and interest of parent(s) to implement care	Promotes plan of instruction that is realistic to ensure compliance of medical regimen; prevents repetition of information
Provide information and explanations in clear, understandable language; use pictures, pamphlets, video tapes, model in teaching about disease	Ensures understanding based on readiness and ability to learn; visual aids reinforce learning
Instruct in administration of medications including action of drugs, dosages, times, frequency, side effects, expected results, methods to give medications; provide written instructions and schedule to follow and inform to administer full course of antibiotic to child	Provides information about drug therapy, which is the most important treatment for the cure of pneumonia, and about prevention of lung complications resulting from the disease; bacterial pneumonia is treated with antibiotic therapy

Interventions	Rationales
Instruct and assist to plan feedings and/or develop menus for appropriate inclusion of nourishing fluids, daily caloric and basic four requirements for age group	Promotes proper diet, which enhances health status, and adequate fluid intake, which prevents dehydration
Inform of importance of activity or activity restrictions and of adequate rest during illness and convalescence	Promotes more rest and possible restriction of activity needed during more acute stages of disease
Instruct in care of used tissues and to cover mouth and nose when coughing or blowing nose, proper handwashing technique for parent and child	Prevents transmission of microorganisms by droplets dispersed into the air or by hands
Instruct parents on the signs and symptoms of impending respiratory distress	Encourages parents to seek prompt medical treatment as necessary

Discharge or Maintenance Evaluation

- Statements of knowledge of disease, medications, dietary and exercise requirements of child
- Adaptation and compliance of parent(s) with medical regimen
- Precautions taken to prevent spread of infection or contraction of other upper respiratory infections
- Secures pneumonia vaccination if underlying chronic conditions exist and risk for recurrence is high for child over 2 years of age
- Verbalized signs and symptoms of disease progression or recurrence
- Parent(s) recognize the signs of impending respiratory failure and seek medical attention, as needed

Pneumonia

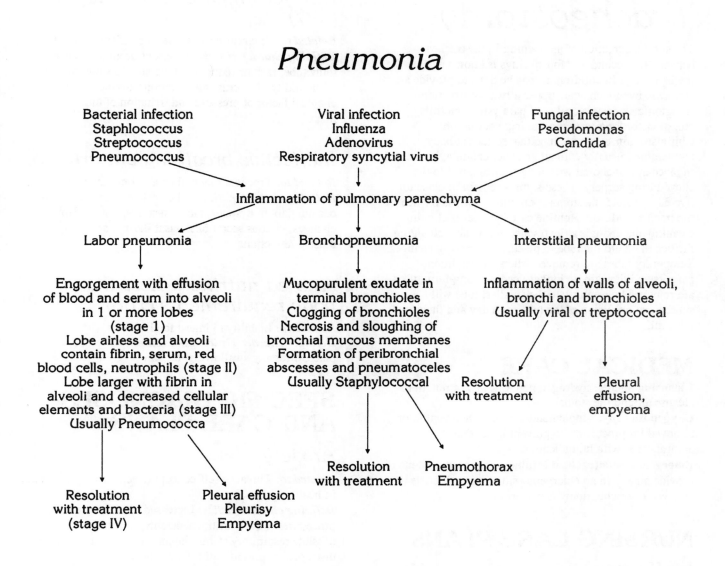

Bacterial infection
Staphlococcus
Streptococcus
Pneumococcus

Viral infection
Influenza
Adenovirus
Respiratory syncytial virus

Fungal infection
Pseudomonas
Candida

Inflammation of pulmonary parenchyma

Labor pneumonia

Bronchopneumonia

Interstitial pneumonia

Engorgement with effusion
of blood and serum into alveoli
in 1 or more lobes
(stage 1)
Lobe airless and alveoli
contain fibrin, serum, red
blood cells, neutrophils (stage II)
Lobe larger with fibrin in
alveoli and decreased cellular
elements and bacteria (stage III)
Usually Pneumococca

Mucopurulent exudate in
terminal bronchioles
Clogging of bronchioles
Necrosis and sloughing of
bronchial mucous membranes
Formation of peribronchial
abscesses and pneumatoceles
Usually Staphylococcal

Inflammation of walls of alveoli,
bronchi and bronchioles
Usually viral or treptococcal

Resolution
with treatment

Pleural
effusion,
empyema

Resolution
with treatment

Pneumothorax
Empyema

Resolution
with treatment
(stage IV)

Pleural effusion
Pleurisy
Empyema

Tracheostomy

The surgical creation of an opening in the trachea between the second and fourth rings is known as a tracheostomy. In children, it may be done to provide an airway to bypass an acute upper airway obstruction (subglottic stenosis, vocal cord paralysis, piglottitis, croup) or for long-term mechanical ventilation administration. A plastic tube that softens at body temperature, usually without an inner cannula, is inserted in place and anchored with long sutures taped to the chest during surgery. These sutures remain in place for five days to hold the stoma open until a tract is formed in the trachea and skin. Routine care includes suctioning, cleaning and changing the tracheostomy tube, changing the ties that hold the tube in place, and dressing changes. Temporary tubes are removed when the condition permits and they are no longer needed. Long-term tubes are removed by weaning to the smallest tube with subsequent occlusion of the tube for a day and then final removal.

MEDICAL CARE

Cleansing agents: hydrogen peroxide at ½ strength to cleanse around the stoma.
Oxygen therapy: supplements oxygen when ventilator removed for procedures to prevent hypoxemia, administered with humidication.
Emergency endotracheal intubation: procedure done to provide airway in an emergency situation until crisis is resolved or tracheostomy is performed.

NURSING CARE PLANS

Ineffective airway clearance (42)

Related to: Tracheobronchial secretion, obstruction
Defining characteristics: Abnormal breath sounds (crackles, wheezes), change in rate or depth or respirations, dyspnea, cyanosis, tube dislodgement or decannulation, tube occlusion, viscous secretion

Impaired gas exchange (47)

Related to: Altered oxygen supply
Defining characteristics: Hypoxia, hypercapnia, inability to move secretions, improper suctioning procedure

Risk for impaired skin integrity (397)

Related to: External factors (presence of tracheostomy)
Defining characteristics: Secretions around tracheostomy tube; rash or redness around site; low environmental humidity; dry, crusting secretions around site; mechanical factor of pressure and irritation of tube movement

Ineffective breathing pattern (45)

Related to: Tracheobronchial obstruction, anxiety
Defining characteristics: Tube occlusion or accidental decannulation, dyspnea, tachypnea, respiratory depth changes, viscous secretions, nasal flaring, accessory muscle retractions

Altered nutrition: Less than body requirements (168)

Related to: Inability to ingest food
Defining characteristics: Poor feeding with tube in place, difficulty swallowing, choking

SPECIFIC DIAGNOSES AND CARE PLANS

Anxiety

Related to: Threat to self-concept (tracheostomy); change in health status
Defining characteristics: Increased apprehension, fear of procedures to care for tracheostomy, uncertainty about possible respiratory status changes, expressed feelings of distress over presence of tracheostomy

Outcome Criteria

Reduced parental and child anxiety verbalized as respiratory status maintained
Adaptation to presence of tracheostomy (long-term)

Interventions	Rationales
Assess level and manifestations of anxiety in parent(s) and child	Provides information needed for interventions and clues to severity of anxiety

Interventions	Rationales
Allow parent(s) and child to express fears and concerns and to ask questions about disease and what to expect	Provides opportunity to vent feelings and secure information to reduce anxiety
Provide supportive and nonjudgmental environment	Promotes trust and reduces anxiety
Inform parent(s) and child of all procedures and treatments	Relieves anxiety caused by fear of unknown
Allow parent(s) to stay with child, allow open visitation and telephone communications; encourage to participate in care that is planned around usual home routines	Reduces anxiety by allowing presence and involvement in care, familiar routines and persons for child
Inform of all procedures and care and any changes in the child's condition	Reduces anxiety caused by fear of the unknown
Provide child with pencil and paper, pictures, slate as age allows	Provides means of communication and interaction with the child
Provide child with medical play objects such as a doll with a tracheostomy, suction catheters, tracheostomy tubes and ties, as applicable	Provides child the opportunity to have hands on experience with supplies; improves their understanding of procedures; gives health care professionals some insight into the child's understanding of the procedure
Allow child to assume position of comfort, provide familiar object (toy or blanket)	Promotes comfort and security
Provide child/parent(s) tours of the PICU and the floor prior to the surgical procedure as applicable	Promotes understanding of what to expect which may help to decrease anxiety

Information, Instruction, Demonstration

Interventions	Rationales
Inform of disease process and behaviors and physical effects and symptoms of tracheostomy; assure parent(s) that tracheostomy will facilitate breathing	Relieves anxiety by knowing what to expect, especially if tracheostomy is long-term
Explain to parent(s) and child in age-related fashion reason for tracheostomy procedure or therapy, effects of presence of tracheostomy, how procedures are performed	Reduces anxiety caused by fear of unknown
Clarify any misinformation with honesty and in simple understandable language	Prevents any unnecessary anxiety resulting from inaccurate information or beliefs
Refer to counseling, community groups or agencies	Reduces anxiety by providing to parent(s) and child support and information from those with similar problems

Discharge or Maintenance Evaluation

- Verbalization that anxiety reduced by parent(s) and child
- Secures information and support from community agencies
- Expresses increased comfort when participating in care and support of child
- Symptoms of anxiety in the child decreasing or controlled
- Child participates in school and social activities

Risk for infection

Related to: Invasive procedures (tracheostomy and care)
Defining characteristics: Stasis of secretions, suctioning tracheostomy, redness, excoriation, swelling and drainage at tracheostomy site, change in breath sounds and sputum, increased temperature, presence of infection of family members

Outcome Criteria

Absence of pulmonary or tracheostomy site infection

Interventions	Rationales
Assess for change in breathing pattern, color of mucus, diminished breath sounds, ability to cough and raise secretions	Indicates presence of respiratory infection
Avoid exposure to persons with respiratory infection, isolate from infectious patients or family members	Prevents increased susceptibility and risk for infection
Utilize hand washing technique before giving care or performing procedures	Prevents transmission of microorganisms to child
Assist to cough or remove secretions by suctioning via sterile technique	Stasis of secretions provide medium for infection
Use medical asepsis techniques or sterile technique when administering tracheostomy and site care	Prevents exposure to infectious agents
Change tracheostomy dressing, tube, and ties when soiled, wet, or encrusted with secretions as needed	Maintains cleanliness of wound and removes risk of contact with infectious agents
Administer antibiotic therapy if ordered	Provides protection from or treatment of infection by destroying or inhibiting growth of microorganisms
Obtain sputum or wound drainage culture	Identifies presence of pathogenic organisms

Information, Instruction, Demonstration

Interventions	Rationales
Demonstrate handwashing technique to parent(s) and child and allow for return demonstration	Prevents cross-contamination by hands
Inform parent(s) of child's high susceptibility to infection and to avoid contact of child with persons or family members with respiratory infections	Provides information that any infection will compromise respiratory status and could be life threatening

Interventions	Rationales
Instruct parent(s) to provide humidity to environment by vaporizer	Liquefies secretions for easier removal
Inform parent(s) to provide adequate fluid and nutritional intake based on age	Maintains fluid and nutritional requirements of infant/child
Inform parent(s) to report any changes in sputum, respiratory status, skin at tracheostomy site to physician	Provides for immediate interventions to control infection
Instruct parent(s) and allow for demonstration of sterile or clean technique	Promotes sterility or cleanliness of procedures based on healing of tracheostomy site

Discharge or Maintenance Evaluation

- Takes measures to avoid exposure to respiratory infections
- Maintains respiratory status
- Mucus effectively removed and of thin consistency and clear color
- Performs hand washing techniques
- Adheres to diagnostic test schedule and interaction with physician when needed
- Provides appropriate fluid and nutritional requirements
- Performs procedures utilizing medical asepsis
- Administers antibiotics correctly, avoids medications not recommended by physician

Risk for aspiration

Related to: Presence of tracheostomy or endotracheal tube
Defining characteristics: Impaired swallowing, vomiting, choking

Outcome Criteria

Absence of aspirations of fluid or food into airway

Interventions	Rationales
Assess ability to swallow, type of food consistency (solid or formula), age of child	Provides information about potential for choking or aspiration

Interventions	Rationales
Offer small amounts of liquids initially and follow with increases as tolerated; add cereal to infant formula or offer thick milkshakes to child	Provides fluids and nutrients of a consistency that is best managed and swallowed to prevent choking
Place in upright or sitting position for feedings or place on lap or in infant seat; allow to remain in position for 30 minutes afterwards	Promotes flow of fluids and foods by gravity
If choking occurs, suction fluids from mouth and airway; avoid suctioning procedure after feedings	Removes fluid or food from airway to prevent aspiration; suctioning after feedings may cause nausea or vomiting

Information, Instruction, Demonstration

Interventions	Rationales
Instruct parent(s) in types of foods and liquids to offer infant/child	Promotes nutrition requirements that are easier to tolerate and swallow with tube in place
Inform parent(s) of actions to take when choking occurs; positions that are most effective, procedure for feeding	Prevents aspiration of fluid or food into airway
Inform parent(s) to suction airway if choking, perform after other measures have failed	Removes fluid or feedings from airway
Inform parent(s) to notify physician in presence of respiratory distress	Prevents life-threatening situation caused by suffocation

Discharge or Maintenance Evaluation

- Maintains feedings without aspiration into airway
- Positions for optimal feedings and/or nutritional intake
- Absence of choking, vomiting during feedings
- Suctions airway if needed to prevent aspirations

Risk for injury

Related to: External factors associated with tracheostomy complications
Defining characteristics: Damage to tracheal mucosa by inappropriate suctioning, excessive movement or dislodgement of tube, accidental decannulation

Outcome Criteria

Absence of respiratory distress with proper tube placement and absence of airway obstruction
Absence of tracheal damage
Tracheostomy tube remains in place and patent

Interventions	Rationales
Assess for proper tube placement, presence of an air leak around tube, patency of tube	Ensures effective tube function to provide airway for ventilation
Assess security of tapes and knots, tightness of tapes by inserting small finger between tape and neck	Promotes safe use of ties to stabilize tube, which should not be frayed and should fit snugly without compromising circulation
Assess need for suctioning by noting change in breath sounds and respiratory rate, depth and ease	Allows for removal of secretions to prevent obstruction and respiratory distress
Assess stay sutures if new tracheostomy by noting security of tapes on side of neck, any movement or dislodgement of tube	Ensures safe placement of tracheostomy tube and prevents dislodgement
Hold tube in place when dressing changed, ointment applied under wings of tube, changing tapes, or suctioning tube	Prevents manipulation of tube which causes mechanical irritation and may dislodge tube
Restrain if appropriate developmentally and if needed; inform parent(s) and child of reason	Prevents child from pulling tube out accidentally
Suction carefully and intermittently, use proper catheter size and technique	Clears airway and tube of secretions without damage to trachea, prolonged suctioning causes vagal stimulation and bradycardia and high pressure may damage mucosa of trachea

Interventions	Rationales
Provide spare tracheostomy tube, scissors, bag and proper sized mask and adaptor, oxygen source and suctioning equipment at bedside	Provides for emergency interventions for airway obstruction or decannulation
Change tapes 3 days after surgery and tube 2 weeks after surgery, with 2 nurses present or respiratory therapist if available	Ensures safety of procedures with help at hand if needed
Change tube if obstructed, reinsert new tube if dislodged; have 2 people present	Maintains effective tube functioning and airway patency

Information, Instruction, Demonstration

Interventions	Rationales
Instruct and demonstrate and allow parent(s) to return demonstration of the tube change (insertion and removal) to be done every month or as needed, tube ties change, suctioning and cleansing of tube if long-term care needed	Promotes continuity of care by parent(s) if able to perform skills and approved by physician; promotes independence and control of family in child's care
Inform parent(s) of positive effects of tracheostomy, such as ease of breathing, improved rest and feeding, progress in developmental tasks	Provides emotional support to parent(s) and family
Inform parent(s) of equipment and supplies to have on hand	Provides support for any emergency
Inform parent(s) to clothe child in loose-fitting clothing around neck with no loose threads or frayed material, remove crumbs, beads or dangerous toys, careful bathing with elimination of water near tube; cover tube with bib when drinking or eating meals	Prevents obstruction of tube or entry of foreign materials

Interventions	Rationales
Instruct parent(s) to report any swelling or bleeding around tube, increased respiratory effort, change in skin color, absence of air moving in and out of tube, inability to insert suction tube, excessive choking during feeding	Prevents complications that may compromise respiratory status

Discharge or Maintenance Evaluation

- Maintains tube placement and patency
- Maintains respiratory status within baseline parameters
- Absence of airway obstruction with effective, safe suctioning
- Absence of unnecessary movement of tube during procedures
- Maintains tube stability
- Change tubes, ties when needed
- Maintains emergency supplies on hand and ready for use
- Contacts social worker if needed
- Removes dangerous objects or materials from area of tracheostomy site
- Verbalized signs and symptoms to report and actions to take

Knowledge deficit (potential or actual)

Related to: Lack of understanding of the care necessary for a child at home with a tracheostomy; impending discharge of child to home
Defining characteristics: Parent(s) request information regarding care of the child at home; child returns to the hospital due to problems encountered during/with caregiving at home

Outcome Criteria

Parent(s) learn to comfortably care for the child at home
Child's care is managed at home, without the necessity of an extended hospitalization or rehospitalization

Interventions	Rationales
Instructions should be in short sessions, tailored to parent(s)' specific learning styles and needs; written	Understanding will be improved when sessions are short and individualized; written materials reinforce

Interventions	Rationales
materials should be given after each session	learning and improve comprehension
Notify local utilities and EMS regarding the child's condition	Response time may be heightened if the appropriate personnel are notified in advance
Facilitate the acquisition of necessary supplies and equipment needed at home, including suction apparatus, oxygen, pulse oximetry, etc.; coordinate the necessary teaching regarding the equipment as applicable	Ensures appropriate supplies and equipment are available at discharge; promotes understanding of how equipment works
Contact local home health nursing agencies, as applicable; facilitate arrangements	Promotes feelings of control and decreases anxiety within parent(s); discharge is often a time of higher stress for parent(s), and they can become easily overwhelmed

Information, Instruction, Demonstration

Interventions	Rationales
Demonstrate all aspects of tracheostomy care for the child (if applicable), family, and other significant caregivers; observe return demonstrations; teaching should include: tracheostomy site assessment, suctioning techniques, tracheostomy site care, tracheostomy changes, and emergency protocols	Including all family members and significant others may help expand the level of support felt by the immediate family; stress will be decreased if they have a sense that they can have some time away, while still leaving the child in good hands
Caregivers must be able to provide all aspects of care regarding the tracheostomy prior to discharge home	Promotes a high level of understanding while simultaneously decreasing anxiety as caregivers are available if necessary
Instruct all caregivers on CPR, with return demonstrations encouraged; reinforce with written materials	Promotes increased understanding of emergency resuscitation needs of patient; prior knowledge of CPR may reduce stress felt by the family

Interventions	Rationales
Teach and encourage the family to treat the child as normally as possible, including information on growth and development, discipline, school, sibling reactions, the importance of play and trips outside the home	Promotes normalcy within the family which facilitates positive adaptation; lessens anxiety and stress
Teach child and parent(s) vocalization techniques as applicable	Promotes communication which enhances self-esteem and facilitates normal growth and development

Discharge or Maintenance Evaluation

- Parent(s)/caregiver(s) verbalize and demonstrate proper care of the tracheostomy
- Parent(s)/caregiver(s) verbalize and demonstrate proper CPR techniques
- Parent(s)/caregiver(s) utilize appropriate supplies and equipment necessary for care of the tracheostomy
- Parent(s) understand the importance of maintaining a sense of normalcy within the home environment
- Child learns to vocalize and communicate with the tracheostomy, as applicable

Tracheostomy

Upper airway obstruction

Croup
Epiglottitis
Enlarged thyroid (goiter)
Subglottic stenosis
Vocal cord paralysis
Foreign body aspiration

Access for prolonged use of
mechanical ventilation

Respiratory distress or failure
Spinal cord injury (quadriplegia)
Cerbral injury (coma)

Tracheostomy
(between 2nd and 4th tracheal rings)

Plastic or Silastic trachesotomy
tube without inner cannula

Metal tracheostomy tube with an
inner cannula

Tuberculosis

Tuberculosis in children is usually contracted from an infected adult by droplets expelled from the respiratory tract and dispersed into the air. Although its incidence and death rate are greater in other parts of the world, there has been an increase of cases in the United States. Most cases are managed at home with drug therapy. Only patients with more serious forms of the disease or who need special diagnostic tests are hospitalized.

MEDICAL CARE

Anti-infectives/Antituberculosis: isoniazid (INH) PO, IM, IV in combination with rifampin (Rifadin) PO or ethionamide (Trecator) PO or ethambutol (Etibi) PO in older children to inhibit bacterial growth (bacteriostatic action).

Skin Tests: purified protein derivative (PPD) by multiple puncture (Aplitest) or old tuberculin (Tine), with verification of a positive reaction by the Mantoux intradermal injection (Tubersol) done to screen for sensitivity to the bacillus as a result of past exposure, or to test for suspected tuberculosis (testing usually done at 12 -15 months, before school entry, and during adolescence; done annually in high-risk areas).

Sputum or gastric washing culture: identifies causative agent in sputum coughed up from lower respiratory tract in children or fasting gastric contents in infants or young children who swallow sputum.

Chest x-ray: reveals tuberculosis lesion if disease is suspected, but radiography results are difficult to differentiate from other diseases.

NURSING CARE PLANS

Essential nursing diagnosis and plan associated with this condition:

Altered nutrition: Less than body requirements (168)

Related to: Inability to ingest food because of biological, economic factors
Defining characteristics: Inadequate food intake, lack of food availability, pyridoxine deficiency as result of drug therapy

SPECIFIC DIAGNOSES AND CARE PLANS

Knowledge deficit of parent(s), caretaker

Related to: Unfamiliarity with disease and treatment
Defining characteristics: Verbalization of need for information about medications, activity and rest, nutritional requirements, and infection transmission prevention

Outcome Criteria
Adequate knowledge for safe and compliant administration of medication regimen and requirements for basic health needs

Interventions	Rationales
Assess knowledge of disease and methods to control and resolve disease; willingness and interest of parent(s) to implement care	Promotes plan of instruction that is realistic to ensure compliance of medical regimen; prevents repetition of information
Provide information and explanations in clear, understandable language; use pictures, pamphlets, video tapes, model in teaching about disease	Ensures understanding based on readiness and ability to learn; visual aids reinforce learning
Instruct in administration of medications, including action of drugs, dosages, times, frequency, side effects, expected results, methods to give medications; provide written instructions and schedule to follow	Provides information about drug therapy which is the most important treatment for the cure of tuberculosis and is administered for at least 9 months during the course of the disease and for 6 months after negative cultures secured; isoniazid alone or in combination with other antituberculosis drugs administered for active tuberculosis and conversion from negative to positive skin testing
Instruct and assist in planning feedings and/or developing menus for appropriate inclusion of meat and milk and daily caloric and basic four requirements for age group	Ensures proper diet that enhances health status, and adequate amounts of meat and milk supply pyridoxine in those receiving isoniazid to prevent peripheral neuritis

Interventions	Rationales
Inform of importance of activity or activity restrictions and adequate rest during convalescence	More rest and possible restrictions of activity needed during active stage of disease, but school or nursery school attendance is encouraged if asymptomatic
Provide information on the importance of limiting competitive and contact sport activities when the disease is active	Promotion of optimal health without injury will enhance complete recovery
Instruct in care of used tissues and to cover mouth and nose when coughing or blowing nose, proper handwashing technique	Prevents transmission of microorganisms by droplets dispersed into the air
Instruct parent(s) on prevention of unnecessary exposure to other infectious diseases, including the importance of maintaining the appropriate immunizations as applicable	Promotes the body's own defenses; prevents secondary infection and/or complications
Inform of importance of testing family members and follow-up skin tests for exposed contacts	Provides early detection of disease and possible source of disease, and prevents potential spread of disease
Provide parent(s) information on isolation procedures, as needed, during the active stage of the illness	Prevents transmission of the disease
Inform parents of importance of maintaining the treatment regimen over long period of time; offer information and support for continued care	Recovery requires extended period of time and support helps to ensure compliance with regimen
Instruct parent(s) on the importance of protecting the child from stressors, such as parental anxieties and pressures regarding eating and nutritional intake	Promotes body's own use of natural defenses; stress may further weaken those defenses

Discharge or Maintenance Evaluation

- Verbalizes knowledge of disease, medications, dietary and exercise requirements
- Adaptation and compliance of parent(s) with medication regimen of daily or twice weekly administration of drugs
- Appropriate growth and development advances for age group
- Maintains follow-up schedule for physician visits, laboratory testing for culture
- Precautions taken to prevent spread of infection or contracting other upper respiratory infections
- Continues with activities (play, school) or limits activities such as contact sports or strenuous games
- Obtains additional educational information from American Lung Association

Tuberculosis

Mycobacterium tuberculosis

↓

Droplet nuclei in air currents

↓

Inhalation into respiratory tract
Organisms deposited in lung periphery

↓

Inflammatory response
Polymorphonuclear leukocytes accumulate

↓

Polymorphonuclear leukocytes replaced by
macrophages that engulf bacteria

↓

Formation of epithelial cells, which join together
to form granular cells that surround foreign cell

↓

Necrosis within giant cell

↓

Calcification of lesion
Formation of granuloma (tubercle)

↓

Scar tissue encapsulates tubercle to separate it from body

Death of microorganisms

↓

Sensitization of T Lymphocytes
Positive tuberculin skin test

Bacilli spread throughout lung
Caseous necrosis

↓

Clinical tuberculosis

Neurologic System

Neurologic System

The neurologic system includes the central nervous system (CNS) consisting of the cerebrum, cerebellum, brain stem and the spinal cord; the peripheral nervous system consisting of the motor (efferent) and sensory (afferent) nerves; and the autonomic nervous system (ADS) consisting of the sympathetic and parasympathetic systems providing the control of vital body functions. Any alterations in the system affects the process of receiving, integrating and responding to stimuli that enters the system. This results in disturbances with signs and symptoms dependent on the type and site of the impairment and the normal functioning of the system. The disturbances may be manifested by alterations in consciousness or muscle function. Changes in the system also occur as the child develops neurologically and completes the growth and development requirements for adulthood with this system one of the last to finish complete development after birth.

GENERAL NEUROLOGIC CHANGES ASSOCIATED WITH PHYSICAL GROWTH AND DEVELOPMENT OF INFANTS AND CHILDREN

Brain and Spinal Cord Structure

- Skull structure is expansible during infancy and young childhood and becomes rigid with growth in older child
- Head circumference at birth 13-24 inches with a slight decrease after birth as molding takes place: size increases to 17 inches at 6 months of age and 18 inches at 12 months
- Cranial sutures close during infancy (by 6 months); posterior fontanel at 6-8 weeks and anterior fontanel at 12-18 months
- Increases in brain size and cell numbers occur between birth and 1 year of age, growth continues with increases primarily in size from 1 year of age until maturity; weight of the brain at birth is approximately 350 g or 12% of total body weight, doubling by 1 year of age and approximately 1000 g or 2/3 of adult size by 2 years of age, followed by continual slower pace until adulthood with a final size of 2% of total body weight
- Cortex is 1/2 of the thickness of the adult brain at birth and continues to develop and mature with growth
- Myelinization of nerves and fiber tracts develop rapidly after birth with sensory pathways earlier than motor pathways; continues to develop with growth of child until reaching completion in late adolescence
- Myelinization of nerve tracts follows a cephalo-caudal and proximodistal sequence which allows for progressive neuromotor function; begins with cranial nerve fibers and spinal cord nerve fibers and then to brainstem and corticospinal nerve tracts
- At birth, spinal nerves are attached to the cord in a horizontal position in relation to the vertebral column; with growth, lower nerves are directed more downward and sacral and coccygeal nerves are directed in a vertical direction while cervical nerves remain in a horizontal position

Sensory and Motor Function

- As neurologic system develops, the integrated functions of consciousness, mentation, language, motor function, sensory function, bowel and bladder function develop to completion
- Infant has reflexive responses and learns to bring responses under conscious control with growth and development of cortex — areas of cerebrum development correspond to the development of intellect, controls attention span and responses to stimuli
- Neuromuscular maturity and myelinization of spinal cord promotes walking and exploration learned by the age of 2 with skills perfected through preschool years
- Gross and fine motor development and coordination developed by age 3 for most activities and continues with growth, physical strength and endurance continue to develop throughout school age
- At birth, response to sound is present with ability to locate and identify sounds as myelinization of auditory pathways beyond the midbrain occurs; corvoture of the external equal develops to adult position by 3 years of age
- Hearing fully developed by 5 months of age and proceeds to listen and react to sounds and understands words by 1 year of age
- Sense of taste, smell and touch are present at birth with responses to strong odors, sour solutions, pin prick apparent

- In the infant, ciliary muscles are immature, which limits accommodation and the ability of the eye to fixate on an object for a period of time
- Macula and muscles develop with growth
- Responds to color by 1-2 months, color vision at 6 months
- Eye movement coordination by 3 months, function matures at 6 months
- Binocular vision by 4 months, tear glands function by 4 months
- Depth perception by 6-9 months, detail perception by 8 months
- Peripheral vision by 1 year of age
- Permanent iris color by 1 year of age
- Visual acuity matures at 6 years of age
Infant:	20/100-20/400
	(technique dependent)
2 years:	20/40
4 years:	20/30
Schoolage:	20/20
- Body temperature regulation unstable at birth with decrements and improved regulation taking place with maturity
Infant:	99.4-99.5 degrees F
Toddler:	99.7-99 degrees F
Preschool:	99-98.6 degrees F
Schoolage:	98.6-97.8 degrees F
- Length of sleep time decreases from infancy throughout childhood; amount of REM sleep is 20% compared to 50% in infancy, non-REM sleep increases with age, length of the sleep cycle increases from 50 minutes in the infant to 90 minutes in later childhood, number of hours decrease with age

ESSENTIAL NURSING DIAGNOSES AND CARE PLANS

Hyperthermia >38° C (100°F)

Related to: Illness or trauma
Defining characteristics: Increase in body temperature above normal range, flushed skin, warm to touch, increased respiratory rate, tachycardia, seizures/convulsions
Related to: Dehydration
Defining characteristics: Increase in body temperature above normal range, flushed, dry skin, warm to touch, increased respirations, pulse, oliguria, poor skin turgor, sunken eyeballs

Outcome Criteria

Return of body temperature to baseline parameters for age
Absence of dehydration with balanced I&O

Interventions	Rationales
Assess temperature via axillary method in infants and children to age 5 years, oral in children 5-6 years and older, depending on the individual child's ability to safely and accurately keep the thermometer in their mouth; check for malaise or lethargy and compare to normal ranges for age or low grade or high elevations associated with specific microorganisms or diseases	Provides information about temperature changes caused by high susceptibility to fluctuations in infants and young children since their regulatory function is unstable (regulated in the hypothalamus); temperature in infant and young child responds to infection with higher and more rapid elevations and may become overheated as environmental temperatures change or from activity, crying and emotional upsets since regulating mechanism immature until age 8
Assess temperature q1-2h for sudden increase in presence of any temperature elevation or illness	Sudden temperature elevation may induce a seizure
No specific level of temperature requires treatment; the main reason for treating a fever is discomfort (not including hyperthermia); two anti-pyretic drugs of choice: Acetaminophen and non-steroidal anti-inflammatory drugs such as Ibuprofen; administer in the form (liquid, tablet) that is appropriate for the age of the child and illness severity. Acetaminophen: dosage based on body weight, given every 4 hours (no more than 5 doses/24 hours); Ibuprofen: 5 mg/kg for temperature greater than 39.1°C	Reduces temperature; (lowers set point); prevents possible toxicity caused by accumulation if given too often, may be administered by tablet, liquid, chewable, suppository

Interventions	Rationales
(102.5°F) and 10 mg/kg for temperatures greater than 39.1°C (102.5°F), duration of action 6-8 hours; recheck temperature 30 minutes after medication given	
Cooling measures such as lightweight clothing, skin exposure, decreasing room temperature and cool, wet compresses to skin are only effective if given one hour after antipyretic	Anti-pyretics lower the set point, enabling cooling measures to be effective
Sponging/tepid baths are not recommended for children with hyperpyrexis (fever)	Utilized only for child with hyperthermia due to elevated set point; hyperthermia is a condition where body temperature exceeds set point — more heat created than eliminated due to internal factors such as hyperthyroidism, cerebral dysfunction, "malignant hyperthermia" (a reaction to anesthesia), or external factors (heat stroke)
Provide additional fluid orally or IV depending on condition of the infant/child	Maintains hydration when fluids are lost through fever or hyperthermia
Treat shivering by warming the body with clothing (especially extremities), increasing room temperature, and warm baths	Shivering increases metabolic demands which produces more heat; it is the body's natural mechanism to maintain the higher set point by producing more heat
Promote rest and provide a stress free environment, hold and rock infant/child if needed	Decreases metabolic requirements
For hyperthermia only: cooling measures such as cooling blankets/mattresses and tepid tub baths are utilized; water temperature should be 1-2 degrees less	Cooling measures are effective due to normal set point in hyperthermia; antipyretics are not effective

Interventions	Rationales
than the child's temperature; recheck temperature 30 minutes after intervention; discontinue if shivering occurs	

Information, Instruction, Demonstration

Interventions	Rationales
Instruct parent(s) and demonstrate taking oral axillary temperature and allow for return demonstration; instruct in use of digital thermometers and plastic strips	Allows parents to monitor temperature for elevation when child feels warm
Inform parent(s) of the difference between fever and hyperthermia and use of antipyretics to reduce fever and cooling baths to treat hyperthermia; instruct in safe use of antipyretics including type, dosage, frequency, form and limitations in 24 hour administration and sponging without use of cold water or alcohol	Antipyretics given to control fever which is an elevation in set point and cooling measures given to control hyperthermia which is a temperature that exceeds the set point
Instruct parents to report to physician immediately if: child is less than 2 months old with any fever; fever greater than 40.5°C. (105°F); presence of excessive crying; decreased level of consciousness; seizures; stiff neck; difficulty breathing; or if child has underlying illness	Prevents severe complications from elevated temperature that persists and is not relieved by medications; physician intervention to initiate or change treatment may be necessary
Inform parent(s) that temperature may become elevated without the presence of a serious illness	Reduces parental anxiety if unduly concerned about fever
Instruct parents to call their physician during office hours if: child is 2-4 months of age (unless related to DPT immuniza-	Fever is the body's normal body defense and does not always warrant immediate attention, depending on child's history and accom-

Interventions	Rationales
tion); fever is 40-40.5°C., especially if child is less than 2 years old; fever present for greater than 72 hours; fever returns after disappearing; history of febrile seizures; fever present for greater than 24 hours without other signs of illness	panying signs and symptoms

Discharge or Maintenance Evaluation

- Absence of temperature elevation above baseline for age
- Takes temperature q2-4h if child ill by proper method and route
- Keeps log of temperature readings and associated signs and symptoms to report
- Administers antipyretic correctly and safely and note temperature decreased; limits 24 hour doses, safe levels and frequencies
- Maintains environmental temperature at acceptable level
- Clothe child in cool, comfortable clothing and light covering
- Maintains hydration by increasing intake to meet losses caused by fever
- Reports temperature elevations that persist over 24 hours to physician with associated symptoms if present
- Use appropriate treatments depending on type and severity of fever or hyperthermia

Sleep pattern disturbance

Related to: Internal factor of illness
Defining characteristics: Interrupted sleep, temperature elevation, irritability, restlessness, listlessness, fatigue, weakness, nightmares
Related to: External factor of environmental changes
Defining characteristics: Hospitalization, interrupted sleep, separation anxiety, stimuli overload, lack of privacy, breaks in bedtime rituals or routines

Outcome Criteria

Restorative, restful sleep appropriate for age requirements
Absence of sleep, nap, rest problems or behaviors that aggravate problems

Interventions	Rationales
Assess sleep patterns and changes, nap times and frequency, sleep problems, pattern of awakenings and reason	Provides information about fulfillment of sleep needs related to age requirements: infants need 10-20 hours/24 hours with a routine and sleep through the night by 5 months of age; toddlers need 12 hours/night and 2 naps which gradually changes to 10 hours/night and 1 nap; preschoolers need 10 hours/night with or without a nap; schoolagers need 10 hours/night; wakenings may be caused by anxiety, nightmares and the absence of good sleep habits may create sleep problems
Assess presence of temperature elevation, restlessness caused by pain, dyspnea, other signs and symptoms of an illness	Provides possible reasons for restlessness, wakenings and sleep/rest deficit
Assess for fatigue, irritability, weakness, lability, yawning	Results of sleep deficit or deprivation, overactivity
Place infant (0-6 months) on back or side-lying position for sleep, utilizing positioning aids such as rolled blankets to maintain desired position; infants with gastroesophageal reflex, premature infants, and infants with specific upper airway problems may sleep in prone position; premature infants benefit developmentally from the prone position as it often facilitates flexion, and is soothing	Recent research has led the American Academy of Pediatrics to recommend these positions which have shown to decrease the incidence of SIDS (Sudden Infant Death Syndrome)
Avoid waking/interrupting sleep for feedings or caregiving	Provides comfort for sleep without interruptions
Offer snack and one toy at bedtime for child, follow home routines for time,	Promotes comfort and familiar bedtime pattern

Interventions	Rationales
night light, reading a story at bedtime, playing, tapes of music	
Allow time for quiet play before bedtime	Avoids overstimulation before bedtime
Provide soothing comfort if child has a nightmare and explain bad dream, stay until child returns to sleep	Provides security and explanation to encourage child to sleep without fear
Promote naps during day if such a routine has been established	Follows usual age dependent nap/rest pattern
Provide environment that is quiet, calm and warm; proper clothing, covers and diaper change as needed	Promotes sleep and/or rest periods
Try to avoid painful procedures prior to bedtime when possible	Decreases stimuli which prevent rest and sleep
Encourage parent to stay with child at night if possible or hold, rock, or stroke child "until" asleep	Promotes sleep and relaxation with a familiar person giving care

Information, Instruction, Demonstration

Interventions	Rationales
Discuss with parent(s) importance of sleep to health and amount of sleep needed by infant/child	Promotes parental understanding of sleep needs which are age dependent
Inform parent(s) that infant/child has specific need: Infant: place in side-lying or supine position, feed, change diaper, dress appropriately Toddler: inform of bedtime or nap in advance, offer snack, allow one toy in bed, allow to prepare for bed independently Preschool: provide own room, night light, story or music	Provides suggestions that may assist to establish bedtime rituals

Interventions	Rationales
Schoolage: provide time before sleep for talk, fear of sleep, activities of day	
Inform parent(s) to maintain same sleep schedule, set limits for inappropriate behaviors, reinforce appropriate behaviors	Promotes sleep pattern and avoids sleep problems
Instruct child in relaxation techniques such as tensing each part of the body and slowly relaxing each part, taking deep breaths, repeating a word that the child associates with relaxation	Promotes rest and induces sleep
Instruct parents on steps to take to solve chronic sleep problems after acute illness is resolved and child is at home; suggestions may include: importance of a bedtime ritual; importance of a consistent bed time and location; encourage use of a favorite blanket or toy to increase feelings of security; avoid use of bed as punishment; avoid feedings/drinks at night; if child consistently awakens at night, implement strategies which promote gradual change such as: entering room without picking up the child, then leaving for progressively longer periods of time until the child falls asleep by him/herself	Routines greatly promote the child's sleep quality and quantity; promotes the child's feelings of security; improves the quality of the parent-child relationship; promotes the child's own natural body defenses

Discharge or Maintenance Evaluation

- Verbalizes amount of sleep needed for infant/child specific to age
- Adequate number of hours of sleep daily appropriate for age
- Establishment of nap and bedtime rituals that are age related

- Verbalizes plan of approaches to take to solve sleep problems
- Takes appropriate actions to resolve nightmares, sleep problems
- Absence of sleep problems, manifestations of sleep deficits

Altered thought processes

Related to: Physiological changes
Defining characteristics: Altered attention span, disorientation to time, place, person, circumstances and events, changes in consciousness, hallucination, cognitive dissonance, inappropriate affect, memory deficit

Outcome Criteria

Maintenance or restoration of mental and psychological functions
Absence of signs and symptoms of encephalopathy and increased intracranial pressure

Interventions	Rationales
Assess history for neurologic conditions or infection, cognitive functioning	Provides information about reason for mentation changes
Assess for increased ICP and effects on orientation mentation, intellectual function, motor function	Provides information about increased ICP which results from brain edema, shift or distortion and brain hypoxia
Perform neurologic checks q2h including PERL, orientation, grip and grasp and pain response, presence of irritability, confusion, memory loss; include cranial nerve function if indicated	Provides data about changes in thought processes that indicate serious pathology
Elevate head of bed 30 degrees and maintain proper head and neck alignment	Promotes blood flow to brain and prevents hypoxia
Provide toys and stimulation that are age appropriate and modified for illness	Promotes developmental level within prescribed limitations to improve orientation and attention span
Limit sensory and motor expectations if unable to maintain thought processes and independence in activities	Prevents frustration and insecure feelings

Information, Instruction, Demonstration

Interventions	Rationales
Inform parent(s) of reason for loss of thought processes and temporary nature of this condition	Relieves doubts and anxiety about mental status of infant/child
Inform to expose infant/child to stimulation, toys and play activities and praise desired behaviors indicating orientation	Promotes developmental task achievement

Discharge or Maintenance Evaluation

- Mental and psychologic function at optimal level
- Absence of increased intracranial pressure
- Awareness of environment and orientation preserved
- Thought processes returned to baseline level
- Absence of residual effects (mental retardation) of brain disease

Hydrocephalus

Hydrocephalus is the enlargement of the intracranial cavity caused by the accumulation of cerebrospinal fluid in the ventricular system. This results from an imbalance in the production and absorption of the fluid causing an increase in intracranial pressure as the fluid builds up. Fluid may accumulate as a result of blockage of the flow (noncommunicating hydrocephalus) or impaired absorption (communicating hydrocephalus). In the infant, as the head enlarges to an abnormal size, he experiences lethargy, changes in level of consciousness, lower extremity spasticity and opisthotones and, if the hydrocephalus is allowed to progress, he experiences difficulty in sucking and feeding, emesis, seizures, sunset eyes and cardiopulmonary complications as lower brainstem and cortical function are disrupted or destroyed. In the child, increased intracranial pressure (ICP) focal manifestations are experienced related to space-occupying focal lesions including headache, emesis, ataxia, irritability, lethargy, confusion. Treatment may include surgery to provide shunting for drainage of the excess fluid from the ventricles to an extracranial space such as the peritoneum or right atrium (in older children) or management with medications to reduce ICP if progression is slow or surgery is contraindicated.

MEDICAL CARE

Diuretics: acetazolamide (Diamox) given PO, IV Lasix (Furosemide) to decrease production of CSF if progress of disease is slow.

Anticonvulsants: phenobarbital (Luminal, Luminal Sodium) given PO or IV to interfere with impulse transmission of cerebral cortex and prevent seizures.

Antibiotics: culture and sensitivity dependent given IV for shunt infections such as septicemia, meningitis, ventriculitis or given as prophylactic treatment.

Skull x-ray: reveals increasing head enlargement, widening of suture lines and fontanelles.

Magnetic Resonance imaging: reveals presence of hydrocephalus.

Echoencephalogram: reveals comparison of ratio of ventricle to cortex.

Ventriculogram: reveals size of ventricles and patency of a shunt if present.

Serial lumbar punctures: draining CSF at intervals to decrease excessive accumulation of CSF.

Surgical management: therapy of choice in almost all cases. Includes use of ventriculo-peritoneal shunt (VP), ventriculo-atrial shunt (VA), temporary ventriculostomy.

Lumbar puncture: relieves intracranial pressure by removing CSF when done with medication regimen.

Electrolyte panel: reveals changes indicating dehydration or losses from diuretic therapy.

Complete blood count: reveals increased WBC if infection presence of dehydration.

NURSING CARE PLANS

Essential nursing diagnoses and plans associated with this condition:

Fluid volume excess (5)

Related to: Compromised regulatory mechanism shunt placement — ventriculoatira or VP

Defining characteristics: Decreased cardiac output, change in respiratory pattern, tachycardia, tachypnea, dyspnea, weight gain, chest pain, cardiac arrhythmias, pulmonary congestion

Risk for fluid volume deficit (222)

Related to: Excessive losses through normal routes

Defining characteristics: Postoperative vomiting or diarrhea, use of diuretics, altered intake, thirst, dry skin and mucous membranes

Altered nutrition: Less than body requirements (168)

Related to: Inability to ingest food/feedings

Defining characteristics: Advanced stage of hydrocephalus, postoperative vomiting, NPO status

Risk for impaired skin integrity (397)

Related to: Physical immobilization and external factor of pressure

Defining characteristics: Decreased movement of head, disruption of skin surface by surgical procedure (shunt insertion) or diagnostic procedure

Hyperthermia (112)

Related to: Illness (infection)

Defining characteristics: Increase in body temperature above normal range

Altered growth and development (419)

Related to: Effects of disorder or disability
Defining characteristics: Altered physical growth, mental retardation, delay or difficulty in performing motor, social skills typical of age, dependence

SPECIFIC DIAGNOSES AND CARE PLANS

Anxiety

Related to: Threat to or change in health status; threat to or change in environment (hospitalization)
Defining characteristics: Increased apprehension that condition of infant might worsen or condition may develop in child as a complication, expressed concern and worry about preoperative preparation and the surgical procedure, possible or actual physical, neurologic and mental deficits

Outcome Criteria

Reduced parental and child anxiety verbalized as understanding of condition and treatment is increased and what can be expected as a result of the condition and/or surgery

Interventions	Rationales
Assess source and level of anxiety and need for information and support about condition and impending surgery	Provides information about severity of anxiety and need for interventions and support; allows for identification of fear and uncertainty about condition and/or surgery and treatments and recovery; guilt about condition, possible loss of infant/child or of parental responsibility
Allow expressions of concern and opportunity to ask questions about condition and recovery of ill infant/child	Provides opportunity to vent feelings, secure information needed to reduce anxiety
Communicate with parent(s) and answer questions calmly and honestly	Promotes calm and supportive environment

Interventions	Rationales
Encourage parent(s) to remain calm and involved in care and decision making regarding infant/child noting any improvement that results	Promotes constant monitoring of infant/child for improvement or worsening of symptoms
Allow parent(s) to stay with infant/child or visit when able if hospitalized, assist in care (hold, feed, diaper) and suggestions for routines and methods of treatment	Allows parent(s) to care for and support child instead of becoming increasingly anxious due to absence from child and wondering about infant/child's condition
When surgery is planned, answer all questions from parent(s) and child with honesty and hope; refer to physician for answers and explanations if needed	Promotes supportive environment and reduces anxiety caused by fear of unknown
Prepare child/parents for diagnostic tests and potential surgical procedures	Promotes reduction in anxiety if they have knowledge of expectations

Information, Instruction, Demonstration

Interventions	Rationales
Explain reason for and what to expect for each procedure or type of therapy; use drawings and pictures, video tapes for child	Reduces fear which causes anxiety
Inform parent(s) and child (age dependent) about reason for and type of surgery to be done, site and dressings, time of surgery and length of time of procedure, preoperative care and treatments	Provides information about surgery and desired effects as well as possible residual effects
Clarify any misinformation and answer all questions honestly and in simple understandable language	Prevents unnecessary anxiety resulting from inaccurate information or beliefs
Inform of shunt placement and reason; possible future revision of shunt place-	Shunt is placed to bypass an obstruction or remove excess cerebrospinal fluid

Interventions	Rationales
ment, signs and symptoms of shunt complication or malfunction	that predisposes to increased ICP; a shunt revision may be done to treat shunt complication such as infection or obstruction or as a result of child growth

Discharge or Maintenance Evaluation

- Expression of reduction in anxiety about condition, therapy and prognosis — participates in care and decision-making regarding infant/child
- Verbalizes positive effect of caring for and supporting infant/child
- Visits or telephones if unable to stay
- Verbalizes understanding of surgical procedure and perioperative care
- Participates in infant/child care following surgery
- Utilizes social services, counseling services, clergy for support

Risk for injury

Related to: Internal factors of sensory, integrative and effector dysfunction preoperatively
Defining characteristics: Neuromuscular changes, neurosensory changes, behavioral changes, increased ICP, CSF accumulation, vital signs changes, seizure activity

Outcome Criteria

Appropriate observations and reporting of signs and symptoms of possible increased ICP
Prevention of effects of complications of condition

Interventions	Rationales
Assess for rapidly increased circumference of head, tense, bulging fontanels, widening suture lines, irritability, lethargy, "cracked pot" sound percussion, sunset sign, opisthotonos, spasticity of lower extremities, seizures, high-pitched cry, distended scalp veins, changes in normal feeding patterns	Indicates increasing ICP in infant/small child

Interventions	Rationales
Assess for early signs including: headache, nausea, vomiting, diplopia, blurred vision, seizures, irritability, restlessness, decrease in school performance, decreased motor performance, sleep loss, weight loss, memory loss progressing to lethargy and drowsiness. Late signs: decreased level of consciousness, decreased motor response to commands, decreased response to pain, change in pupils, posturing, papilledema	Indicates increasing ICP in children with symptoms related to cause of hydrocephalus
Perform neurologic and vital sign assessment q4h or as needed	Provides data indicating an increasing ICP causing decreased respirations, increase blood pressure and pulse
Position with head elevated 30° and support head when handling or changing position; monitor skin integrity with position change	Promotes drainage of CSF and reduces accumulation of CSF; infant may not be able to lift and move head
Carry out seizure precautions including padding of crib/bed, remove toys and objects from bed, maintain suction and oxygen at bedside, note and report characteristics of seizure	Prevents injury to self during seizure activity caused by increased ICP and to treat apnea during seizure activity
Support an enlarged head by cradling it in an arm when holding, place infant on a pillow when moving, move head and body of infant at the same time	Protects infant's head from trauma and neck from strain

Information, Instruction, Demonstration

Interventions	Rationales
Inform parent(s) of signs and symptoms of increased ICP and changes to report to physician	Promotes knowledge of risk of developing increased ICP and encourages preventative measures

Interventions	Rationales
Inform parent(s) that condition is life-long and monitoring and follow-up care on a regular basis is required	Provides realistic and honest information that promotes optimal health and function for the infant/child

Discharge or Maintenance Evaluation

- Identification of signs and symptoms of increasing ICP
- Maintains stable neurologic status
- Prevents injury resulting from seizure activity or enlarged head positioning
- Complies with follow-up care and visits to physician and other professionals

Risk for injury

Related to: Internal factor of shunt placement and potential complications of shunt functioning
Defining characteristics: Increased ICP, kinking or plugging of shunt tubing, separation of tubing, changing of position of tubing, obstruction of shunt, displacement with growth

Outcome Criteria

Proper functioning shunt
Relief of hydrocephalus signs and symptoms
Absence of signs and symptoms of shunt blockage or infection

Interventions	Rationales
Assess for signs and symptoms of increased ICP, swelling along shunt tract; note presence/severity of headache and neck pain; behavior changes (lethargy, irritability), physical changes (full fontanel, nausea, vomiting, edematous eyes, tender, swollen abdomen)	Provides data that indicates shunt malfunction
Note vomiting, drowsiness, irritability, swelling at pump site, redness, exudate and temp of child	Indicates shunt blockage

Interventions	Rationales
Position carefully on non-operative side postoperatively; maintain bed position and activity level as ordered depending on shunt dynamics	Prevents trauma to surgical site; maintain shunt patency

Information, Instruction, Demonstration

Interventions	Rationales
Instruct parent on hydrocephalus and shunt placement; teaching should include: definition of hydrocephalus (brain anatomy), causes, diagnostic tests, treatments, signs of shunt malfunction and infection, interventions and proper notification of health professionals, and documentation; supplemental written materials are important; emphasize the importance of early identification of infection/malfunction and prompt notification	Promotes understanding of illness/treatments which may decrease anxiety; knowledge of prompt treatment of complications often life-saving
Instruct parent(s) of need for bowel elimination at least every 2 days and steps to take to ensure bowel movement	Prevents complications associated with ventriculoperitoneal shunt
Inform parent(s) of agencies for guidance and support such as National Hydrocephalus Foundation	Provides assistance with management of child with hydrocephalus
Discuss and encourage parent(s) to treat child as member of family and instruct in activities to be avoided such as rough contact sports	Promotes growth and development and feeling of belonging

Discharge or Maintenance Evaluation

- Absence of shunt malfunction
- Recognizes signs and symptoms of increased ICP and shunt malfunction
- Maintains and supports postoperative measures to ensure success of surgery and decrease infection
- Utilizes community agencies for information and support
- Maintains follow-up appointments with physician and diagnostic procedures to monitor condition and shunt function
- Parent promptly contacts appropriate health care professional with questions/concerns as they arise

Risk for infection

Related to: Invasive procedure of shunt insertion
Defining characteristics: Elevated temperature, swelling, redness at shunt tract or operative site, nausea, vomiting, lethargy, excessive drainage on dressing, poor feeding

Outcome Criteria

Infection at shunt site prevented or absent
Progressive healing of incision site

Interventions	Rationales
Assess site for inflammatory process, temperature for elevation, WBC for increases, characteristics of drainage on dressings	Provides data indicating presence or potential for infection which affects shunt function
Follow principles of asepsis when performing procedures such as dressing changes	Prevents transmission of microorganisms to shunt site
Monitor temperature q4h	Elevation of temperature indicates infection
Avoid positioning head of valve site for at least 2 days postoperatively	Alleviates the risk of infection

Information, Instruction, Demonstration

Interventions	Rationales
Instruct about signs and symptoms of infection of site and shunt tract and to notify physician if noted	Promotes early detection of infection which may occur for up to 1-2 months after shunt insertion
Instruct and demonstrate wound care and dressing change, emphasize importance of good handwashing techniques	Provides clean, sterile dressings when soiled or wet

Discharge or Maintenance Evaluation

- Measures taken to prevent infection
- Preventative antibiotics administered for 2 days postoperatively
- Protects site and shunt from contamination and trauma
- Absence of infection leading to shunt malfunction and externalization of shunt

Hydrocephalus

Increased production of cerebrospinal fluid	Obstruction of flow of cerebrospinal fluid	Failure of cerebrospinal fluid to be reabsorbed

Choroid plexus tumor

Congenital malformation
Tumors
Post infection

Congenital anomalies
Post hemorrhage
Meningitis
Maternal infections

Obstruction of flow of
CSF through ventricles

Occlusion of villi by
scarring, blood fragments
or infection debris

Enlargement of ventricular
system

CSF not absorbed into
arachnoid villi

Noncommunicating hydrocephalus

Communicating hydrocephalus

Increased volume of CSF

Ventricular dilatation

Increased intracranial pressure

Grossly enlarged head
Separated cranial sutures
Bulging fontanels
Protruding eyes

Increased head size
Irritability
Feeding difficulty
Delayed motor skills
Setting sun eyes

Blindness
Paralysis
Mental retardation

Developing hydrocephalus

Shunting procedure

Death

Return CSF to circulation

Intracranial Tumor

A brain tumor is a solid tumor that may be benign, malignant or a metastatic growth from a tumor in another part of the body. Most central nervous system tumors occur in the cerebellum or brainstem causing increased intracranial pressure and the symptoms associated with it. Other tumors occur in the cerebrum. A malignant brain tumor is the second most common type of cancer in children and has a poor prognosis since the tumor usually enlarges and becomes advanced before signs and symptoms appear or are detected as they are easily missed. Signs and symptoms are site and size dependent. Brain tumors are most prevalent in children 3-7 years of age. Treatment includes surgery, although total removal is not usually possible, chemotherapy and radiation, which may be done to decrease the size of the tumor before surgery. One or a combination of these procedures may be done with each resulting in possible residual neurologic deficits.

MEDICAL CARE

Analgesics/Antipyretics: acetaminophen (Tylenol tablets, Pedric wafers, elixir, Liquiprin solution drops) given PO for headache and to reduce fever, Ibuprofen PO, Codein PO to decrease pain.

Diuretics (osmotic): mannitol (Osmitrol) given IV to induce diuresis with a hypertonic solution to prevent reabsorption of water by the glomeruli and decrease cerebralede.

Antibiotics: specific to microorganisms identified by culture and sensitivities to treat infection or given to prevent infection.

Anti-inflammatories: hydrocortisone (Cortef) given PO or prednisolone sodium phosphate (Hydeltrasol) given IV; Dexamethasone (Decadron) to reduce inflammation process in brain.

Saline solution: given as eye drops or eye irrigation to prevent corneal ulceration.

Stool softeners: docusate calcium (Surfak) given PO to lower surface tension in bowel to allow for water and fats to mix with stool for easier elimination to prevent constipation and Valsalva's maneuver which increase intracranial pressure.

Computerized tomography scan (CT): reveals changes in position of brain parenchyma, ventricles and subarachnoid space caused by tumor growth.

Stereotactic surgery: use of CT/MRI to reconstruct brain tumor three-dimensionally to accurately remove it surgically.

Laser therapy: vaporization of tumor tissue.

Radiotherapy: use of radiation to shrink tumor size.

Chemotherapy: used to treat malignant tumors.

Cerebral angiogram: reveals vascularity and blood supply to the tumor before surgery.

Magnetic resonance imaging (MRI): reveals tumor growth and size before, during and after treatment.

Electrolyte panel: reveals changes indicating dehydration or losses from diuretic therapy.

Complete blood count: reveals increased WBC if infection present.

Urinalysis: reveals increased Sp.gr. in presence of dehydration.

NURSING CARE PLANS

Essential nursing diagnoses and plans associated with this condition:

Hyperthermia (112)

Related to: Illness

Defining characteristics: Increase in body temperature above normal range, presence of infection (meningitis or upper respiratory), surgical procedure (anesthesia, brainstem or hypothalamus area)

Sleep pattern disturbance (114)

Related to: Sensory alternations caused by internal factors of illness

Defining characteristics: Lethargy, restlessness, irritability, disorientation, coma, frequent napping

Risk for fluid volume deficit (222)

Related to: Excessive losses through normal routes

Defining characteristics: Vomiting, altered intake, diuresis with use of diuretic, diabetes insipidus development, thirst, dry skin and mucous membranes

Altered nutrition: Less than body requirements (168)

Related to: Inability to ingest food

Defining characteristics: Vomiting, nausea, choking and possible aspiration with facial paralysis or edema, refusal to eat or drink, gavage feedings, depressed gag reflex

Impaired physical mobility (278)

Related to: Neuromuscular impairment
Defining characteristics: Inability to purposefully move within physical environment, impaired coordination, loss of balance, decreased muscle strength and control spasticity, hypo or hyperreflexia, paralysis, general weakness, ataxia following surgery

Altered growth and development (419)

Related to: Effects of disorder or disability following surgery/other
Defining characteristics: Delay or difficulty in performing skills typical of age group (motor, social or expressive), inability to perform self-control activities appropriate for age behavior and/or intellectual deficits, presence of somnolence syndrome

SPECIFIC DIAGNOSES AND CARE PLANS

Pain

Related to: Biologic injuring agents
Defining characteristics: Verbal descriptor of pain, headache in frontal or occipital area that is worse in the morning and becomes worse if head lowered or with straining, increased VS, restlessness, hostility, inability to relax

Outcome Criteria

Relief or control of headache
Absence of progressively increased headache

Interventions	Rationales
Assess severity of headache, recurrence and progressive characteristics, precipitating factors and length of headache	Provides information regarding presence of tumor as headache is a most common symptom in child
Administer analgesic to treat or anticipate headache based on assessment	Relieves headache and promotes rest and comfort
Provide toys, games for quiet play	Provides diversionary activity to detract from pain
Apply cool compress to head for low to moderate pain	Provides comfort and relief from headache, decrease facial swelling, if present

Interventions	Rationales
After surgical intervention, opioids (Morphine Sulfate) may be initially used. Assess for side effects such as sedation and respiratory depression; use Naloxone to reverse	Side effects occur rarely, opioids can be given safely with appropriate monitoring
Determine the child's understanding of the word "pain" and ask family what word the child normally uses. Use a pain assessment tool appropriate for age and developmental level to identify intensity of pain	Promotes better communication between child/family and nurse
Plan a preventative approach to pain management around the clock; observe for signs of pain, both physiologic and behavioral	Promotes early identification of pain which enhances pain relief measures

Information, Instruction, Demonstration

Interventions	Rationales
Inform parent(s) and child of need for analgesics, to administer in anticipation of headache and type to give (sustained release) and that it will help to control headache	Controls pain before it becomes severe
Inform parent(s) and child to restrain from coughing, sneezing, straining during defecation	Prevents straining that precipitates or intensifies headache
Assist parent(s) to develop activities that will not precipitate or increase headache pain	Promotes stimulation for child's development needs

Discharge or Maintenance Evaluation

- Pain is absent or relieved
- Complies with analgesic regimen to prevent or control headache

- Limits activities that initiate or increase headache
- Participates in quiet play

Risk for injury

Related to: Internal factors of sensory, integrative and effector dysfunction
Defining characteristics: Neuromuscular changes, neurosensory changes, behavioral changes, increased ICP, seizure activity, vital signs changes

Outcome Criteria

Appropriate observations and reporting of signs and symptoms difficult to do — how is this related to diagnosis?
Preventative measure taken to ensure safety during diagnostic period of illness

Interventions	Rationales
Assess head circumference in the infant/small child for increases as fluid obstruction caused by tumor will increase head size	Provides data indicating an increase in ICP as tumor grows with a poorer prognosis because tumor size becomes large before diagnosis is made
Assess vital signs including increased BP, decreased pulse pressure, pulse and respirations; take for 1 full minute when monitoring pulse and respirations	Provides changes indicating presence of brain tumor depending on type and location of tumor
Assess changes in gross and fine motor control, weakness, ataxia, spasticity, paralysis or change in balance, coordination	Provides changes in neuromuscular status indicating presence of brain tumor
Assess changes in vision (visual acuity, strabismus, diplopia, nystagmus), head tilt, papilledema	Provides changes in neurosensory status indicating presence of brain tumor
Assess for irritability, lethargy, loss of consciousness or coma, fatigue, napping	Provides changes in behavior indicating presence of brain tumor
Assess for increased ICP including irritability, poor feeding, vomiting, head enlargement, lethargy, high-pitched cry (infant) or	Provides information about ICP change caused by brain distortion or shifting caused by tumor

Interventions	Rationales
vomiting, diplopia, behavioral changes, change in VS, seizure activity	
Alter environment by padding bed or crib, reduce light and stimulation	Prevents injury if seizure activity possible
Place in position of comfort with head elevated	Promotes comfort and decreases increased ICP by gravity

Information, Instruction, Demonstration

Interventions	Rationales
Inform parent(s) and child of diagnostic procedures done to evaluate tumor presence; base information on child's age and past experiences	Promotes understanding of procedures to reduce
Inform parent(s) that surgery may be performed to remove the tumor as a reinforcement of physician information and that radiation and chemotherapy may be administered after surgery	Prepares for surgery and possible postoperative therapy with information limited to sensitive, hopeful explanation; information about postoperative therapy should be postponed until this decision is made after surgery

Discharge or Maintenance Evaluation

- Symptoms of brain tumor assessed and identified
- Prepares for diagnostic and surgical procedures
- Maintains safe environments with absence of injury

Anxiety

Related to: Change in health status and threat to self-concept
Defining characteristics: Increased apprehension as diagnosis is confirmed and condition worsens, expressed concern and worry about postoperative residual tumor and effects, hair removal before surgery, insomnia, social isolation

Outcome Criteria

Reduced parental and child anxiety verbalized as information is given
Ability to cope with appearance following surgery

Interventions	Rationales
Assess level of anxiety and need for information that will relieve it following surgery	Provides information about degree of anxiety and need for interventions and support; allow for identification of fear and uncertainty about surgery and treatments and recovery, guilt about illness, possible loss of child, parental role and responsibility
Allow expression of concerns and inquire about condition of ill child and possible consequences and prognosis	Provides opportunity to vent feelings, secure information needed to reduce anxiety
Prepare family and/or child for diagnostic tests and surgery. Encourage child to draw a picture of the brain to clarify any misconceptions; encourage use of medical play (dolls, puppets, equipment) after procedures	Promotes understanding which decreases anxiety; may clarify misconceptions and increase feelings of control
Encourage parent(s) to stay with infant/child; encourage participation in care of infant/child	Promotes care and support of child by parent(s)
If surgery planned, orient to special care unit, equipment and staff	Reduces anxiety caused by fear of unknown

Information, Instruction, Demonstration

Interventions	Rationales
Inform parent(s) and child of hair clipping and that hair will grow back in short period of time, to cover head with cap or scarf temporarily; that	Promotes understanding of postoperative appearance to maintain self-image; support self-concept

Interventions	Rationales
there is edema of the face and eyes after surgery; that a dressing will be applied that completely covers the head; use of a doll with head wrapped in a bandage may be useful in explaining the post-surgical dressing	
Inform parent(s) and child that after surgery a headache and sleepy feeling may be present for a few days or even lethargy and coma may be present	Provides an explanation of what to expect after surgery
Explain reason for and type of surgery to be done and possible serious effects of surgery	Provides information about surgery and desired and residual effects or damage
Clarify any information in lay terms and use aids that are age related if helpful to child	Prevents unnecessary anxiety resulting from misunderstanding or inconsistencies in information

Discharge or Maintenance Evaluation

- Expresses reduction in anxiety and adjustment to diagnosis and treatments
- Participates in care and supports infant/child
- Maintains child's self-concept and body image
- Asks questions, expresses concern about treatment and prognosis

Intracranial Tumor

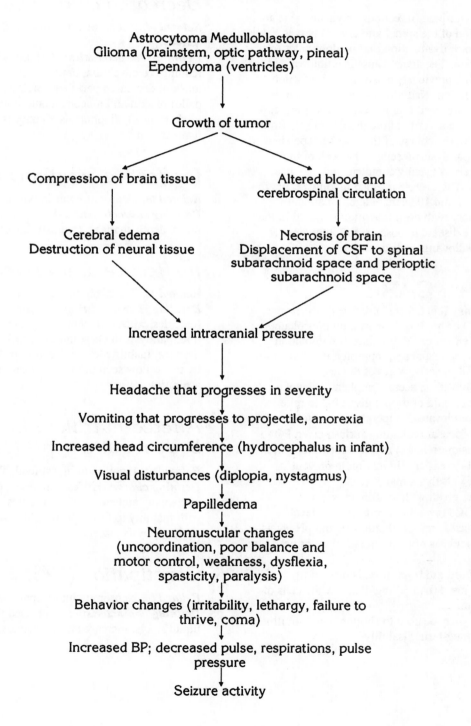

Astrocytoma Medulloblastoma
Glioma (brainstem, optic pathway, pineal)
Ependyoma (ventricles)

Growth of tumor

Compression of brain tissue

Altered blood and
cerebrospinal circulation

Cerebral edema
Destruction of neural tissue

Necrosis of brain
Displacement of CSF to spinal
subarachnoid space and perioptic
subarachnoid space

Increased intracranial pressure

Headache that progresses in severity

Vomiting that progresses to projectile, anorexia

Increased head circumference (hydrocephalus in infant)

Visual disturbances (diplopia, nystagmus)

Papilledema

Neuromuscular changes
(uncoordination, poor balance and
motor control, weakness, dysflexia,
spasticity, paralysis)

Behavior changes (irritability, lethargy, failure to
thrive, coma)

Increased BP; decreased pulse, respirations, pulse
pressure

Seizure activity

Guillain-Barré Syndrome

Guillain-Barré Syndrome (infectious polyneuritis) is an acute inflammation of the spinal and cranial nerves manifested by motor dysfunction that predominates over sensory dysfunction. The actual cause is unknown, but it is associated with a previously existing viral infection or vaccine administration. Neurologic symptoms include muscle cramps and paresthesia with weakness progressing to paralysis. The severity of the disease ranges from mild to severe with the course of the disease dependent on the degree of paralysis present at the peak of the condition. Recovery is usually complete and may take weeks or months. The disease most commonly occurs in children between 4 and 10 years of age. Treatment is symptom dependent with hospitalization required in the acute phase of the disease to observe and intervene for respiratory or swallowing complications.

MEDICAL CARE

Anti-inflammatory (corticosteroids): hydrocortisone (Cortef) given PO or prednisolone sodium phosphate (Hydeltrasol) given IM or IV to reduce inflammation process and immune responses; Ibuprofen PO may or may not be helpful in early stages of disease.

Analgesics/Antipyretics: acetaminophen (Tylenol tablets, Liquiprim liquid or drops) given PO to relieve pain in muscles or elevated temperature if present.

Stool softeners: docusate calcium (Surfak) given PO to lower surface tension in bowel to allow for water and fats to mix with stool for easier elimination to prevent constipation and Valsalva's maneuver.

Oxygen therapy: given with ventilatory support depending on ABGs revealing decreased PO_2 level.

Arterial blood gases: reveals O_2 and CO_2 and pH levels as indication of acidosis or respiratory failure or need for oxygen therapy.

Cerebrospinal fluid analysis: reveals protein concentration of more than 60 mg/dl and white cells of less than 10/cu mm.

Plasmapheresis: may be used to shorten length of illness and/or to lessen long-term disability.

NURSING CARE PLANS

Essential nursing diagnoses and plans associated with this condition:

Decreased cardiac output (3)

Related to: Effects of autonomic dysfunction on cardiac activity

Defining characteristics: Variations in hemodynamic readings (tachycardia, bradycardia, hypotension, hypertension) decreased peripheral pulses, oliguria, cyanosis, pallor of skin and mucous membranes, ECG changes (arrhythmias), diaphoresis, dizziness, orthostatic hypotension

Ineffective breathing pattern (45)

Related to: Neuromuscular impairment

Defining characteristics: Altered chest expansion, respiratory depth changes, cyanosis, abnormal ABGs

Ineffective airway clearance (42)

Related to: Tracheobronchial obstruction, secretions

Defining characteristics: Abnormal breath sounds (crackles, wheezes), changes in rate or depth of respiration, paralysis in chest muscles, tachypnea, cough, dyspnea, inability to clear secretions from airway, inability to swallow secretions, weakness in speech, gag reflex, aspiration

Altered nutrition: Less than body requirements (168)

Related to: Inability to ingest food, absorb nutrients

Defining characteristics: Anorexia, diarrhea, weakness of chewing and swallowing muscles, dysesthesia of hands with inability to feed self, weight loss, loss of muscle tone, paralysis (ascending)

Constipation (173)

Related to: Neuromuscular impairment

Defining characteristics: Increased frequency, loose, liquid stools, increased bowel sounds, steatorrhea

Impaired physical mobility (278)

Related to: Neuromuscular impairment
Defining characteristics: Paralysis, inability to purposefully move within physical environment including bed mobility, transfer and ambulation, limited ROM, decreased muscle strength and control, trauma from falls

Hyperthermia (112)

Related to: Illness causing autonomic instability
Defining characteristics: Increase in body temperature above normal range or decrease below normal range, warm or cool to touch

SPECIFIC DIAGNOSES AND CARE PLANS

Altered urinary elimination patterns

Related to: Neuromuscular impairment
Defining characteristics: Paralysis, retention

Outcome Criteria

Return of optimal urinary elimination as disease is resolved
Absence of retention of urine

Interventions	Rationales
Assess continuing extent of paralysis and effect on urinary elimination	Provides information about effect of motor weakness which travels upward from extremities
Assess for I&O q4-8h and palpate bladder q2h; assess for cloudy, foul-smelling urine	Provides monitoring for I&O ratio and presence of urinary retention, UTI as paralysis progresses
Provide urinary elimination rehabilitation program; perform Crede maneuver in gentle fashion if indicated	Promotes urine elimination and return to normal pattern as soon as possible
Catheterize as last resort; maintain indwelling catheter if needed to maintain elimination	Relieves distention and retention

Information, Instruction, Demonstration

Interventions	Rationales
Instruct parent(s) in program to rehabilitate urinary function	Promotes urinary elimination and return to baseline pattern without retention and possible urinary bladder infection
Instruct to maintain fluid intake and monitor output in relation to intake	Maintains I&O balance and enough intake to encourage urinary output
Inform to report any reduction or absence of urinary elimination	Prevents complication of neuromuscular impairment of disease and effect on urinary bladder function

Discharge or Maintenance Evaluation

- Maintains I&O ratio within baseline
- Promotes urinary elimination program
- Monitors presence of retention and reports to physician
- Absence of urinary retention and signs of increased infection

Pain

Related to: Biological injuring agent (inflammation of nerves)
Defining characteristics: Communication of pain descriptors of discomfort in hands and feet, guarding behavior, alteration in muscle tone, autonomic responses of diaphoresis, VS changes

Outcome Criteria

Absence or control of pain in extremities

Interventions	Rationales
Assess pain and ability to participate in activities	Provides information about degree of pain or presence of progressive paralysis
Reposition q2h, support extremities and maintain clean, comfortable bed with eggcrate mattress and padding to bony prominences as needed; use good	Promotes comfort and reduces risks for skin impairment

Interventions	Rationales
postural alignment, provide passive ROM	
Administer analgesics based on pain assessment and respiratory status; evaluate effect	Eliminates or controls pain and promotes comfort
Apply moist heat to painful areas as ordered	Promotes circulation to area and relieves pain

Information, Instruction, Demonstration

Interventions	Rationales
Inform parent(s) and child of reason for pain, what will be done to relieve pain	Allows for a decrease in anxiety which increases pain and more control over the situation
Inform parent(s) and child that pain decreases as motor changes become resolved or improve	Provides information about length of time pain might be expected to continue
Determine the child's understanding of the word "pain" and ask family members what word the child uses at home; use pain assessment tool appropriate for the child's age and developmental level to identify the intensity of pain	Promotes better communication between the child/family and nurse
Plan a preventative approach to pain around the clock; observe for signs of pain, physiological and behavioral	Promotes early identification of pain which enhances effective pain relief

Discharge or Maintenance Evaluation

- Absence of pain in extremities
- Control of pain sensation with proper use of analgesics
- Participates in ADL and other activities
- Distracts child from dwelling on pain

Anxiety

Related to: Change in health status and threat to self-concept

Defining characteristics: Increased apprehension as condition worsens and paralysis spreads, expressed concern and worry about permanent effects of disease, treatments during hospitalization, expressed feeling of increased helplessness and uncertainty

Outcome Criteria

Reduced parental and child anxiety verbalized as illness is resolved

Interventions	Rationales
Assess source and level of anxiety, how anxiety is manifested and need for information that will relieve it	Provides information about degree of anxiety and need for interventions, sources may include fear and uncertainty about treatment and recovery, guilt about presence of illness, possible loss of parental role and responsibility while hospitalized
Allow expression of concerns and opportunity to ask questions about condition and recovery of ill child	Provides opportunity to vent feelings, secure information needed to reduce anxiety
Communicate with parent(s) and child and answer questions calmly and honestly	Promotes supportive environment
Encourage parent(s) and child to note improvements resulting from treatments	Promotes positive attitude and optimistic outlook for recovery
Encourage parent(s) to stay with child and telephoning and allow to assist in care of child	Allows for care and support of child instead of increasing anxiety that is caused by absence and lack of knowledge about child's condition
Allow child to participate in own care depending on ability and/or paralysis; allow to make choices about ADL as soon as possible	Promotes independence and control and preserves developmental status

Information, Instruction, Demonstration

Interventions	Rationales
Inform parent(s) and child of disease process and behaviors, physical effects	Provides information to relieve anxiety by knowledge of what to expect
Explain reason for and what happens for each procedure or type of therapy, effects of any diagnostic tests to parent(s) and child as appropriate to age	Reduces fear of unknown which may increase anxiety
Inform parent(s) and child that degree of severity varies but motor weakness and paralysis start with extremities and move upward with the peak reached in 3 weeks and improvement seen by 4-8 weeks	Provides information about usual course of disease and length of illness
Clarify any information and answer questions in lay terms and use aids for visual reinforcement if helpful	Prevents unnecessary anxiety resulting from inaccurate knowledge or beliefs or inconsistencies in information

Discharge or Maintenance Evaluation

- Expresses reduction in anxiety concerning disease process, therapy and prognosis
- Participates in care and decision-making regarding child
- Visits or calls hospital if unable to stay
- Verbalizes that anxiety decreases as resolution of disease begins
- Maintains child's self-concept and developmental status
- Allows for optimal self-care by child

Risk for altered parenting

Related to: Lack of knowledge
Defining characteristics: Verbalization of decreased interactions with hospitalized child and inability to provide care, lack of control over situation, request for information about parenting skills for long recovery period or permanent residual disability

Outcome Criteria

Verbalizes readiness to deal with long-term recovery and consequences
Adapts to loss of function

Interventions	Rationales
Assess for presence of permanent disability or possibility of long-term recovery and effect on parent(s)	Identifies factors associated with long recovery period
Encourage parent(s) to express feelings and unmet needs and ability to meet and develop self-expectations	Identifies potential for social deprivation of parent(s) and development of strategies to achieve realistic expectations
Encourage touching and play activities between parent(s) and child	Enhances comfort and positive parental behaviors
Encourage and praise positive parental behaviors; support any participation in care or decision-making on behalf of the child	Reduces anxiety for and enhances learning about child's needs and care

Information, Instruction, Demonstration

Interventions	Rationales
Inform of parental tasks and child's developmental tasks to be encouraged	Provides reference to task achievement for both child and parent(s)
Instruct in parenting skill needed for long-term recovery period	Promotes parental knowledge and awareness of skills to be learned and implemented
Inform of possibility of progressive deterioration even with treatment	Prevents depression as disease peaks and promotes hope for improvement
Instruct in an active physical therapy program including ROM, exercises, gait training, bracing	Facilitates muscle recovery and prevents contractures and permanent disability, promotes sense of confidence and control
Continue to inform and support parent(s) during recovery period	Provides reassurance that recovery is slow and conserves parental emotional reserves

Interventions	Rationales
Inform to contact Guillain-Barré Syndrome Support Group for assistance or community agencies for support	Provides information and support from those with experience with the disease

Discharge or Maintenance Evaluation

- Maintains parental role as illness is resolved
- Participates in care and physical rehabilitation
- Verbalizes positive effects of treatment and participation in care
- Adapts to long-term therapy and any loss of function
- Attends parenting classes if appropriate
- Maintains decision-making and control over care and child rearing practices
- Participates in agency for assistance and support in dealing with long-term recovery

Guillain-Barre Syndrome

Virus infection   Vaccination   Autoimmune reaction

Measles
Mumps
Infectious mononucleosis
Febrile condition

Attack on peripheral nerves

Inflammation and edema of spinal
and cranial nerves
Peripheral and spinal nerve root demyelination
Axon destruction

Sensory impairment   Impaired nerve conduction   Autonomic dysfunction

Muscle tenderness

Bilateral facial paresis
Symmetric weakness of
extremities and areflexia
Hypotonia
Paresthesia
Bowel and bladder dysfunction
Partial or complete paralysis

Tachycardia
Orthostatic
hypotension

Total paralysis of
respiratory muscles, swallowing
and gag reflexes

Return of muscle function
within 2 weeks

Pneumonia

Death

Complete resolution within a
few weeks or months depending
on severity of paralysis

Meningitis

Meningitis is the inflammation of the meninges and is the most common infection of the central nervous system (CNS). It may be bacterial or viral in origin and may be caused by a bacterial infection such as Haemophilus influenzae (type B), Streptococcus pneumoniae, Neisseria meningitidis, or Stephlococcus aureus. Those at greatest risk for this disease are infants between 6 and 12 months of age with most cases occurring between 1 month and 5 years of age. The route of infection most commonly is vascular dissemination from an infection in the nasopharynx or sinuses or may be implanted as a result of wounds skull fracture, lumbar puncture or surgical procedure. It may be also viral (aseptic) and caused by a variety of viral agents and usually associated with measles, mumps, herpes, enteritis. This form of meningitis is self-limiting and treated symptomatically for 3-10 days. Treatment includes hospitalization to differentiate between the two types of meningitis, isolation and management of symptoms and prevention of complications.

MEDICAL CARE

Antipyretics: acetaminophen (Tylenol tablets, Pedric wafers or elixir, Liquiprin solution drops) given PO to reduce fever, Ibuprofen PO, PR.

Antibiotics: penicillin G potassium (Pfizerpen), methicillin (Staphcillin), oxacillin sodium (Bactocill, Vancomycin, Gentamycin) given IV to treat the infection, or other specific to identified microorganism as a result of culture and sensitivity tests.

Anticonvulsants: phenobarbital (Luminal, Luminal Sodium) given PO or IV to prevent seizure activity; Dilantin PO, IV.

Computerized tomography scan: reveals subdural effusion.

Cultures of blood, urine, cerebrospinal fluid, nasopharynx: reveals causative organism.

Lumbar puncture: reveals cloudy or purulent appearance, increased WBC predominant polymorphonuclear leukocytes, increased protein, decreased glucose in bacterial type; clear, normal or slight elevation of WBC with predominant lymphocytes, slight increased glucose, slight protein, normal lactate dehydrogenase in viral type.

Electrolyte panel: reveals decreased K and increased Na, changes indicating dehydration.

Serum osmolality: reveals increase if antidiuretic hormone secretion increased.

Complete blood count: reveals increased WBC.

Urinalysis: increased osmolarity if antidiuretic hormone secretion increased, increased Sp.gr.

NURSING CARE PLANS

Essential nursing diagnoses and plans associated with this condition:

Hyperthermia (112)

Related to: Illness

Defining characteristics: Increase in body temperature above normal range, warm to touch, increased respiratory and pulse rate

Risk for fluid volume deficit (222)

Related to: Excessive losses through normal routes

Defining characteristics: Vomiting, diarrhea

Related to: Deviations affecting intake of fluids

Defining characteristics: Decreased intake, fluid restrictions, change in level of consciousness

Related to: Failure of regulatory mechanisms

Defining characteristics: Secretion of antidiuretic hormone, increased Sp. gr. and osmolality, reduced output, dehydration

Altered thought processes (116)

Related to: Physiological changes

Defining characteristics: Disorientation to time, place, persons, events, changes in consciousness, behavior changes also important to monitor fluids and ventilation

SPECIFIC DIAGNOSES AND CARE PLANS

Anxiety

Related to: Threat to or change in health status of child; threat to or change in environment (hospitalization of child)

Defining characteristics: Increased apprehension that condition of child might worsen, expressed concern and worry about actual hospitalization of child and seriousness of illness

Outcome Criteria

Reduced parental anxiety with understanding of disease and what can be expected until illness is resolved

Interventions	Rationales
Assess sources and level of anxiety, how anxiety is manifested and need for information and support	Provides information about the need for interventions to relieve anxiety and concern; sources may include fear and uncertainty about treatment and recovery, guilt for presence of illness, possible loss of parental role and loss of responsibility when hospitalization necessary
Allow to express concerns and ask questions regarding condition of ill child	Provides opportunity to vent feelings, secure information needed to reduce anxiety
Encourage to remain calm and involved in care and decision-making regarding child's needs and noting any improvements that result	Promotes constant monitoring of child's condition for improvements or worsening of symptoms
Allow parent to stay with child or visit when able and call when concerned if hospitalized; assist in care (hold, feed, bathe, clothe and diaper) and provide information about child's daily routines	Allows parent to care for and support child instead of increasing anxiety if not with child

Information, Instruction, Demonstration

Interventions	Rationales
Assess parental feelings of guilt from not suspecting the seriousness of the illness sooner; encourage them to openly discuss feelings	Prevents or minimizes feelings of blame or guilt
Inform of disease process and behaviors, physical effects and symptoms of disease	Relieves anxiety of parent(s)

Interventions	Rationales
Explain reason for each procedure or type of therapy, effects of any diagnostic tests	Reduces fear of unknown which increases anxiety
Inform parents of reason for isolation precautions for at least 24 hours or until diagnosis is made and antibiotic therapy begins to take effect	Provides opportunity to validate type of meningitis and to take measures to prevent transmission to others in contact with child
Clarify any misinformation and answer questions in lay terms when parent(s) able to listen, give same explanation as other staff and/or physician gave regarding disease process and transmission	Prevents unnecessary anxiety resulting from inaccurate knowledge or beliefs or inconsistencies in information

Discharge or Maintenance Evaluation

- Expresses a reduction in anxiety with explanations of disease process and therapy
- Verbalizes the positive effect of caring for and supporting their sick infant/small child
- Participates in care and decision-making regarding infant/small child
- Visits and/or telephones the hospital if unable to stay

Risk for injury

Related to: Internal factor of altered neurologic regulatory function

Defining characteristics: Increased intracranial pressure; early signs of lethargy, restlessness, increased head circumference, headache, vomiting, personality changes or late signs of decreased level of consciousness, change in posturing, widening of pulse pressure, projectile vomiting, decreased pulse and respirations, seizure, abnormal PERL, shrill cry, bulging fontanel, changes in vision

Outcome Criteria

Improved and/or stabilization of neurologic status within normal or baseline parameters for infant/child

Interventions	Rationales
Assess neurologic status to include VS pattern, changes in consciousness, behavior patterns and pupillary/ocular responses appropriate for age; measure head circumference in infant	Provides information that offers clues to possible change in intracranial pressure caused by inflammation of the brain and associated edema
Attach cardiac and respiratory monitor to assess for bradycardia and hypoxia	Increased intracranial pressure will decrease pulse and respirations, widen the pulse pressure with pulse becoming irregular and respirations rapid and shallow as ICP progresses and the body attempts to decrease blood flow to brain
Reposition q2h, positioning child to optimize comfort with HOB slightly elevated, no pillow in bed, side-lying position if nuchal rigidity present, avoid sudden movements such as lifting the head; have oxygen and suctioning equipment on hand to be administered when needed	Maintains airway patency and prevents obstruction by secretion which increases CO_2 retention and ICP
Provide quiet environment free from bright lighting, minimize gentle handling and care of infant/child, allow for rest periods between care or procedures, restrict visiting if irritable	Promotes comfort and rest and reduces irritability
Administer antibiotics as prescribed as soon as ordered based on analysis of CSF, throat cultures	Manages existing infection and prevents further spread of infection
Note any seizure activity including onset, frequency, duration and type of movements before, during or after seizure; pad bed and remove objects/toys from bed and administer any ordered anticonvulsants	Prevents injury during seizure which is a complication of meningitis

Interventions	Rationales
Administer stool softeners, avoid use of restraints and prevent or reduce crying episodes	Prevents Valsalva's maneuver which will increase ICP
Position with head elevated up to 30 and maintain head alignment with sand-bag	Decreases intracranial pressure by allowing blood flow from brain by gravity or any obstruction of jugular drainage
Stay with infant/child and sit near and speak in a low voice	Provides limited stimulation to infant/child during acute stage of disease

Information, Instruction, Demonstration

Interventions	Rationales
Inform parent(s) of changes in condition, reasons for physical and mental changes and effects of the disease	Promotes knowledge about possible manifestations of the disease and causes
Explain causes of increased ICP and importance of preventing any further increases in ICP	Allows for understanding of increased ICP and life-threatening nature of such a complication
Inform of reason for seizure activity and other signs and symptoms of the disease and treatment necessitated by them	Provides knowledge of seizure complications and actions and responsibility in prevention and or treatment of this activity
Inform parent(s) of risk for complications and need for monitoring for increased ICP; review signs and symptoms of increased ICP	Allows for ongoing care and responsibility in preventing change in neurologic status

Discharge or Maintenance Evaluation

- Verbalizes signs and symptoms of complications to report
- Absence of complications associated with the disease
- Resolution of the disease with minimal or no long-term effects
- Monitors neurologic status for changes or deviations from baselines
- Maintains safe environment for resolution of disease and convalescent

Knowledge deficit of parent(s), caretaker

Related to: Lack of exposure to information
Defining characteristics: Request for information about medications, signs and symptoms and behaviors to report, general care during convalescence of infant/child

Outcome Criteria

Adequate knowledge for safe and compliant administration of medication regimen and developmental needs of infant/child, adequate knowledge of potential risk for changes that require physician attention and intervention

Interventions	Rationales
Assess knowledge of disease and method to control and resolve disease; willingness and interest of parent(s) to implement care	Promotes plan of instruction that is realistic to ensure compliance of medical regimen; prevents repetition of information
Provide information and explanations in clear language that is understandable; use pictures, pamphlets, video tapes, model in teaching about disease	Ensures understanding based on readiness and ability to learn; visual aids reinforce learning
Instruct in administration of medications including action of drugs, dosages times frequency, side effects, expected results, methods to give medications; provide written instructions and schedule to follow and inform to administer full course of antibiotic to child	Provides information for compliance in medication therapy to prevent or treat infection and seizure activity resulting from the disease; bacterial meningitis is treated with antibiotics, and viral meningitis may be treated with antibiotics until diagnosis is established
Instruct and assist to plan feedings and/or develop menus to include nourishing fluids, caloric and basic four groups for age group	Promotes optimal nutrition in a progressive manner as tolerable
Instruct parents regarding importance of follow up to assess for potential hearing impairment	Promotes identification of hearing loss (injury to 8th cranial nerve due to meningitis)
Inform parents as to the benefits of routine immunizations with H.	May prevent the disease; data suggests the incidence of this form of meningitis

Interventions	Rationales
Influenzae type B vaccine, beginning at 2 months of age for a total of 3 doses	has decreased since the vaccine was introduced; may decrease the spread of infection to unvaccinated infants
Inform of importance of adequate rest and activities that provide age appropriate play and stimulation	Rest important for convalescence and stimulating activities needed for continued development or to promote stimulation if developmental lag is present
Inform to isolate other children in family for 24 hours if respiratory infection present or until culture is negative	Prevents transmission of bacteria to others in family
Inform to report elevated temperature, poor feeding or anorexia, irritability or other changes in behavior or level of consciousness, decrease in hearing acuity	Reveals signs and symptoms of presence of or spread of infection

Discharge or Maintenance Evaluation

- Statements of knowledge of medication regimen, dietary and activity requirements of infant/child
- Appropriate precautions taken to prevent spread or recurrence of infection
- Performs developmental activities related to the age and needs of the infant/child — statement of signs and symptoms to report to physician
- Adaptation to appropriate care during convalescence within prescribed requirements and limitations
- Maintains follow-up visits to physician as scheduled
- Appropriate growth and development advances for age group

Meningitis

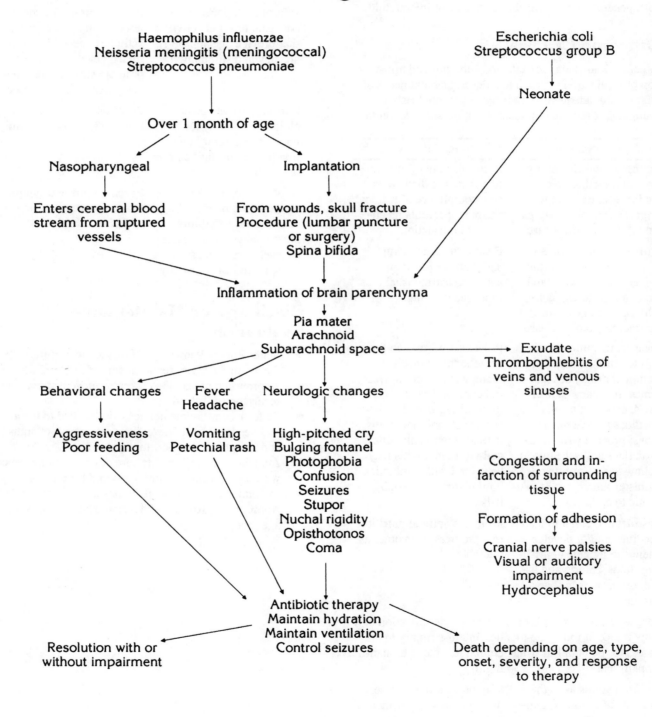

Haemophilus influenzae
Neisseria meningitis (meningococcal)
Streptococcus pneumoniae

Escherichia coli
Streptococcus group B

Neonate

Over 1 month of age

Nasopharyngeal

Implantation

Enters cerebral blood
stream from ruptured
vessels

From wounds, skull fracture
Procedure (lumbar puncture
or surgery)
Spina bifida

Inflammation of brain parenchyma

Pia mater
Arachnoid
Subarachnoid space

Exudate
Thrombophlebitis of
veins and venous
sinuses

Behavioral changes

Fever
Headache

Neurologic changes

Aggressiveness
Poor feeding

Vomiting
Petechial rash

High-pitched cry
Bulging fontanel
Photophobia
Confusion
Seizures
Stupor
Nuchal rigidity
Opisthotonos
Coma

Congestion and in-
farction of surrounding
tissue

Formation of adhesion

Cranial nerve palsies
Visual or auditory
impairment
Hydrocephalus

Antibiotic therapy
Maintain hydration
Maintain ventilation
Control seizures

Resolution with or
without impairment

Death depending on age, type,
onset, severity, and response
to therapy

Neurosensory Deficits

Sensory deficits or impairments lead to auditory and/or visual deprivation that place a child at risk for cognitive, perceptive, communication and socialization development skills that affect the way he or she relates to his or her environment and result in disability and disadvantage in achieving long-term goals. Vision disorders are common in children with the most prevalent problems of a refractive type (myopia or hyperopia) and others that include amblyopia, strabismus, cataracts and glaucoma. Trauma from injury with balls or sticks, use of contact lenses or improper eye care may result in conjunctivitis, keratitis or loss of an eye that may result in visual loss or even blindness. Auditory disorders are classified as conductive, sensorineural or mixed conductive-sensorineural hearing loss. Causes include damage to the inner ear structures or the auditory nerve from congenital defects, infection, ototoxic drugs, long-term excessive exposure to noises (sensorineural) or middle ear infection such as otitis media (conductive). Hearing and vision screening vary with the age of the infant/child and is performed as part of physical assessment of all children. Treatment focuses on the correction and rehabilitation of any actual or potential impairment.

MEDICAL CARE

Anti-inflammatories: prednisolone sodium phosphate (Inflamase) given TOP to eye to reduce inflammation if present.

Antibiotics: bacitracin (Bacitracin Ophthalmic) given TOP to treat infection by interfering with bacterial cell wall synthesis.

Vision tests: Lighthouse Vision test or Blackbird Preschool Vision Test for children 3-4 years of age; Snellen E vision chart for children 5-6 years of age; Snellen vision chart for children 7 years and older who are familiar with the alphabet; Corneal Light Reflex test and Cover/Uncover test to reveal malalignment; visual tracking to identify muscle movement abnormalities; tests for peripheral vision and amblyopia reveals objection to cover over eye or inability to see at a 90 degree angle from straight line of vision.

Hearing tests: audiometry reveals degree of hearing loss and possible locale of defect in child 2-5 years of age based on behavior modification and over 5 years if child is able to cooperate; reaction to noise in infant; conductive tests (Rinne and Weber) in children of school-age reveals auditory acuity; tympanometry reveals middle ear air pressure and abnormalities but not reliable in young children; brain stem-evoked audiometry reveals hearing acuity in the infant or child by computer analysis of electrical or brain wave potentials that are initiated by the hearing process.

NURSING CARE PLANS

Essential nursing diagnoses and plans associated with these conditions:

Altered growth and development (419)

Related to: Effects of physical disability
Defining characteristics: Delay or difficulty in performing skills (motor, social, expressive) typical of age group, behavior and/or intellectual deficits, poor academic performance, reduced independence in performance of ADL

SPECIFIC DIAGNOSES AND CARE PLANS

Sensory/perceptual alteration: Auditory

Related to: Altered sensory reception, transmission and/or integration of neurologic disease or deficit, altered state of sense organ, inability to hear (partial or complete deafness)
Defining characteristics: Change in behavior pattern, anxiety, change in usual response to stimuli, altered communication pattern, auditory distortions, reduced auditory acuity, inappropriate responses

Outcome Criteria

Effects of auditory impairment controlled
Facilitation and maximization of auditory function

Interventions	Rationales
Assess history of chronic otitis media, brain infection, use of ototoxic drugs, rubella or other intra-uterine infections (viral), congenital defects of ear or nose, presence of deafness	Provides information about possible risks for conductive or sensorineural hearing loss

Interventions	Rationales
in family members, hypoxemia and increased bilirubin levels in low birth weight infants	
Assess for auditory acuity: • Infant: failure to waken to sounds; no response to loud noise; no response to sound made out of visual field; lack of startle and blink reflexes; failure to turn head to localize sound by 6 months; absence of babble by 7 months; lack of response to spoken words/failure to follow simple commands (older infant) • Child: failure to respond to name or to locate sound; failure to respond to being read to or to sound of music; failure to respond to verbal speech; requesting repeat of message; gesturing instead of speech; shy, timid, inattentive; poor performance in school; failure to develop understandable language by 24 months; vocal play, head banging for increased vibratory sensation; stubborn attitude related to decreased comprehension; appear to be "in their own world"	Provides information of infant/child ability to hear using techniques that are age dependent
Perform audiometry or other tests depending on age and preparation of technician	Evaluates degree of hearing acuity and/or loss and type of hearing loss
Face infant/child when speaking, speak distinctly and slowly without shouting to gain child's attention	Provides opportunity to develop lip reading

Interventions	Rationales
Assist with use of hearing aid	Promotes maximum benefit from aid
Encourage use of sign language, lip reading, cued speech, speech therapy and as much verbal communication as possible	Promotes communication with others
Provide for play and social interactions, self-care in all activities for age group, continued attendance at school	Promotes independence for age group and security in interacting with peers
Anticipate grief reaction after the diagnosis; facilitate expression of feelings and concerns	Grief reaction is normal part of early adjustment phase; promotes adjustment to diagnosis
Help child focus on sounds in the environment	Maximizes child's hearing potential
Recommend closed-captioned TV	Provides enjoyment for the child; facilitates feelings of normalcy
Encourage child to read books and practice responding to cues with language development or use of aids or methods	Promotes effective communication and corrects or prevents impairments
Encourage child to take responsibility for the care and use of the aid as soon as possible	Promotes independence and self esteem

Information, Instruction, Demonstration

Interventions	Rationales
Instruct parent(s) and child in type of tests to be performed and procedure to be followed by child	Prevents anxiety caused by test and possible results if not done as part of normal child assessment and screening
Inform parent(s) of behavioral cues indicating hearing impairment	Promotes identification of hearing loss for correction before development is affected
Inform parent(s) of hearing aid resources, types available and instruct in clean-	Assists with hearing aid selection if loss is conductive type

Interventions	Rationales
ing and care of aid and the proper adjustment for optimal benefit	
Instruct child in methods to conceal hearing aid	Prevents negative effect of self-concept and image
Inform parent(s) and child of resources to learn lip reading or signing or speaking	Promotes a method of communication with others and especially those with hearing impairment
Instruct parent(s) and family to provide stimulation through language	Promotes developmental process and language use
Refer to appropriate community resources and support groups, as needed	Provides support to parents
Inform parents of the importance of socialization with peers; promote these relationships when possible	Promotes feelings of normalcy and self-esteem
Inform parents of the importance of vision testing	Poor sight may decrease the ability to learn lip reading or sign language
Discuss with the family the importance of maintaining normalcy, including discipline and limit setting	Promotes normal growth and development
Inform parent(s) and child to adjust environment and select toys that promote social interactions and increase hearing potential	Encourages social interactions, development of friendships and sense of belonging
Inform parent(s) to notify school nurse and teacher of degree of hearing loss and methods of communications use by child	Provides information that encourages a positive school experience and opportunity for learning in a regular classroom and socialization with classmates

Discharge or Maintenance Evaluation

- Optimizes auditory acuity
- Uses assistive aid to maximize hearing (hearing aid)
- Learns lip reading and/or signing and use for communication

- Corrects any language or speech impairment for optimal effect
- Maintains independence in learning and activities
- Maintains and/or progress in developmental tasks
- Participates in play and other social interactions with others
- Attends school regularly
- Adapts to hearing loss
- Utilizes any helpful devices or signaling aids
- Participates in formal rehabilitation program or home training program
- Contact national associations for information and assistance for hearing aids, signing, lip reading, rehabilitation programs

Sensory/perceptual alteration: Visual

Related to: Altered sensory reception, transmission and/or integration of neurologic disease or deficit, altered state of sense organ, inability to see (partial or complete loss of sight)

Defining characteristics: Change in behavior pattern, anxiety, change in usual responses to stimuli, visual distortions, reduced visual acuity, myopia, hyperopia, lazy eye, cross-eye, cataracts, glaucoma, trauma to eye, frequent injury by walking into objects

Outcome Criteria

Effects of sensory deficit controlled
Facilitation and maximization of visual function

Interventions	Rationales
Assess history of rubella or syphilis of mother before birth of child, presence of genetic disorders in the family, excessive oxygen given to infant, congenital conditions that cause blindness, impairment caused by strabismus, cataract or glaucoma	Provides information about risks for or presence of sight impairment or blindness
Assess for risk of trauma to an eye from toys, missiles or projectiles into eye during games or play, excessive sunlight to eyes	Eye trauma caused by accidents is most common cause of blindness in children and information provides safety education plan to prevent eye injury

Interventions	Rationales
Assess for visual acuity: • Infant: failure to follow light or object with eye movement and cessation of body movement; failure to fixate on mother's face; delay in posture and in developmental tasks; absence of binocularity; failure to move eyes together • Child: failure to respond to visual stimuli; squinting, blinking, rubbing of eyes; eye crossing after 6 months of age; headache after using eyes; failure to initiate eye contact, nystagmus, head tilt, holding reading material close to face, bumps into objects when walking or crawling; poor performance in school	Provides information of infant/child ability to see using techniques that are age dependent
Perform visual tests for acuity peripheral vision and muscle balance depending on age and intellectual development level; include tests for strabismus, amblyopia	Evaluates degree of acuity and/or loss and possible causes with consideration for improving visual acuity with age
Face infant/child when speaking, explain sounds and what is happening in the environment	Promotes comfort and security with environment
State name when approaching and explain any procedure before starting, use touch if acceptable	Reduces anxiety and sudden contact that is unexpected
Assist with use and care of glasses or patching one eye and encourage wearing of these as prescribed	Promotes independence in use of aids for refractive disorders and strabismus
Provide for age related toys and social interactions within secure environment	Promotes stimulation and development

Interventions	Rationales
Provide well lit environment and familiar placement of objects to orient child to environment	Promotes safety and security in the environment and prevent possible trauma from bumping into furniture or falling
Emphasize the abilities and praise attempts and/or accomplishments	Promotes self-esteem of child
Talk softly to infant before contact; learn to read total body cues, not just eyes and visual cues; use gentleness of touch when interacting with infant	Promotes association of human voice with anticipated changes; prepares infant for changes
Tell the child exactly what you will be doing before you do anything; reinforce this as you perform the procedure; warn of discomfort	Promotes understanding and feelings of security and trust
Allow the child to touch instruments and equipment whenever possible	Promotes increased understanding through speech
Use the child's name specifically when you want a response from him/her	Promotes communication since visually impaired children lack the input of visual cues

Information, Instruction, Demonstration

Interventions	Rationales
Instruct parent(s) and child of type of tests to be performed, what is being tested and procedure to be followed by child	Prevents anxiety and promotes cooperation
Inform parent(s) of child's abilities and impairment and what might be expected of child; behaviors that might indicate a decrease in visual acuity	Provides a realistic appraisal of visual ability of the child
Inform parent(s) to explore the possibility of rehabilitation to accomplish ADL skills, use of Braille, mobility aids, trained dogs	Provides assistance to gain independence for the child

Interventions	Rationales
Inform parent(s) to treat child as others in family, setting limits, encouraging play and relationships with family members	Promotes integration into the family and creates a sense of belonging
Instruct in eye care, administration of eye medications	Promotes health of eye and compliance with medical regimen
Emphasize the importance of wearing glasses or eye patch; attach a strap that fits around head to hold in place	Enhances visual acuity or corrects eye problem
Inform parent(s) to notify school of sight deficit and to place in a front row, use large printed materials, proper lighting	Encourages learning with optimal consideration for impairment
Instruct parent(s) of need for regular vision screening	Monitors visual acuity for improvements or need for change in treatment; screening is often done in schools
Initiate and inform parent(s) of a referral to an ophthalmologist for evaluation if acuity is not normal for age or if indication of a disorder is present	Permits thorough examination of eyes to identify and treat any disorder
Inform of national and community agencies and associations that supply educational materials, services for blind or partially sighted children	Provides information and support for families of child with impaired vision

- Absences of injury to eye, removal of hazards in the environment
- Complies with visual testing schedule
- Participates in rehabilitation or special programs for child
- Contacts agencies for information and assistance for books, records, tapes, visual aids

Discharge or Maintenance Evaluation

- Provides and functions in safe environment
- Optimizes visual acuity
- Uses assistive aids to maximize vision, development and independence
- Maintains and/or progress in developmental tasks
- Attends school regularly
- Adapts to visual loss and maintains activities, play and social interactions
- Administers ophthalmic medications correctly

Neurosensory Deficits

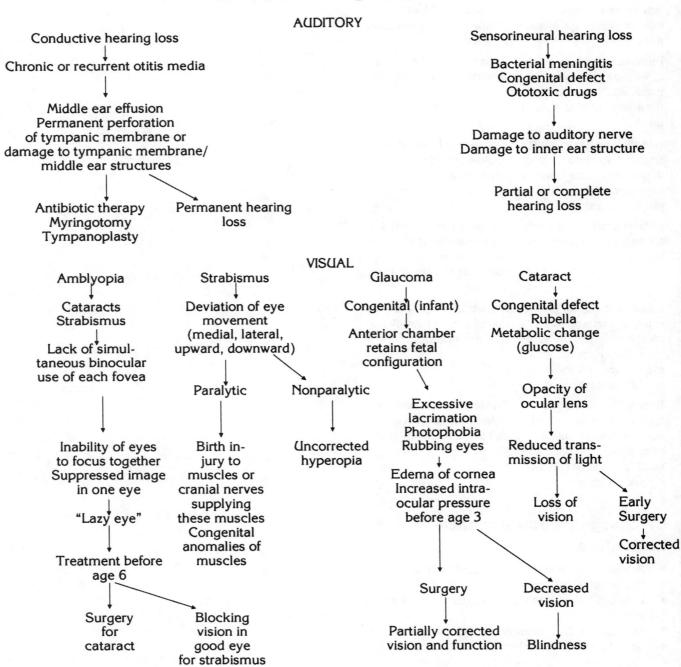

AUDITORY

Conductive hearing loss
↓
Chronic or recurrent otitis media
↓
Middle ear effusion
Permanent perforation
of tympanic membrane or
damage to tympanic membrane/
middle ear structures
↓
Antibiotic therapy   Permanent hearing
Myringotomy   loss
Tympanoplasty

Sensorineural hearing loss
↓
Bacterial meningitis
Congenital defect
Ototoxic drugs
↓
Damage to auditory nerve
Damage to inner ear structure
↓
Partial or complete
hearing loss

VISUAL

Amblyopia
↓
Cataracts
Strabismus
↓
Lack of simul-
taneous binocular
use of each fovea
↓
Inability of eyes
to focus together
Suppressed image
in one eye
↓
"Lazy eye"
↓
Treatment before
age 6
↓
Surgery   Blocking
for   vision in
cataract   good eye
                 for strabismus

Strabismus
↓
Deviation of eye
movement
(medial, lateral,
upward, downward)
↓
Paralytic   Nonparalytic
↓   ↓
Birth in-   Uncorrected
jury to   hyperopia
muscles or
cranial nerves
supplying
these muscles
Congenital
anomalies of
muscles

Glaucoma
↓
Congenital (infant)
↓
Anterior chamber
retains fetal
configuration
↓
Excessive
lacrimation
Photophobia
Rubbing eyes
↓
Edema of cornea
Increased intra-
ocular pressure
before age 3
↓
Surgery   Decreased
↓   vision
Partially corrected   ↓
vision and function   Blindness

Cataract
↓
Congenital defect
Rubella
Metabolic change
(glucose)
↓
Opacity of
ocular lens
↓
Reduced trans-
mission of light
↓
Loss of   Early
vision   Surgery
                 ↓
                 Corrected
                 vision

Reye's Syndrome

Reye's syndrome is an acute encephalopathy, often including fatty infiltration of organs such as the liver, heart, lungs, pancreas and skeletal muscle. It has been associated with a viral condition such as influenza or varicella and the use of aspirin as an analgesic/antipyretic, but the exact cause is not known. Serious complications of the disorder can include increased intracranial pressure from cerebral edema, high levels of ammonia from organ involvement and mental dysfunction from progressive coma. Recovery is complete in most depending on severity of the condition but some neurologic and mental residual disability may occur. The most common group affected by this condition are those between 6-11 years of age although all ages are susceptible. Hospitalization with close observation is required with therapy to monitor and treat all vital functions affected by the condition and state of consciousness.

MEDICAL CARE

Sedatives/anticonvulsants: phenobarbital (Luminal, Luminal Sodium) given PO or IV to promote CNS depression for sedation or to prevent or treat seizures.
Muscle relaxants: pancuronium bromide (Pavulon) given IV as a neuromuscular blocking agent to induce sedation and relax muscles if mechanical assistive ventilation used.
Diuretics (osmotic): mannitol (Osmitrol) given IV to induce diuresis by increasing osmotic pressure of glomerular filtrate to prevent reabsorption of water.
Antibiotics: neomycin sulfate (Mycifradin) given PO to treat infection if present or specific antibiotic dependent on culture and sensitivities.
Vitamins: phytonadione (Vitamin K) given IM or SC to assist with hepatic biosynthesis of clotting factors in presence of liver dysfunction.
Anti-inflammatories: dexamethasone (Decadron) given PO to reduce inflammatory process, capillary dilation and permeability.
Antacids: magaldrate (Riopan) given PO via nasogastric tube to maintain pH of over 4.0 to prevent gastrointestinal bleeding.
Liver biopsy: reveals histologic results of impaired liver or pathology.
Lumbar puncture: reveals infection (meningitis) if present for disease differentiation.

Enzymes: reveals increased glutamic oxaloacetic transaminase (SGOT), glutamic pyruvic transaminase (SGPT), lactic dehydrogenase (LDH), creatine phosphokinase (CPK), amylase and lipase.
Ammonia: reveals increases of twice the normal level (hyperammonimia).
Glucose: reveals decreases with this disease (hypoglycemia) which may lead to brain damage.
Prothrombin/Partial thromboplastin times (PT, APPT): reveals prolonged times.
Cholesterol: reveals decreased level.
Uric acid: reveals increased level.
Arterial blood gases (ABGs): reveals levels that may indicate possible increases in cerebral edema or respiratory distress.

NURSING CARE PLANS

Essential nursing diagnoses and plans associated with this condition:

Decreased cardiac output (3)

Related to: Mechanical or electrical effect on the heart
Defining characteristics: Variations in hemodynamic readings, ECG changes, arrhythmias, decreased peripheral pulses, oliguria, diuretic therapy, changes in perfusion of vital organs

Impaired gas exchange (47)

Related to: Assistive ventilatory use and oxygen supply
Defining characteristics: Hypercapnia, hypoxia, confusion, restlessness, irritability, inability to move secretions, cyanosis, retractions, changes in ABGs

Altered thought processes (116)

Related to: Physiological changes, encephalopathy
Defining characteristics: Cognitive dissonance, disorientation, changes in consciousness, hallucination, altered sleep patterns, coma, altered attention span and memory, lethargy, drowsiness

Hyperthermia (112)

Related to: Illness
Defining characteristics: Increase in body temperature above normal range, increased respiratory and pulse rate, warm to touch

Risk for fluid volume deficit (222)

Related to: Medications
Defining characteristics: Diuretic therapy, altered intake, NPO status, increased urinary output, loss via nasogastric tube suctioning

Risk for impaired skin integrity (397)

Related to: External factor of physical immobilization, hypothermia blanket, invasive procedures
Defining characteristics: Disruption of skin surfaces, redness, edema, discharge, warmth at insertion sites for IV, monitoring devices, redness or excoriation at pressure points

SPECIFIC DIAGNOSES AND CARE PLANS

Anxiety

Related to: Threat of death; change in health status; change in environment (hospitalization)
Defining characteristics: Apprehension and uncertainty about child's condition, feelings of inadequacy and increased helplessness about child cared for in intensive care unit, fear associated with severe acuity of condition, possible sequelae as a result of the disorder

Outcome Criteria

Reduced anxiety verbalized as understanding of condition and treatments is increased
Acceptance of emotional support to assist in management of anxiety

Interventions	Rationales
Assess level of anxiety, need for information and support about severity and life threatening nature of the illness	Provides information about severity of stress and anxiety, guilt about responsibility of delay in diagnosis and loss of parental role, fears and feelings about possible complications
Allow expression of concerns and opportunity to ask questions about condition and recovery of child	Provides opportunity to vent feelings, secure information needed to reduce anxiety

Interventions	Rationales
Encourage parent(s) to remain with child and participate in care if appropriate; if parent(s) unable to stay, allow open visitation and frequent telephoning	Promotes parent involvement and interaction with the child
Encourage parent(s) to bring a favorite toy, book or other items	Promotes contact with familiar objects outside the hospital environment
Provide for space to rest, bathe and relax if staying with child; provide quiet room if desired	Promotes emotional support to parent(s) to reduce anxiety
Refer to clergy or social services as appropriate	Provides support and assistance in dealing with severely ill child

Information, Instruction, Demonstration

Interventions	Rationales
Explain reason for and what to expect for each procedure or type of therapy (lumbar puncture, IV lines, urinary catheter, N/G tube, respirator)	Reduces fear and promotes understanding
Provide honest information in understandable language and reinforce physician	Prevents unnecessary anxiety resulting from inaccurate information or beliefs
Inform parent(s) of state of consciousness of child, stage of disease and signs and symptoms to expect	Reduces fear and anxiety

Discharge or Maintenance Evaluation

- Expression of reduction in anxiety about condition, therapy and need for care in intensive care unit
- Participates in care of child when possible
- Maintains emotional stability with utilization of support system
- Supports and contributes to decisions regarding care of child

Risk for injury

Related to: Internal factors of regulatory function, abnormal blood profile

Defining characteristics: Altered clotting factors, changes in orientation and consciousness, increased ICP, altered sleep pattern, cognitive dissonance, inability to close or blink eyes, hypoglycemic seizure activity, coma

Outcome Criteria

Maintenance and stability of neurologic status in each stage of disease
Prevention of effects of complications of the disorder

Interventions	Rationales
Assess for stage by noting signs and symptoms associated with the condition which range from vomiting and lethargy and liver dysfunction to disorientation, deepening coma, loss of reflexes and seizures	Indicate stage as a basis for expected behaviors and need for specific care and preventative measures
Assess vomiting, papilledema, ataxia, irritability, lethargy, apathy, confusion, change in level of consciousness, increased pulse and decreased BP q1h; if ICP monitor in place, note elevation above 20 mm Hg or any gradual increases for physician	Indicates increasing ICP caused by cerebral edema and advancing stage of disease
Elevate head of bed 30 degrees and maintain head and neck alignment	Promotes cerebral circulation and reduces venous pressure; prevents neck flexion
Administer osmotic diuretic, diretic, sedative, anti-convulsants, neuromuscular blocking agent IV separately or in combination as ordered	Administered to promote fluid output to reduce edema, prevent seizure activity and induce sedation to reduce agitation and activity which increases ICP
Provide spacing of care and procedures	Decreases stimuli which increases ICP
Carry out seizure precautions of padding bed, removing objects from bed, maintain suction and oxygen at bedside	Prevents injury during seizure and treats apnea if it occurs

Interventions	Rationales
Monitor laboratory tests of increased prothrombin or partial thrombin time, fibrin split products, decreased platelets and serum glucose, decreased electrolyte levels (K)	Provides information about coagulation defects from liver dysfunction, hypoglycemia metabolic dysfunction and loss of electrolytes from diuretic therapy
Monitor for occult blood in stool, gastric aspirate, skin for petechiae, hematoma, oozing or frank bleeding from any orifice or mucous membranes	Provides information about possible bleeding from impaired liver function
Administer antacid, vitamin K and/or blood as ordered	Replaces blood loss and increases blood clotting capabilities; antacids are given to discourage gastrointestinal irritation and bleeding
Instill eye drops (methylcellulose) or tape eyelids closed if paralyzed	Provides moisture to eyes if unable to blink or close eyes to prevent corneal damage

Information, Instruction, Demonstration

Interventions	Rationales
Inform parent(s) of every aspect of care and equipment used including comatosed status, effects of medications, IV therapy, N/G tube care, use of catheter, use of monitoring devices (ICP, cardiac, CVP), intubation and ventilation	Assist parent(s) to deal with their child that is acutely ill
Inform parent(s) that mild stimulation is allowed and that speaking and touching child is permitted	Provides stimulation as child may be able to perceive tactile and auditory stimuli when unresponsive
Inform parent(s) that child will be reoriented to person, time and place when awakened from the coma	He or she may not be aware of the environment and realize that he or she has been hospitalized
Inform parent(s) that child will be moved to room on the regular unit as soon as condition warrants	Increases comfort as having child in intensive care unit is traumatic to both child and parent(s)

Interventions	Rationales
Instruct parent(s) in reading labels for aspirin (salicylate) content and to avoid using these drugs (e.g., Pepto-Bismol) when child is ill	Promotes prevention of syndrome as aspirin considered to be a causative factor
Inform parent(s) that deficits usually improve and resolve in 6-12 months during recovery and evaluation and rehabilitation may be needed	Provides guidance as to what to expect as child progresses to wellness

Discharge or Maintenance Evaluation

- Identification of signs and symptoms associated with specific stages of the disease
- Maintains stable neurologic, liver and metabolic function
- Monitors blood and urine tests related to organ function
- Administers medications PO or IV accurately and safely
- Performs care and monitoring procedures for comatose child
- Absence of increased ICP, seizures, bleeding, eye injury, cardiac or respiratory complications
- Parent(s) participate in care and support of child
- Complies with follow-up care and rehabilitation if needed
- Parents agree to give children acetaminophen for fever instead of aspirin

Reye's Syndrome

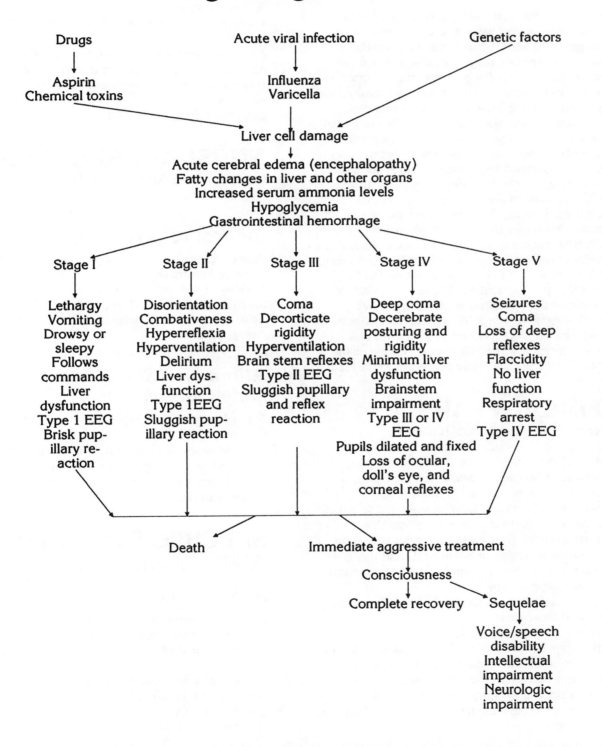

Drugs → Aspirin / Chemical toxins

Acute viral infection → Influenza / Varicella

Genetic factors

Liver cell damage

Acute cerebral edema (encephalopathy)
Fatty changes in liver and other organs
Increased serum ammonia levels
Hypoglycemia
Gastrointestinal hemorrhage

Stage I
Lethargy
Vomiting
Drowsy or
sleepy
Follows
commands
Liver
dysfunction
Type 1 EEG
Brisk pup-
illary re-
action

Stage II
Disorientation
Combativeness
Hyperreflexia
Hyperventilation
Delirium
Liver dys-
function
Type 1 EEG
Sluggish pup-
illary reaction

Stage III
Coma
Decorticate
rigidity
Hyperventilation
Brain stem reflexes
Type II EEG
Sluggish pupillary
and reflex
reaction

Stage IV
Deep coma
Decerebrate
posturing and
rigidity
Minimum liver
dysfunction
Brainstem
impairment
Type III or IV
EEG
Pupils dilated and fixed
Loss of ocular,
doll's eye, and
corneal reflexes

Stage V
Seizures
Coma
Loss of deep
reflexes
Flaccidity
No liver
function
Respiratory
arrest
Type IV EEG

Death

Immediate aggressive treatment

Consciousness

Complete recovery

Sequelae

Voice/speech
disability
Intellectual
impairment
Neurologic
impairment

Seizure Disorders

A seizure is a central nervous system (CNS) condition characterized by an excessive level of neuronal electrical discharges in the brain. Seizures may be idiopathic or chronic and recurrent (epilepsy or acute acquired and nonrecurrent). Seizures can be partial or generalized with signs and symptoms dependent on the areas involved and ranging from varying degrees of motor, sensory and sensorimotor changes and altered consciousness. Partial seizures may be classified as partial or complex partial and generalized seizures as tonic-clonic, absence, atonic or akinetic, myoclonic and infantile spasms. Seizures occur at any age in children with epilepsy, mostly occurring in children over 3 years of age. Infantile spasms occur in infants between 3-9 months of age. Treatment focuses on prevention of subsequent seizure activity with medication regimen or surgical removal of a focal lesion, tumor or hemorrhage. Febrile seizures occur in children between 3 months and 5 months and the younger the age of the first episode, the more likely of recurrence. Status epilepticus is characterized by a seizure lasting more than 30 minutes or repeated seizures without regaining consciousness and is viewed as a medical emergency with a prognosis dependent on the length of the seizure activity and the effect on the brain.

MEDICAL PLANS

Anticonvulsants: phenobarbital (Luminal), carbamazepine (Tegretol), phenytoin (Dilantin), primidone (Mysoline), Valproic Acid (Depakene), ethosuximide (Zarotine), Clonazepam (Klonopin), clorazepate (Tranxene) given PO singly or in combination to decrease or limit impulses and spread of electrical discharges in the brain. Diazepam (Valium), lorazepam (Ativan) given IV to treat status epilepticus.
Amphetamines: dextroamphetamine (Dexadrine) given PO to stimulate CNS and counteract drowsiness caused by anticonvulsant therapy.
Diuretics: acetazolamide (Diamox) given PO as adjunct to remove fluid by diuresis.
Electroencephalogram (EEG): reveals abnormal electrical impulses to the brain in initial stage of seizure and characteristic patterns identifying type of seizure.
Skull x-rays: reveals head trauma if present.
Computerized tomography scan (CT): reveals abnormalities such as brain tumor, trauma or infection as causes of seizure.

Ultrasound: reveals intraventricular hemorrhage if present as cause of seizure.
Brain scan: reveals abnormality as source of seizure if present.
Lumbar puncture: reveals abnormality in cerebrospinal fluid caused by bleeding trauma or infection responsible for seizure activity.
Complete blood count: reveals increased WBC if infection present.
Electrolyte panel: reveals abnormal levels of calcium or phosphorus as cause of seizure if levels decreased.
Blood glucose: reveals metabolic cause for seizure if decreased.
Lead level: reveals increased level as cause of seizure.

NURSING CARE PLANS

Essential nursing diagnoses and plans associated with this condition:

Ineffective breathing pattern (45)

Related to: Neuromuscular impairment, perception or cognitive impairment
Defining characteristics: Dyspnea, tachypnea, changes in respiratory depth, cyanosis, cessation of breathing in status epilepticus, obstruction of airway by secretions during a seizure

Altered nutrition: Less than body requirements (168)

Related to: Inability to ingest food because of rejection of diet
Defining characteristics: Weight under ideal for height and frame, poor eating patterns, anorexia, rejection of decrease in protein and carbohydrate and increase of fat in dietary intake

SPECIFIC DIAGNOSES AND CARE PLANS

Risk for injury

Related to: Internal factors of biochemical regulatory function (seizure, tissue hypoxia), physical trauma (broken skin, altered mobility), psychological changes (orientation)
Defining characteristics: Seizure activity with change in consciousness, falls, muscle flaccidity or rigidity, aspiration of secretions, cyanosis, change in sensation in a body part, muscle weakness, presence of aura before seizure

Outcome Criteria

Resolution of seizure without physical injury or complication

Interventions	Rationales
Assess seizure activity including type of activity before, during and after seizure, movements and parts of body involved (tonic and clonic), site of onset and progression of seizure, duration of seizure, pupillary changes, bowel or bladder incontinence, paralysis, sleep or alertness or confusion after seizure, presence of aura	Provides information that prepares environment for prevention of trauma or complications as a result of seizure
Assess skin for color (pallor, flushed or cyanosis), respiratory rate, depth and ease for signs of distress; have oxygen, suctioning equipment on hand	Provides information about possible obstruction or aspiration of secretions if seizures are prolonged and affect ventilation
Maintain sidelying position with side-rails up, bed or crib padded and articles removed from area near child	Allows for secretions to drain and maintains airway patency; padding protects child from injury during seizure
Avoid attempts to restrain any movements or putting anything in child's mouth; provide gentle support to head and arms if harm might result	Restraint may result in fracture and inserting object in mouth increases stimuli
Loosen clothing, assist child to floor if not in bed and place pad under head	Prevents injury from fall
Stay with child during seizure, reorient when awake and allow to rest or sleep after seizure	Provides support and prevents any injury to child
Administer and evaluate anticonvulsants obtaining blood levels as ordered	Prevents subsequent seizures as medications are most effective in prevention of seizures

Information, Instruction, Demonstration

Interventions	Rationales
Inform parent(s) to remain calm during seizure activity of child	Allows parent(s) to function appropriately to protect the child from injury
Instruct in information to record about seizure activity should it occur	Provides physician with important information needed to prescribe medical regimen
Instruct parent(s) in care of child during seizure and precautions to take	Ensures safe and effective actions to prevent injury
Inform parent(s) and child of importance of compliance of medication regimen	Provides information about importance of compliance as use of anticonvulsants are best preventative therapy

Discharge or Maintenance Evaluation

- Verbalizations of understanding of condition and preventative measures to take to comply with medical regimen
- Supports child during seizure with calm, effective actions
- Prevents any injury caused by seizure activity
- Acts to maintain respiratory function and ventilation
- Records and reports seizure activity to physician

Ineffective family coping: Compromised

Related to: Situational crisis faced by the parent(s) and family members
Defining characteristics: Preoccupation of significant persons with anxiety, guilt, fear regarding child's disorder, display of protective behaviors by significant persons that are disproportionate to child's needs (too much or too little), recurrence of seizure activity, lack of support by family members to child
Related to: Inadequate or incorrect information or understanding by a primary person and/or significant persons
Defining characteristics: Verbalizations by significant persons of inadequate knowledge base that interferes with care and support of infant/child

Outcome Criteria

Development of family coping skills in dealing with infant/child's illness

Adaptation of family members to infant/child's disorder and stigma attached to this disorder

Interventions	Rationales
Assess anxiety, fear, erratic behavior, perception of crisis situation by family members	Provides information affecting family ability to cope with infant/child's recurring disorder
Assess coping methods used and effectiveness; family ability to cope with ill member of family, stress on family relationships, developmental level of family, response of siblings, knowledge and attitudes about disorder and health practices	Identifies coping methods that work and need to develop new coping skills; family attitudes and coping abilities directly affect child's health and feeling of wellness, members of family may develop emotional problems when stressed and ill member may strengthen or strain family relationships
Encourage expression of feelings and questions in accepting, non-judgmental environment and assist family members to express problems and explore solutions responsibly	Reduces anxiety and enhances family's understanding of infant/child's condition and provides opportunity to express feelings, problems and problem solving strategies by whole family
Encourage family involvement in care during hospitalization and after discharge	Provides for reduction of anxiety and fear
Allow for open visitation, encourage telephone calls to hospital by family members	Encourages bonding and assists in coping with infant/child's hospitalization
Provide place for family members to rest, freshen up	Promotes comfort of family
Suggest social worker referral if needed	Provides support and resources for financial or infant/child's care relief
Give positive feedback and praise family efforts in developing coping and problem solving techniques and caring for infant/child	Encourages parent(s) and family to participate in care and gain some control over the situation

Interventions	Rationales
Assist to establish short- and long-term goals in maintaining child care and family integration of child into home routing	Promotes inclusion of ill child in family routines and activities

Information, Instruction, Demonstration

Interventions	Rationales
Inform and reinforce appropriate coping behaviors	Promotes behavior change and adaptation to care of infant/child prone to seizures
Inform that overprotective behaviors may hinder growth and development	Knowledge will enhance family understanding of condition and adverse effects of behavior
Inform of need to maintain health of family members and discuss needs of all family members and inform of methods to provide care and attention to all members	Chronic anxiety, fatigue will affect health and care capabilities of family
Inform family of methods to maintain child's independence and role in the family	Ensures acceptance of child into family routines
Inform parent(s) that they do not pass this disorder directly onto their offspring, that intellectual functioning is not affected, that the child is not considered violent or insane, that the disorder is not contagious	Explodes the many myths associated with the disorder
Inform parent(s) that child should attend school and participate in activities with friends and peers	Normalizes life of child as much as possible
Instruct in ketogenic diet if prescribed	Provides a high fat diet that prevents development of ketones which is thought to increase seizure threshold

Interventions	Rationales
Inform parent(s) and child to wear or carry identification and treatment information	Provides information that may be needed in an emergency
Refer to Epilepsy Foundation	Provides information and support to family for chronic, long-term care

Discharge or Maintenance Evaluation

- Verbalizes and clarifies family and child's knowledge about seizures and emotional responses to disorder
- Supports child and participates in care by family members
- Verbalizes that improved coping skills practiced by family
- Verbalizes that adaptations and inclusion of child into family maintained
- Maintains positive and proper behaviors toward child without preferential treatment
- Maintains social responsibilities and health of family
- Secures genetic counseling if appropriate, services of social worker if needed
- Family relationships preserved and stressors minimized with differences resolved
- Maintains social and school activities of child
- Wears or carries identification information about condition

Knowledge deficit of parent(s), child

Related to: Lack of exposure to information about ongoing care

Defining characteristics: Expressed request for information about medication regimen, causes of seizures and when to report to physician

Outcome Criteria

Verbalizes accurate medication administration and importance of compliance, reasons why frequency of seizures may increase prevention or control of seizure activity

Interventions	Rationales
Assess parent(s) and child perceptions and knowledge about disorder, fears and misconceptions about disorder, nature and frequency of seizures and factors that initiate seizures	Provides information regarding long-term care of child with a seizure disorder and how to deal with seizures and the stigma attached to this disorder
Instruct in administration of anticonvulsants including name of drug(s), action of drug(s) and when given in combination, times, frequency, side effects, expected results, methods to give drugs and provide written instructions to follow related to age group and a schedule to follow; give at most convenient times with meals or at bedtime with as few disruptions in routines and activities as possible; give in tablets, liquid extracts, emulsions or crushed in syrup or jelly; avoid milk if giving phenytoin or phenobarbital and supplement vitamin D; replace prescription before running out of drug(s) and avoid skipping doses	Promotes compliance to drug regimen which is the most important treatment to prevent seizure
Instruct parent(s) and child to report lethargy, ataxia, nausea, vomiting, hyperactivity, blood dyscrasia, stomatitis, tremor, nystagmus	Indicates side effects of sedatives and anticonvulsants
Inform parent(s) of need to have blood testing for therapeutic levels, blood count, liver function tests when instructed	Prevents toxicity and other severe side effects of drug therapy by adjusting dosage or changing medication(s)
Inform that seizures may be provoked by omission of medication administration, an illness or infection, too much activity, lack of sleep, excessive alcohol or drug intake, emotional stress or other causes specific to child	Promotes knowledge and understanding of causes of increased frequency of seizures

Interventions	Rationales
Inform parent(s) to supervise child in bathroom, avoid dangerous play and toys, avoid exposure to incidents that trigger seizure, pad areas in bed or wear protective clothing if needed	Provides precautions to prevent injury as a result of a seizure
Inform parent(s) to notify school nurse and teacher of disorder and actions to take including telephone number to call	Promotes knowledge and understanding to prevent injury and embarrassment to child
Instruct and assist to plan menus for ketogenic diet to manage seizures	Increases seizure threshold
Inform of any activity restrictions such as sports, rough play, need for someone in attendance	Promotes knowledge of activity based on individual child and seizure activity and response to therapy
Alert parent(s) of possible changes in behavior, activity or personality or changes in school performance or interactions with family and peers	Indicates effects of anticonvulsants on behavior and learning
Inform parent(s) and child of resources offering assistance such as Epilepsy Foundation of America, community support groups	Provides educational materials, employment, legal services, support and counseling to families and children

Discharge or Maintenance Evaluation

- Statements of knowledge of disorder, causes of seizure activity
- Adaptation and compliance of parent(s) and child with medication regimen including all aspects of dosage and form, time and frequency, side effects
- Complies with recommended visits to physician and laboratory for ongoing care and testing
- Continues with activities and limits those that are to be avoided that may be harmful or initiate seizure
- Provides ketogenic diet and varies inclusions according to preference
- Reports signs and symptoms of medication side effects or changes in learning or behavior

- Obtains information and support from community agency, National Epilepsy Foundation of America
- Verbalizes understanding of need for long-term therapy and support for child to comply with medical regimen

Seizure Disorders

Recurrent seizure activity
↓
Epilepsy (idiopathic/secondary)
Migraine
Uremia
Allergies
Hypoglycemic disorders
Brain damage
Congenital anomalies
Phenylketonuria
Retarded psychomotor development

Nonrecurrent seizure activity
↓
Febrile episode
Tumor or edema
Toxins
Intracranial infection/
hemorrhage
Metabolic disorders

Spontaneous paroxysmal electrical
discharges from cortical centers

Neuronal excitation in centrencephalic
or focal area of the brain
↓
Partial seizure

Spread of neuronal excitation to
brain stem
↓
Generalized seizure

Simple
↓
Involves one
hemisphere
↓
Local motor move-
ment related to
involved area of
brain
Sensory
manifestations
related to involved area
of brain (numbness,
tingling, crawling
sensation, foul
taste in mouth)
Autonomic manifest-
ations (tachycardia,
diaphoresis, blood
pressure or pupillary
changes)
Unfamiliarity with
events or environment

Complex
↓
Involves both
hemispheres
↓
Loss of
consciousness
Hallucinations
Automatism
Unusual sensations

Infantile spasms
↓
Jackknife posture
Eyes roll upward
or downward
May have loss of
consciousness
Flush, pallor
or cyanosis
↓
Drowsiness or
sleep

Absence
↓
Brief loss
of contact
with envir-
onment
Blank stare
Unresponsive
Change in
postural tone
Lip smacking

Tonic-clonic
↓
Unconscious
Tonic con-
traction
of muscle
Rigidity
Falls to
ground
Incontinent
↓
Clonic
convulsive
movements
↓
Muscle
relaxation
Deep res-
pirations
Deep sleep

Spina Bifida

Spina bifida is a defect of the central nervous system involving the failure of neural tube closure during embryonic development. There are two types of spina bifida: spina bifida occults and spina bifida cystica. Spina bifida occults is a defect in the closure without the herniation and exposure of the spinal cord or meninges at the surface of the skin in the lumbosacral area. Spina bifida cystica (meningocele or myelomeningocele) is a defect in the closure with a sac and herniated protrusion of meninges, spinal fluid and some part of the spinal cord and nerves at the surface of the skin in the lumbosacral or sacral area. Hydrocephalus is often associated with spina bifida cystica. The neurologic effects are related to the anatomic level and nerves involved in the defect and range from varying degrees of sensory deficits, to partial or total motor impairment resulting in flaccidity, partial paralysis of lower extremities, and loss of bladder and bowel control. Children with spina bifida cystica, especially myelomeningocele, are commonly afflicted with orthopedic abnormalities that may include hip dislocation, spinal curvatures, clubfeet and may require assistive devices such as braces, special crutches or wheelchairs for mobility. Treatment includes surgical repair of defect as well as other anomalies depending on severity of the neurologic deficit and may be done during infancy or later. Other treatment focuses on prevention of complications, bowel and urinary management, and promotion of optimal growth and development.

MEDICAL CARE

Antibiotics: given PO or IV to prevent or treat infection with selection specific to identified microorganisms from culture and sensitivities.

Stool softeners: docusate calcium (Surfak) given PO for easier elimination to prevent constipation and promote bowel rehabilitation. Laxatives: bisacodyl (Dulcolax), glycerin (Sand Supp) given REC as support for bowel rehabilitation by producing irritating effect and removing water from bowel mucosa to encourage mass formation of feces and elimination.

Antispasmodics: flavoxate hydrochloride (Urispas) given PO as urinary smooth muscle relaxant to increase capacity or urinary bladder in treatment of bladder spacticity.

Cholinergics: neostigmine methylsulfate (Prostigmin) given SC or IM to increase urinary bladder tone and prevent retention.

Cultures: urine, stool, throat, sputum examination to identify presence of infection and sensitivity to specific antibiotic therapy.

Complete blood count (CBC): reveals increased WBC in presence of infection.

NURSING CARE PLANS

Essential nursing diagnoses and plans associated with this condition:

Risk for impaired skin integrity (397)

Related to: External factors of excretions and secretions
Defining characteristics: Urinary and/or fecal incontinence, redness and irritation of perineal and anal areas, disruption of skin in perineal and anal areas, leakage of CSF from sac, rupture of sac, use of diapers
Related to: External factors of physical immobilization and pressure
Defining characteristics: Redness, excoriation at bony prominences or other pressure areas, skin breakdown at pressure points, inability to change position, paralysis
Related to: Internal factors of altered sensation, circulation and skeletal prominence
Defining characteristics: Loss of tactile perception in extremities, pressure on bony prominences, lack of padded protection and massage of bony prominences, improper application of hot or cold

Impaired physical mobility (278)

Related to: Neuromuscular impairment
Defining characteristics: Inability to purposefully move within physical environment, including bed mobility, transfer, and ambulation, imbalance, impaired coordination, partial or complete paralysis of lower extremities, flaccidity, spasticity, skeletal abnormalities (hip, feet, spine)

Altered nutrition: Less than body requirements (168)

Related to: Inability to ingest food
Defining characteristics: NPO status following surgery, inadequate swallowing or sucking in presence of ICP, reduced muscle tone, abnormal eating pattern development

Constipation (173)

Related to: Neuromuscular impairment
Defining characteristics: Frequency less than usual, hard-formed stool, palpable mass, inability to maintain normal bowel elimination pattern, poor anal sphincter tone and ability to feel urge to defecate

Risk for trauma

Related to: Internal factors of weakness, balancing difficulties, lack of safety precautions, cognitive or emotional difficulties, reduced muscle coordination, skeletal abnormalities
Defining characteristics: Injury from falls, improper use of assistive aids, fractures, mental impairment, loss of tactile sensation, paralysis of extremities

Altered growth and development (419)

Related to: Effects of disorder or disability before or after surgery
Defining characteristics: Frequent hospitalizations, delay or difficulty in performing skills typical of age group (motor, social or expressive), inability to perform self-care or self-control activities appropriate for age, behavior and/or intellectual deficits

SPECIFIC DIAGNOSES AND CARE PLANS

Risk for infection

Related to: Inadequate primary defenses (broken skin, inadequate bladder emptying)
Defining characteristics: Breaks or leaks in meningeal sac, abrasion or irritation of sac, contamination of sac or surgical repair by urinary or stool incontinence

Outcome Criteria

Sac intact, moist and free of infectious process
Surgical wound intact, free from infectious process and healing
Absence of residual urine in bladder and absence of signs and symptoms of urinary tract infection

Interventions	Rationales
Assess sac for breaks or leakage of CSF, irritation of sac redness, swelling, purulent drainage at or around sac area, fever, irritability, nuchal rigidity, cloudy, foul smelling urine	Provides information about potential for infection of the sac site meningitis if sac is ruptured, or is present
Maintain the infant in prone position or sidelying, as permitted, with head lower than buttocks or hips slightly flexed with a pad between the knees; anchor position with sandbags	Reduces pressure on the sac to prevent possible rupture and prevents rolling on side or back
Apply a moist sterile dressing over the sac, use sterile saline or antibiotic solution; ointment if ordered may be applied	Prevents drying of sac membrane which could predispose to break, or rupture of sac and contamination
Reinforce moist dressing with dry sterile dressing and change when needed being careful to avoid damage to sac by removing moist dressing after it has dried	Prevents contamination by capillary action through moisture
Apply a shield over the sac dressing and tape a plastic sheet below the defect; following surgical closure on the defect, apply a transparent occlusive dressing over the area below the sac site	Protects the sac from contamination by urine or feces
Alter routine nursing care activities such as feedings, changing linens and comforting as needed	Prevents trauma to sac
Perform handwashing before any care or procedure involving the site before or after surgery and carry out sterile technique for all sac and wound care	Prevents transmission of microorganisms to site
Maintain cleanliness of anal area and apply a sterile shield between anus and sac or wound site	Prevents contamination by feces caused by poor anal sphincter control which allows for dribbling and incontinence of stool

Interventions	Rationales
Administer antibiotics as ordered	Prevents or treats infection
Following surgical repair of defect, note any changes in wound including redness, swelling, warmth, drainage, fever	Indicates wound infection
Following surgery, cleanse wound with antiseptic and change dressings when needed using sterile technique for at least 24 hours	Promotes cleanliness of wound and prevents infection
Avoid ureteral contamination with stool, perform thorough perianal hygiene as needed	Prevents urinary tract infection

Information, Instruction, Demonstration

Interventions	Rationales
Instruct parent(s) in positioning of infant, application of protection around sac (shield, foam rubber doughnut)	Prevents damage to the sac and possible infection
Instruct parent(s) in cleansing the sac gently with moist cotton balls if soiled, avoid diapering the infant until after surgery and healing has taken place	Protects sac from contaminants and maintains cleanliness
Handle infant gently, hold and support back above the defect or place on pillow in prone position to move from place to place	Prevents pressure on the sac area
Inform parent(s) of signs and symptoms of infection of sac or surgical site, whichever is applicable that should be reported	Promotes early detection of infectious process for early treatment
Instruct in handwash technique, dressing change, use of clean or sterile linens, gloves, supplies when caring for sac area	Prevents transmission of infectious organisms; sterile technique may not be needed in giving care after surgery is performed

Discharge or Maintenance Evaluation

- Maintains sac or surgical wound integrity
- Absence of infection in sac or wound area or CNS
- Protects sac or wound from contamination
- Performs sterile or clean technique in care of sac or wound
- Administers or applies antibiotic therapy systemically or topically
- Reports changes and signs and symptoms of infection to physician
- Complete bladder emptied with assistance and absence of signs and symptoms of infection

Hypothermia

Related to: Illness and abnormal presence of sac
Defining characteristics: Fluid and heat loss from large area of exposed sac, cool skin, body temperature lower than normal range

Outcome Criteria

Temperature stabilized and maintained within normal range

Interventions	Rationales
Assess temperature q2-4h and note lack of stability; assess temperature of extremity	Provides information as to source of temperature changes which may be low if infection is present
Place infant in an isolette or provide radiant warmer based on hypothermia evaluation keeping sac moist postoperatively	Provides warmth and reduces the heat loss causing hypothermia

Information, Instruction, Demonstration

Interventions	Rationales
Instruct parent(s) to take temperature and report any decreases or increases	Monitors for temperature instability detection for early intervention
Instruct parent(s) in proper amount of clothing and room temperature for infant/child	Provides optimal environmental temperature

Discharge or Maintenance Evaluation

- Maintains temperature within normal range for age
- Monitors temperature for increases or decreases and report changes

Bowel incontinence

Related to: Neuromuscular involvement
Defining characteristics: Constant dribbling or involuntary passage of stool, reduced anal sphincter tone and control, skin integrity breakdown due to continuous contact with liquid stool

Outcome Criteria

Bowel elimination pattern established with control of incontinence, skin around perianal area is kept as clean, dry and free from irritation as possible

Interventions	Rationales
Assess presence of neurogenic bowel, degree of incontinence, potential for rehabilitation	Provides information about condition for use in plan of establishing bowel elimination routine
Change diapers as quickly as feasible; cleanse perianal area carefully	Dry, clean skin resists breakdown
Apply barrier creams as ordered to perianal area during diapering	Prevents skin breakdown
Place child on a toilet or potty chair at the same time each day; use stimulation and suppository if helpful	Establishes a routine for elimination to empty bowel
Maintain fluid intake of up to 2000 ml/day depending on age; include fiber and roughage in diet at regular times of the day	Promotes bulk for easier and more manageable passage
Apply padding in waterproof undergarments but avoid use of diapers	Prevents embarrassment for the child if bowel elimination not controlled

Information, Instruction, Demonstration

Interventions	Rationales
Instruct parent(s) and child in program for control of bowel incontinence (fluids, diet, routine toileting, use of stimulation)	Promotes success in bowel training
Inform of behavior modification as a method to be used for bowel rehabilitation	Promotes compliance with routine to control bowel incontinence
Suggest clothing and undergarments to protect from staining accidents	Promotes self-image and prevents embarrassing incidents
Instruct parents on proper cleansing and diapering techniques of infant/toddler	Promotes understanding to maintain good skin integrity

Discharge or Maintenance Evaluation

- Reduces episodes of bowel incontinence
- Maintains bowel elimination pattern with control over incontinence
- Prevents embarrassing situations caused by incontinence
- Complies with rehabilitation regimen established to control bowel incontinence
- Skin integrity of perianal area is maintained

Altered urinary elimination patterns

Related to: Neuromuscular impairment
Defining characteristics: Incontinence, retention, neurogenic bladder with increased or decreased tone (flaccid or spastic), absence of awareness of bladder fullness, passing of urine or ability to stop flow of urine (reflex incontinence)

Outcome Criteria

Urinary elimination pattern established with control or absence of incontinence
Absence of renal complications and urinary bladder infection

Interventions	Rationales
Assess presence of neurogenic bladder, degree of incontinence, potential for rehabilitation, age of child	Provides information about condition for use in plan of establishing urinary elimination routine
Assess urine for cloudiness, foul odor, fever, lethargy, dysuria, retention	Indicates urinary bladder infection caused by urinary retention or residual resulting in urinary stasis and medium for bacterial growth
Offer and encourage intake of 30 ml/lb/day including acid containing beverages and dietary inclusion of foods high in acid content	Promotes renal blood flow and acidifies urine to prevent infection
Maintain clean genital and anal area after each elimination episode or as needed if incontinent	Controls introduction of microorganisms into urethra and urinary bladder
Catheterize after urination if indicated and ordered	Moves residual urine if unable to empty bladder completely
Perform scheduled rehabilitation program of placing child on toilet or potty chair at same times each day	Establishes a routine for urinary elimination if this is a possibility
Perform intermittent catheterization q3-4h if indicated to resolve incontinence	Ensures emptying of bladder to prevent incontinence and infection
Perform Crede maneuver if indicated	Promotes emptying of bladder
Administer antispasmodic, smooth muscle relaxant, anticholinergic as ordered	Improves bladder storage and continence by increasing bladder

Information, Instruction, Demonstration

Interventions	Rationales
Instruct parent(s) and child (age dependent) in use of external urinary device or procedure for intermittent self-catheterization; demonstrate and allow for return demonstration	Provides method for emptying bladder routinely or managing incontinence by use of collecting device connected to a closed system

Interventions	Rationales
Instruct in rehabilitative program of toileting and using Crede method	Provides an alternate method of controlling incontinence although may be temporary
Inform parent(s) to avoid use of diapers for child over 3 years of age; suggest pad and waterproof undergarment as an alternative	Causes embarrassment for child
Inform parent(s) of other methods available including implantation of an artificial sphincter, creation of an artificial reservoir or creation of a urinary diversion to control incontinence	Provides information about procedures that can be done if intermittent catheterization is not successful
Instruct parent(s) and child about changes in urine characteristics indicating bladder infection and measures to take to prevent this complication	Allows for early interventions to control infection and eventual renal complications
Instruct in fluid intake/day, weights and changes to report, foods and fluids that are acidic including citrus fruits, meat, eggs, cheese, prunes, breads	Maintains a monitoring system to ensure control of possible complications

Discharge of Maintenance Evaluation

- Maintains urinary elimination pattern with control over incontinence
- Complies with rehabilitation regimen established to control urinary incontinence
- Performs necessary procedures to attain continence
- Prevents urinary bladder infection
- Prevents embarrassing situations caused by incontinence
- Complies with long-term medication regimen
- Verbalizes changes, signs and symptoms to report to physician

Body image disturbance

Related to: Biophysical, psychosocial factor of child
Defining characteristics: Urinary/bowel incontinence, partial or complete paralysis, recurring hospitalizations,

change in social, verbal expression of negative feelings about body and functional disabilities, feelings of helplessness and hopelessness, inability in performing ADL

Outcome Criteria

Preservation of body image with optimal body functioning
Participation in ADL independently within limitations imposed by defect
Verbalization of progressively positive feelings about progress and social acceptance

Interventions	Rationales
Assess child for feelings about abilities and disabilities in ADL, social interaction, effect on self-concept	Provides information about potential for independence in thinking and functioning
Encourage independence and maximize functioning with use of aids for bathing, grooming, dressing, eating, mobility, toileting and praise any attempts at self-care activities	Promotes ADL capability by use of assistive aids as needed depending on disability
Encourage expression of feelings and concerns and support communication of child with parents and peers	Provides opportunity to vent feelings to reduce anxiety and negative feelings
Provide touch and hugging, age appropriate activities with other children	Conveys caring and concern for child and enhances socialization
Stress and mention positive accomplishment; avoid negative comment	Enhances body-image and confidence

Information, Instruction, Demonstration

Interventions	Rationales
Instruct in use of assistive aids for ADL	Promotes independence and enhances body-image
Inform parent(s) to maintain support and care for child	Encourages acceptance of child
Advise parent(s) to maintain same behavior rules for child as other members	Provides sense of belonging to family

Interventions	Rationales
of family and to integrate care and activities into family routines	
Teach child how to catheterize self when age permits and importance of positioning of assessment of lower extremities	Promotes independence and self-care

Discharge or Maintenance Evaluation

- Verbalizations of improved body-image and sense of well being
- Participates in ADL with or without assistive aids as needed
- Verbalizes feelings about disabilities in positive terms
- Parent(s) support and care for child and allows for maximal independence

Altered family processes

Related to: Situational crisis of long-term condition of child
Defining characteristics: Family system unable to meet physical, emotional needs of its members, inability to express or accept wide range of feelings, family unable to deal with or adapt to chronic condition and disabilities of child in a constructive manner, excessive involvement with child by family members, guilt expressed by family members, lack of support from family and friends, irritability and impatience as a response by family members to child

Outcome Criteria

Progressive adaptation and acceptance of family members to care for child with long-term condition while retaining individual and family functions
Improved coping and problem solving skills of family members

Interventions	Rationales
Assess family ability to cope with child, stress on family relationships, developmental level of family, response of siblings, knowledge of health practices, family role behavior	Provides information about family attitudes and coping abilities which directly affect the child's health and feeling of well-being; chronic condition affecting a child in a family may

Interventions	Rationales
and attitude about long-term care, economic pressures, resources to care for long-term condition and grieving process, signs of depression, feelings of powerlessness and hopelessness	strengthen or strain relationships and members may develop emotional problems when family is stressed
Assess anxiety level of family and child, perception of crisis situation, coping and problem solving methods used and effectiveness	Identifies need to develop new coping skills and realistic behaviors in goal setting and interventions necessary for family and child to adapt to crisis
Encourage expression of feelings and provide factual, honest information about care with or without surgical repair, abilities and disabilities	Allows reduction in anxiety and enhances family understanding of condition and child's needs
Assist to identify helpful techniques to use to problem solve and cope with problem and gain control over the situation	Provides support for problem solving and management of situation
Provide anticipatory guidance for crisis resolution	Assists family to adapt to situation and develop new coping mechanisms
If hospitalizations frequent, assign same personnel to care for child if appropriate	Promotes trust and communication with family members
Support and encourage parental and family caretaking efforts	Provides positive reinforcement of roles and reduces stress in family members
Allow family members to express feelings and reaction to appearance and condition of infant/child	Relieves anxiety and concern and allows a show of acceptance for their responses
Communicate empathy for patient and family	Promotes coping and positive adjustment to illness
Be aware of cultural differences in coping behaviors; needs differ according to cultural and ethnic backgrounds	Promotes cultural and developmental normalcy
Assist family with identifying realities of disabilities	Provides support, information and assistance

Interventions	Rationales
and suggest contact with community agencies, clergy, social services, physical and occupational therapy including Spina Bifida Association of America	

Information, Instruction, Demonstration

Interventions	Rationales
Inform and discuss family dynamics and need to tolerate conflict and individual behaviors	Assists to understand the family behaviors leading to resolution
Inform and reinforce appropriate coping behaviors	Promotes behavior change and adaptation to care of child
Inform that overprotective behavior may hinder growth and development and that child should have limits and rules to live by	Enhances family understanding of condition and need for integration of child into family activities
Inform of need to maintain health of family members and social contacts	Prevents adverse effect of chronic anxiety, fatigue and isolation on health and care capabilities of family
Explain causes, treatment and prognosis of condition; inform parent(s) that they are not at fault for development of the congenital defect	Reduces guilt and provides information about condition
Inform parent(s) that surgery may be performed within 48 hours after birth or be delayed to age of 3 months or until further neurologic function is assessed and to allow for better epithelialization to occur and to reduce the possibility of the development of hydrocephalus; use this information as reinforcement of physician information	Provides information to assist family in decision about surgical procedure

Interventions	Rationales
Inform need for follow-up appointments with physician and therapists	Ensures compliance with medical regimen

Discharge or Maintenance Evaluation

- Family has open discussions and identifies problem areas
- Family develops and uses problem solving techniques to resolve differences
- Family health and social responsibilities met
- Child integrated into family life with care becoming a part of family routines
- Family displays supportive behaviors for each other and constructive responses to problems
- Family relationships preserved and stressors minimized
- Family secures assistance from community agencies
- Complies with daily care and therapy regimens
- Statements by family members of adjustment and progressive adaptation to child's disabilities
- Verbalization of knowledge of normal growth and development of child and family

Risk for injury

Related to: Repeated exposure to latex products and development of latex allergy

Defining characteristics: Child exhibits symptoms such as: sneezing, coughing, rashes, hives, wheezing when handling products made of rubber (balloons, tennis balls, Bandaids™) or when exposed to hospital products that contain latex such as gloves, catheters, etc.

Outcome Criteria

Minimize exposure to latex products
Early identification of latex allergy in children
Proper notification of latex allergy to health professionals in all settings
Prompt and appropriate treatments of affected individuals

Interventions	Rationales
Identify children with latex allergy, children with this allergy should wear a form of identification such as a medical bracelet	Promote expediency in treatment if a reaction occurs; may prevent an allergic reaction

Interventions	Rationales
Maintain an environment that is latex-free, especially with high-risk populations (children with spina bifida, for example)	Prevent development of latex allergy; prevent allergic reaction in those who are already sensitized
Keep emergency equipment nearby, including equipment needed to treat an anaphylactic reaction	Promote prompt emergency treatment
If latex-free products not available and child is allergic, cloth can sometimes be placed between the latex product and the skin; examples include cotton gloves under latex gloves, cloth under a tourniquet or BP cuff	Decreases contact of skin with latex; may decrease allergic reactions
Ask all patients admitted about reactions to latex allergy during all initial interviews	Promotes screening of all patients which may prevent severe allergic reactions in otherwise low-risk patients

Information, Instruction, Demonstration

- Instruct family members/caregivers about latex allergy risks and items with which to avoid contact
- Signs of an allergic reaction
- Emergency treatment, including use of an anaphylactic kit and notification of emergency services

Discharge or Maintenance Evaluation

- Children with allergy are identified properly
- Precautions taken to eliminate or decrease latex exposure
- Allergic reactions are treated promptly and effectively
- Family verbalizes understanding of latex allergy, products to avoid, and treatment measures

Spina Bifida

In utero fetal development

Failure of spinous process
to join lumbosacral area

Defect in closure of neural tube

Spina bifida occulta

Protruding sac through
defect containing -
meninges

Complete nonclosure of
neural tube with pro-
truding sac through
defect containing parts
of spinal cord

Skin depression or dimple
Port wine angiomatous
Tufts of hair
Subcutaneous lipomas

Meningocele

Myelomeningocele

Bowel and bladder sphincter
weakness (persistent or
intermittent enuresis)
Foot weakness, gait dis-
turbance (late walking

Hydrocephalus
Flaccid paralysis of
lower limbs
Absence of sensation
Loss of bowel and bladder
Sphincter control

Surgical repair and hydrocephalus
correction based on type and extent
of defect and deficit

Resolution of defect and
minor deficits

Immobility or
mobility with braces
and crutches

Gastrointestinal System

Gastrointestinal System

The gastrointestinal tract is a common site of disorders and illnesses in infants and children. It begins in the mouth and ends with the anus and is concerned with ingestion, digestion, and absorption of nutrients and the elimination of solid waste materials from the body. It consists of the mouth (tongue and teeth), esophagus, stomach, small intestine, pancreas, liver, gallbladder, large intestine, and anus. Alterations in this system include defects in structure and abnormalities causing obstruction which affects ingestion and the transport or movement of nutrients or disturbances caused by inflammation, malabsorption, and maldigestion that results in gastrointestinal dysfunction. Because of the system's multiple functions and overlapping of symptomology resulting from an alteration in any one function, additional complications may occur. Also, as in the adult, gastrointestinal function is affected by psychological factors (e.g., anxiety) and physiological factors (e.g., diseases of other systems). The physiologic and biochemical functions of the system are present at birth to take over digestion, absorption and elimination that had been performed by the placenta. With growth and maturity of the tract, the system progressively functions within adult parameters.

GENERAL GASTROINTESTINAL CHANGES ASSOCIATED WITH PHYSICAL GROWTH AND DEVELOPMENT

Ingestion, digestion and absorption organ structure/anatomy

- Tooth eruption develops in order of need for swallowing, biting and chewing beginning in infancy at 6-8 months with the primary set of teeth completed at approximately 2 years of age
- Sucking is a reflex activity and tongue may thrust forward until it becomes smaller in relation to buccal cavity with growth and increased motility; it is positioned behind the central incisors
- Striated muscles in the throat develop by 6 weeks of age and cerebral connections are developed at 6 months of age to assist in swallowing which is a reflex activity up to 3 months of age and is stimulated by the flow of milk into the mouth; a coordinated muscular action of swallowing and sucking is developed
- The extrinsic reflex of the tongue disappears by 4 months of age
- The passageway from the mouth to the pharynx is smaller in the infant and small child than in the older child
- A longer posterior soft palate allows milk to be held in the mouth until swallowed for the first 6 months
- Sucking pads present in cheeks to assist sucking and remain until sucking not needed to obtain nutrition
- Stomach is round in shape until 2 years of age, elongates until 7 years of age when it assumes shape and position of an adult
- Stomach becomes larger to hold larger amount of food with ability to eat 3 meals/day and 1 bottle of milk at bedtime by 1 year of age
- Stomach capacity increases:

Newborn:	10-20 ml
1-3 weeks:	30-100 ml
1-3 months:	90-200 ml
1-2 years:	200-500 ml
10 years:	750-900 ml

- Cardiac sphincter immature and relaxed in infant causing regurgitation; as digestive system matures, this "spitting up" is outgrown by 6-7 months of age
- The intestinal tract in the infant and young child is longer than in the older child and the musculature and sphincters are underdeveloped with a deficiency of elastin fibers in the very young child
- Growth of the intestines increases between 1-3 years of age as diet changes take place
- Normal frequency of bowel sounds is 5-20/minute
- Digestive and absorptive surfaces are completely developed at birth
- Liver palpation changes:

up to 6 months:	0-3 cm below costal margin
6 months-4 years:	1-2 cm below costal margin
Over 6 years:	1-2 cm or not palpable below right costal margin

  Liver and spleen percussion changes:
  Liver: tympany louder in children than adults
  Lower liver border: up to 5 years: 2-3 cm lower than costal margin

5-7 years:	7 cm lower than costal margin
12 years:	9 cm lower than costal margin

  Spleen: dullness may extend 1-2 cm below costal margin in infant/child

Gastrointestinal function and height/weight patterns

- Sucking and swallowing are reflex activities after birth without voluntary control until 3 months of age; capable of swallowing, holding food in the mouth and spitting food out of mouth by 6 months of age; swallowing becomes more coordinated and solid foods more acceptable with growth
- Chewing begins with eruption of primary teeth at about 6 months; a sense of taste with response to sugar, salt, sour and bitter solutions by 3 months; sweet taste increases sucking and other tastes decrease sucking
- Stomach empties in 3-4 hours (breast milk faster than formula) in infant and 3-6 hours in older infant and child; begins to enter small intestine in 1-2 minutes after ingestion
- Begins entering cecum in 3-6 hours after reaching stomach and appears in stool 8 hours from time of ingestion
- Immature system allows food to be propelled through system rapidly resulting in bowel elimination frequency and watery stools as water not absorbed as well as in older child; stool less frequent and more regular and becoming firmer as system becomes more efficient during the first year
- Bowel movements reduced to 2/day by 1 year of age
- Intestinal flora introduced through the mouth and established by 2 days of life
- Stool changes from meconium to greenish black, greenish brown, greenish yellow (transitional stools) and then become yellowish and pasty in breast fed infants and paler yellow in infants fed formula
- By 4-6 months, gastrointestinal tract able to handle different nutrients
- Salivary glands increase in size and mature in function by 3 years of age
- Gastric juices increase in acidity with composition the same as an adult by 10 years of age
- Pancreatic amylase and lipase is deficient in infant and affects utilization of complex carbohydrates; absorption of fats until 3 months of age with all fats digested by 1 year of age
- Liver function increases as growth takes place and liver matures; limited ability to conjugate bilirubin which may result in jaundice, but able to conjugate bilirubin and secrete bile by 2 weeks of age with bile composition mature at 6 months of age
- Decreased ability of liver to form plasma proteins which may cause edema; inadequate gluconeogenesis causing decreased blood sugars; unable to form adequate prothrombin and coagulation factors causing a lack of vitamin K needed for blood clotting
- Gluconeogenesis, formation of plasma proteins and ketones, storage of vitamins and the breakdown of amino acids by the liver achieved by 1 year of age
- Basal metabolism rate is highest in infant and decreases as body increases in size; usually higher in boys than girls
- Appetite decreases by 2 years of age as growth and metabolic rate slows and food requirements are reduced
- Caloric requirement of child:

Infant:	110-120 cal/kg
Toddler:	1300 cal/day
Preschool:	1800 cal/day
Schoolage:	2400 cal/day

- Approximate weights (varies with sex, age frame, height):

  Birth: 5 1/2-10 lb (2500-4600 Gm) at full term
  Birth weight doubled by 5 months, tripled by 1 year
  Gains approximately 30 Gm/day

- Length at birth for full-term infant: 18-22 in (45-55 cm)

  Growth rate/year:

2nd year:	11 cm
3rd year:	8 cm
4th year:	7 cm
up to 10 years:	5-6 cm

ESSENTIAL NURSING DIAGNOSES AND CARE PLANS

Altered nutrition: Less than body requirements

Related to: Inability to ingest or digest food or absorb nutrients because of biological or psychological factors

Defining characteristics: Loss of weight with adequate intake, lack of interest in food, anorexia, nausea, vomiting, diarrhea, congenital defect of gastrointestinal system, regurgitation, abdominal pain, dysphagia, inability in infant to suck and swallow, failure to thrive, malabsorption syndromes, growth and developmental changes (food jags, fads, ritualisms, rejection of solid foods), vitamin deficiency, increased metabolic demand, chronic illness, poor nutrient quality of food

Outcome Criteria

Adequate intake of appropriate nutrients for normal growth and development
Height and weight parameters met and maintained based on individual determinations

Interventions	Rationales
Assess history of food intake (24 hour recall, amounts and basic 4 inclusion formula or breast milk), financial and cultural influences, vitamin/mineral supplement, food allergies	Provides information needed to evaluate nutritional pattern, habits and adequacy (deficiency or excess)
Assess appetite changes (poor or excessive), presence of illness and diagnosis, effect of nutrition on skin, hair, eyes, mouth, head, muscles, behavior	Indicates health status and effect of illness which requires an increase in nutritional needs and appetite which is affected by illness and may result in malnutrition
Assess height and weight, head circumference, skinfold thickness and arm circumference and compare with previous values and standard charts	Provides anthropometric information about body's fat and protein content and general nutritional status
Assess difficulty in sucking, swallowing, chewing, gag reflex, teeth, oral mucous membrane, lips, and palate for abnormalities, presence of oral pain or infection	Provides information about ability to ingest foods or formula necessary for normal growth and development; inadequate dental care, oral inflammatory disorders, congenital defects (cleft lip/palate) interferes with feeding
Assess presence of nausea, vomiting and if spitting up, projectile; related to activity or intake or tension/stress; characteristics of vomits (bloody, bile, digested or undigested food), frequency and persistence, amount, associated conditions (diarrhea, fever, headache, motion sickness, anger, conflict with parent)	Provides information about emesis which affects nutrition and is controlled by the vomiting center in the medulla; causes include: blockage of the pylorus, reflex from incompetent esophageal sphincter, gastroenteritis, duodenal and gastric spasm, increased ICP, bowel obstruction, drugs and allergens; persistent losses may lead to fluid and electrolyte imbalance

Interventions	Rationales
Assess abdominal girth, stool characteristics (odor, appearance), presence of diarrhea, bowel sounds for increased motility	Provides information about ability to absorb foods; stool may be bulky and fatty in cystic fibrosis if bile flow obstructed and fats are not digested; diarrhea may cause carbohydrate malabsorption as motility increases and moves nutrients through the bowel before absorption takes place
Place infant/child in position of comfort for feeding/meals: hold infant in arms or upright as condition indicates (cleft defect); child in sitting position at table within easy reach of food and with appropriate sized utensils	Provides most appropriate position to enhance movement of formula/solid food by gravity and peristalsis and to prevent vomiting and/or aspiration
Offer feedings/meals as near usual to normal routine as possible; provide amounts (small when indicated) and frequency (infant feedings q4h and progress to 3 meals/day with introduction of solid foods at proper age); if ill, spread over 6 meals/day	Promotes feedings/meals that are similar to established pattern and adjusted to special needs caused by specific illness or increased metabolic demand (fever, infection, chronic illness, malnutrition)
Request parent to bring foods from home and serve in age appropriate quantities; allow child to eat in a community setting with other children	Promotes appetite and increased independence and familiar types and preparation of foods
Offer age appropriate food consistency and foods that are not irritating to oral, stomach, bowel mucosa; thicken formula with cereal when necessary; modify other foods specific to disorder	Promotes ingestion and retention of foods and prevents exacerbation or increased severity of gastrointestinal disorders
Maintain NPO status if prescribed, provide infant with non-nutritional sucking	Provides rest for gastrointestinal tract needed because of vomiting, diarrhea, preoperative preparation

Interventions	Rationales
Initiate and monitor IV administration of nutrients as prescribed	Provides short-term fluid and nutritional support via peripheral vein in those who are unable to ingest or retain nourishment (vomiting, diarrhea postoperative care)
Initiate and monitor IV total parenteral nutrition as prescribed	Provides long-term fluid and nutritional support via a right atrial catheter in a large vein in those who are nutritionally deficient as a result of a chronic disease (Crohn's disease) or negative nitrogen balance
Insert nasogastric tube and initiate and monitor tube feedings as prescribed; initiate and monitor feedings and insertion site of gastrostomy if present	Provides nutritional support for those with persistent weight loss; unable to chew, swallow, suck; who need an increase in nutrients while ill, but with intact digestive and absorption activity
Avoid excessive handling of an infant after feeding	Prevents possible vomiting from increased stimuli
Administer vitamin/ mineral supplements, digestive enzymes, antispasmodics, antibiotics	Provides or replaces necessary substances that may be deficient if absorption impaired, or be the cause of impaired digestion absorption; reduces peristalsis and infectious process affective nutritional status
Consult with nutritionist if needed	Provides support for the infant/child's special dietary needs

Information, Instruction, Demonstration

Interventions	Rationales
Instruct parent(s) in the different food intake at different ages, the basic 4 food groups and amount and types of foods appropriate to age, how food intake relates to growth and development	Promotes knowledge of needs that will ensure nutritional adequacy of child

Interventions	Rationales
Instruct parent(s) to avoid including sugar and salt in diet; offer nutritious between-meal snacks	Maintains and promotes health status
Instruct parent(s) in caloric needs for age of child and in weight and height measurement techniques	Promotes knowledge to ensure stable weight and gains proportionate to growth
Instruct in proper preparation and storage of foods; handwash before preparing or handling food	Prevents spoiling and contamination of foods that may cause gastrointestinal symptoms
Instruct parent(s) in use of special devices or utensils for feeding or for self-feeding by child	Promotes food intake
Inform parent(s) of need for food supplements and that the quality of food is more important than the quantity of food ingested	Ensures nutritional status and provides parent(s) with realistic information about food intake
Explain method of providing nutrition via IV or N/G or gastrostomy tube	Reduces anxiety by understanding of alternate method of supplying nutrients to infant/child
Inform parent(s) of methods to wean child from breast or bottle, when to add solid foods to diet	Provides information if needed about infant's diet changes
Instruct parent(s) in menu planning that is age appropriate with inclusions of basic four, food preferences, proper consistency and texture, finger and raw foods and allow child to participate in planning	Encourages inclusion of necessary foods and acceptance of foods offered

Discharge or Maintenance Evaluation

- Maintains nutritional status for growth and development
- Complies with and tolerates daily intake of nutrient requirements (caloric and basic 4) for optimal health
- Promotes nutritional intake via method in accordance with disease limitations, presence of gastrointestinal symptoms
- Return to baseline parameters of gastrointestinal function related to ingestion, digestion, absorption

- Absence of anorexia, nausea, vomiting, diarrhea, bowel distention, weight loss
- Offers feedings/meals appropriate for specific age and disorder
- Administers nutrients via IV, tube feedings, feeding device safely and with desired results
- Verbalizes caloric and special nutritional needs for infant/child, methods of preparation and storage, factors that encourage and discourage food intake
- Promotes optimal environment for nutritional health
- Maintains acceptable weight for height and frame

Diarrhea

Related to: Dietary intake
Defining characteristics: Abdominal pain, cramping, increased frequency of bowel elimination and bowel sounds, loose, liquid stools, urgency, intake of high fiber, spicy foods
Related to: Inflammation, irritation or malabsorption of bowel
Defining characteristics: Abdominal pain and cramping, increased frequency of bowel elimination and bowel sounds, loose, liquid, unformed stools, urgency, blood, mucus or pus in stools
Related to: Toxins, contaminants
Defining characteristics: Abdominal pain, increased frequency of bowel elimination and bowel sounds, loose, liquid stools, urgency, fever and malaise
Related to: Medications, radiation
Defining characteristics: Abdominal pain, increased frequency of bowel elimination and bowel sounds, loose, liquid stools, urgency, chemotherapeutic agents, external radiation treatments

Outcome Criteria

Resolution of diarrhea with establishment of pattern of soft formed stool elimination
Absence of precipitating factors causing diarrheal episodes

Interventions	Rationales
Assess normal pattern of bowel elimination and characteristics of stool (frequency, amount, consistency, presence of blood, pus, mucus, color change), presence of diseases or contact with contaminants, infective organisms, medications being taken	Provides information about baseline parameters for comparison, reason for changes; diarrhea may be acute caused by an inflammation, toxin or a systemic disease and last about 72 hours, or chronic caused by inflammation, allergy, malabsorption, bowel
	motility changes or disease and last longer than 72 hours; antibiotic therapy may cause diarrhea as it destroys the normal flora in the bowel
Assess abdomen for distention palpation and bowel sounds for increases in auscultation	Indicates a distended bowel with fluid and hypermotility of bowel which reduces the amount of material that is absorbed by the bowel mucosa
Assess for temperature elevation, irritability, flaccidity, lack of expression, whiny cry, lethargy, anorexia, vomiting, eyes lackluster	Provides information about signs and symptoms associated with diarrhea
Assess for fluid loss with a light weight loss, dry skin and mucous membranes, poor skin turgor, serum potassium, sodium for decreases	Indicates possible dehydration associated with fluid/electrolyte loss from frequent watery stools and vomiting and insensible fluid loss from fever that leads to metabolic acidosis
Obtain stool specimen for laboratory examination for toxins, ova and parasites, number of calories of infective organisms present; fecal analysis for occult blood, fat content; repeat specimen examination as needed to confirm presence of organism	Indicates possible cause of diarrhea
Place on enteric isolation and explain reasons why this is necessary until diagnosis is confirmed; maintain precautions if cause is identified as an infective organism	Prevents undue anxiety and transmission of disease to others since bacterial and viral infections are the most common causes of diarrhea in children
Place on NPO, administer and monitor IV fluids and electrolytes	Allows bowel to rest and IV replaces lost fluids and electrolytes
Administer oral rehydration fluids q4-6 hours and increase or decrease depending on hydration sta-	Provides therapy of choice for mild or moderate dehydration in infants

Interventions	Rationales
tus; volume should equal stool losses and as prescribed, and maintenance therapy includes the addition of 1 bottle of plain water for every 2 bottles of rehydration fluid	
Gradually reintroduce fluids and solid foods orally; begin with clear fluids followed by full liquid diet and then to dry foods without milk or fats followed by low residue diet; eventually allow a general diet or return to previous pattern of foods/fluids ingested	Allows for graduated, slow return to dietary intake based on decrease or cessation of diarrhea and as stool increases in firmness
Administer anti-infective therapy and antidiarrheals	Destroys or inhibits growth of microorganisms; decreases bowel motility in children over 2 years of age
Change diaper frequently as needed in infant, expose buttocks to air and apply skin protective ointment to buttocks and perianal area in infants and anal area in children if irritated and sore; wash area with warm water after each diarrhea episode (commercial wipes may be used if skin not irritated)	Protects skin from excretions and secretions that are irritating and cause excoriation and skin breakdown

Information, Instruction, Demonstration

Interventions	Rationales
Instruct parent(s) and child on enteric precautions including handwashing technique after bowel movement and before meals, disposal of and laundering of linens and articles contaminated by excrement, demonstrate and allow for return demonstration of handwash	Prevents transmission or spread of microorganisms causing diarrhea to others

Interventions	Rationales
Inform parent(s) of signs and symptoms of dehydration or changes in characteristics of diarrhea and to report them to physician; diarrhea that becomes chronic or returns or diet that is not tolerated should be reported	Provides for immediate treatment and prevention of severe complication of acidosis; diarrhea that persists longer than 12-24 hours in infant or longer than 48 hours in child should be reported
Instruct parent(s) and child in reintroduction of fluids at room temperature (avoid citrus fruit juices), then offer small, frequent feedings of soft foods when fluids are tolerated and stools have decreased number (gelatin, broths, bananas, rice, crackers, toast) and continue to gradually add foods as tolerated	Provides for resumption of nutritional intake usually completed in a week
Discuss proper refrigeration and handling of foods	Preserves foods properly to prevent spoiling and possible source of diarrhea
Instruct parent(s) on procedure to collect stool specimen and take to laboratory labeled properly	Provides specimen examination to identify cause of diarrhea
Instruct parent(s) to stop milk and solid foods if diarrhea starts again and begin with sips of fluid and advance diet as before	Prevents recurrence of severe diarrhea or chronic type caused by intolerance to foods or effect of foods on diseased bowel
Instruct parent(s) in medication administration if prescribed and avoidance of medications in children under 12 years of age (absorbents, antidiarrheals)	Promotes correct administration of antibiotics for some types of diarrhea and avoidance of medications that may cause toxicity or mask fluid losses and prolong diarrhea caused by infectious agents by decreasing motility

Discharge or Maintenance Evaluation

- Absence of diarrhea with return to baseline bowel elimination pattern — dietary and fluid modifications to treat diarrhea and prevent recurrence of episodes
- Appropriate administration of medications

- Corrects fluid/electrolyte imbalance potential
- Maintains nutritional status and skin integrity
- Maintains enteric precaution measures (e.g., good handwashing, etc.)
- Collects stool specimens for testing
- Relieves discomfort associated with diarrheal episodes
- Verbalizes proper preparation and storage of foods
- Cooperates with follow-up care instructions and reporting of signs and symptoms of potential complications

Constipation

Related to: Less than adequate dietary intake and bulk
Defining characteristics: Frequency less than usual pattern, hard, dry formed stool, decreased bowel sounds, straining at stool, decreased amount of stool, change from human to cow's milk in infancy
Related to: Personal habits
Defining characteristics: Environmental changes (school), stool withholding in young children, lack of privacy, inability of leisurely use of bathroom, not using bathroom when urge is felt by school age children
Related to: Less than adequate physical activity or immobility
Defining characteristics: Frequency less than usual pattern, hard, dry formed stool, decreased bowel sounds, absence of stool, abdominal distention or rigidity or cramping, postoperative bed rest and immobility, bed rest status
Related to: Medications
Defining characteristics: Administration of diuretics, antacids, anticonvulsives, iron preparation to treat other conditions, diagnostic procedure using barium, hard, dry, less frequent stools
Related to: Neuromuscular or musculoskeletal impairment
Defining characteristics: Inability to feel urge to defecate, fecal impaction, hard, dry formed stool, locomotion impairment, inability to exert force necessary to defecate, painful defecation, mental retardation, poor anal sphincter tone, paralysis, autonomic dysreflexia
Related to: Gastrointestinal obstructive lesions
Defining characteristics: Ribbon-like stools, less frequent or absence of stools, abdominal distention and pain, diminished or absence of bowel sounds

Outcome Criteria

Resolution of constipation with establishment of pattern of soft formed stool elimination depending on age
Bowel elimination alteration (constipation) relieved and return of preoperative or prehospitalization pattern

Interventions	Rationales
Assess normal pattern of bowel elimination and characteristics of stool (frequency, amount, shape and consistency), presence of diseases, abnormalities of the bowel caused by congenital defects	Provides information that indicates baseline parameters for comparison; frequency varies among children depending on age and foods ingested, but may be as few as 3-5/day in infant, as few as 6/week in child less than 3 years of age, and few as 4/week in older child; presence of constipation may be associated with disorders in children that lead to obstruction
Assess abdomen for hard mass or distention, measure abdominal girth, auscultate for bowel sounds that are diminished or absent	Indicates accumulation of stool in bowel or reduction in peristalsis
Assess for toilet training techniques, change in diet, change in environment	Provides information that may lead to reasons for constipation
Assess for intentional stool withholding, discomfort in defecation, word the child uses to indicate need to defecate	Provides information about reason child might have for suppressing the urge to defecate
Assess parent(s) attitude about bowel habits and toilet training	Provides information about child's reaction to parental attitudes and may cause bowel elimination suppression
Provide privacy during bowel elimination	Promotes elimination by preserving privacy which a child considers important for a very private and intimate activity
Allow child to sit up during bowel elimination on a bedpan if necessary or on a commode or toilet if possible	Provides a normal position for easier bowel elimination; a bedpan may eliminate possibility of elimination
Encourage fluid intake and activity within limitations imposed by illness; add fiber, prune juice to diet	Provides fluid and exercise for bowel motility and prevents hard, dry stool if water is reabsorbed because of lack of fluids, bulk in stool provided by fiber in the diet promotes motility

Interventions	Rationales
Add sugar in formula of infant; administer stool softeners, suppositories or isotonic enema as ordered for child; explain procedure and what to expect to the child before administering	Promotes bowel evacuation when unable to control by fluids and diet; preparation by explanation encourages cooperation

Information, Instruction, Demonstration

Interventions	Rationales
Inform parent(s) that daily bowel elimination is not necessary for a child and that straining is not always a symptom of constipation; that changes in bowel elimination pattern may be caused by illness	Provides accurate information to replace beliefs or misinformation by expecting results that will frustrate child
Inform parent(s) that child may suppress defecation as a result of bad experiences during toilet training if punished for accidental soiling of clothing; that an illness or discomfort when defecating may cause a child to suppress defecation	Provides information about behavior common to toddlers and preschool age children and constipation is developed and perpetuated when bowel contents are retained-
Instruct parent(s) and child in dietary inclusion of syrup or corn for infant; high fiber foods including popcorn, cereals, grain foods, fruit and vegetables, or add fiber to foods for child	Provides bulk to increase motility in child and sugar for infant to relieve constipation; fiber absorbs water to soften stool
Instruct parent(s) and child to avoid milk products, rice, apples and apple juice, bananas, gelatin which are constipating foods	Provides information about foods that prevent resolution of constipation
Instruct parent(s) and child to increase fluids, age appropriate, and as child gets older and milk amount is reduced, replace with other fluids	Provides adequate fluid intake to soften stool and maintain bowel elimination

Interventions	Rationales
Inform parent(s) that stool softeners, suppositories may be administered judiciously and instruct in use; instruct in administration of isotonic solution enema if medication is not successful in promoting defecation	Provides information to prevent abuse and possible overuse causing dependence and chronic diarrhea
Inform parent(s) and child to maintain activity and instruct child in abdominal and rectal exercises	Promotes peristalsis and muscle strength involved in bowel elimination especially if child is ill and on bedrest or has poor anal sphincter control

Discharge or Maintenance Evaluation

- Absence of suppression of bowel elimination and relief of constipation
- Return of baseline bowel elimination pattern with soft formed stool
- Appropriate administration of oral or rectal relief measures
- Dietary, fluid and activity modifications for prevention of constipation or resolution of existing constipation
- Modifies bowel elimination pattern to establish regularity and comfort

ESSENTIAL NURSING DIAGNOSES AND CARE PLANS

Fluid volume deficit (related to nausea and vomiting)

Related to: Chemosensitive triggers medication, anesthesia, chemotherapy, toxins, increased ICP, inner ear disturbances, cerebral hypoxia, food intolerances, allergens, motion sickness)

Defining characteristics: Nausea, vomiting, perspiration, weight loss or gain, pallor, dehydration, fluid and electrolyte imbalance, anxiety, hopelessness, loss of control, tachycardia, abdominal cramping, early morning vomiting (ICP and metabolic disease), fever and diarrhea (infection), decreased urine output, fatigue, hypotension, thirst

Related to: Emotional stimuli triggers (unpleasant sights, odors, fright, anorexia, eating disorders)

Defining characteristics: Weight loss, change in level of consciousness or headache, malnutrition, weight gain (overeating), psychogenic vomiting (after meals), nausea, perspiration, pallor, dehydration, fluid and electrolyte imbalance, anxiety, tachycardia

Related to: Visceral stimuli triggers (irritation, inflammation, mechanical disturbance in GI tract or other related viscera, or GI pain)

Defining characteristics: Chronic intermittent vomiting (malrotation), green bilious vomiting (bowel obstruction), curdled mucus or food, vomiting many hours after eating (poor gastric emptying or high intestinal obstruction), constipation (anatomical or functional obstruction), forceful vomiting (pyloric stenosis), localized abdominal pain, vomiting soon after meals (peptic ulcer disease), weight loss, nausea, perspiration, tachycardia, anxiety, pallor, dehydration, fluid and electrolyte imbalance, fatigue, decreased urinary output

Outcome Criteria

Resolution of nausea and vomiting with adequate fluid volume

Absence of participating factors causing nausea and vomiting episodes

Interventions	Rationales
Assess food frequency and 24 hour recall, oral fluids, medications, food likes and dislikes, financial and cultural influences, food allergies, food preparation methods	Provides information to evaluate nutritional status, patterns, habits, and environmental influences on diet
Assess onset of nausea and vomiting, quality, quantity and presence of blood, bile, food and odor	Provides information about emesis and defining characteristics
Assess relationship of nausea and vomiting to meals, time of day or activities, and associated triggers	Provides information to identify factors related to time of fluid deficit
Assess for presence of associated symptoms: diarrhea, fever, ear pain, UGI symptoms, vision changes, headache, seizures, high pitched cry, polydipsia, polyuria, polyphagia, anorexia, etc.; record intake	Provides information to identify associated medical conditions; indicates fluid status; increased output and decreased intake indicate a fluid deficit and need for replacement

Interventions	Rationales
and output, including all body fluid losses, IVs and oral fluids	
Assess skin turgor, mucous membranes, weight, fontanelles of an infant, last void, and behavior changes	Provides information about hydration status; including extracellular fluid losses, decreased activity levels, malaise, weight loss, poor skin turgor, concentrated urine
Maintain NPO status, if prescribed	Provides rest for the gastrointestinal tract because of nausea and vomiting and associated medical conditions
Initiate and monitor IV administration of nutrients as prescribed	Provides fluid and nutritional support to replace active fluid loss and prevention of fluid overload
Assess vital signs, including apical pulse	Provides monitoring of cardiovascular response to dehydration (weak, thready pulse, drop in blood pressure, and increased respiratory rate contribute to fluid loss)
Initiate small amounts of clear liquids, as tolerated when nausea and vomiting subside; offer oral hydration fluids; i.e., water and ice chips; breast-fed babies need frequent short feedings at the breast: Infant: 70-100 ml/kg in 24 hours, toddler: 50-70 ml/kg in 24 hours, school age: 20-50 ml/kg in 24 hours	Provides fluids in minimal amounts until nausea and vomiting resolved
Gradually reintroduce other fluids and solid foods slowly beginning with clear liquids followed by full liquids, and then to dry foods followed by appropriate diet as tolerated by the child, or as needed for the medical condition	Allows for the gradual return to the expected dietary intake

Interventions	Rationales
Monitor urine specific gravity, color, and amount every voiding or as ordered	Concentrated urine with an increased specific gravity indicates lack of fluids to dilute urine
Monitor laboratory data results, as ordered (electrolytes, BUN, CBC, pH, etc.)	Allows identification of fluid losses and electrolyte imbalances
Administer medications (anti-infectives, anti-emetics) as ordered and evaluate effects/side effects	Destroys or inhibits the growth of microorganisms and alleviates nausea and vomiting, allows detection of improved status
Position child on side or sitting up when vomiting; keep suction available	Prevents swallowing or aspiration of emesis
Provide comfort measures (e.g., cool cloth, clean linens, etc.)	Promotes maximal comfort level
Administer or assist with good oral hygiene (brushing teeth, mouthwash or oral swabs)	Provides moisture and comfort for drying oral mucosa
Explain all interventions to child and parent(s) and provide psychological support	Provides comfort, information, relieves anxiety, and decreases feeling of powerlessness
Assist child with activity and position changes	Prevents injury and provides safety due to possible postural hypertension

Information, Instruction, Demonstration

Interventions	Rationales
Instruct parent(s) regarding causes of nausea and vomiting, signs of dehydration, and when to report them to the physician	Provides information for immediate treatment of excessive loss of fluids and electrolytes caused by nausea and vomiting
Instruct parent(s) and child on the reintroduction of food and fluids slowly until symptoms subside, offering ice chips, water or commercial electrolyte solution first, then progress to a regular diet	Provides measure for self-care for early intervention of fluid deficit

Interventions	Rationales
Instruct parent(s) and child on the importance of a balanced diet and adequate fluid intake on a daily basis	Provides information for health promotion and illness prevention
Reinforce importance of adhering to medical regimen, post discharge, and medication administration, if prescribed	Provides information to maintain fluid status and prevent further deficits
Instruct parent(s) to position child safely during vomiting episodes and to provide oral hygiene	Provides information to promote safety, oral hydration and hygiene

Discharge or Maintenance Evaluation

- Absence of nausea and vomiting with return to baseline fluid intake and output pattern
- Dietary and fluid modifications to treat nausea and vomiting
- Appropriate administration of medications
- Corrects fluid/electrolyte imbalance potential
- Maintains nutritional status and oral hygiene
- Maintains safety measures during nausea and vomiting episodes
- Relieves discomforts associated with nausea and vomiting episodes
- Verbalizes understanding of food groups, serving sizes and fluids needed for balanced diet
- Cooperates with follow-up care instructions and reporting of signs and symptoms of potential complications

Appendicitis

Appendicitis is the inflammation of the appendix, a blind sac connected to the end of the cecum. It is caused most commonly by a fecalith (hard feces) and may result in obstruction which leads to ischemia, necrosis, perforation and peritonitis. Surgical removal of the appendix (appendectomy) is performed as treatment for this disorder, preferably before rupture for a positive outcome. Surgery after rupture requires external drainage and management to reduce the spread of peritonitis. The condition commonly occurs in children over 2 years of age.

MEDICAL CARE

Analgesics (narcotic analgesics): codeine (Methyl-morphine), sulfate (MS) given SC, IM after diagnosis has been made and postoperatively.

Analgesics (non-narcotic analgesics): acetaminophen (Tylenol) given PO postoperatively to control moderate pain.

Antibiotics: ampicillin sodium (SK-Ampicillin-N) given IV, IM or other anti-infectives to prevent or treat peritonitis.

Abdominal x-ray: reveals presence of fecalith or other material in the appendix.

Abdominal ultrasound: reveals abscess location if present.

Complete blood count: reveals increased WBC of 15,000-20,000/cu mm and increased neutrophils.

NURSING CARE PLANS

Essential nursing diagnoses and plans associated with this condition:

Risk for fluid volume deficit (222)

Related to: Excessive losses through normal routes, NPO status postoperatively
Defining characteristics: Vomiting, deviations affecting intake of fluids, elevated temperature, reduced urinary output, diaphoresis

Hyperthermia (112)

Related to: Illness (presence of infectious process)
Defining characteristics: Increase in body temperature above normal range, warm to touch, increased pulse and respiratory rate, flushing, abrupt rise in temperature with rupture of appendix

Altered nutrition: Less than body requirements (168)

Related to: Inability to ingest food
Defining characteristics: Vomiting, anorexia, nausea, abdominal pain, presence of nasogastric function postoperative

Constipation (173)

Related to: Less than adequate physical activity
Defining characteristics: Bedrest following surgery, decreased or absent bowel sounds, frequency less than usual pattern, hard formed stool, abdominal pain

SPECIFIC DIAGNOSES AND CARE PLANS

Pain

Related to: Biological injuring agents, inflammation
Defining characteristics: Verbal descriptor of pain, guarding and protective behavior of painful area, irritability, refusal to move or change position, crying, muscular rigidity, clinging behavior, sidelying position with knees flexed

Outcome Criteria

Relief of acute pain pre and postoperatively and associated symptoms

Interventions	Rationales
Assess severity of pain, generalized abdominal pain descending to lower right quadrant and localized at McBurney's point with rebound tenderness, reduced bowel sounds; behaviors indicating pain with psoas and/or obturator signs positive	Provides information symptomatic of appendicitis with pain being the most common presenting complaint; behaviors manifested by pain vary with age with infant responding with crying, facial expression of pain and physical resistance; young children responding with crying loudly, clinging, irritability, uncooperation, rigid position, sidelying position with knees flexed up to abdomen, refusal to move

Interventions	Rationales
Assess for severity of post-operative pain	Provides information needed to administer most effective analgesic therapy
Assess for acuteness of abdominal pain that progresses to abdominal rigidity, abdominal distention, tachycardia, shallow respirations, fever, pallor	Indicates rupture of appendix and peritonitis
Administer narcotic or non-narcotic analgesic PO or IV preoperatively or postoperatively as ordered	Promotes relief of pain depending on severity, age and general condition, NPO status
Avoid palpation of abdomen and unnecessary movements and care procedures of child	Prevents increased pain and possible rupture of appendix
Apply ice packs to abdomen	Provides relief of pain
Place in position of comfort; right sidelying or low to semi-Fowler's	Promotes comfort to reduce pain; postoperatively will facilitate drainage if appendix has ruptured and prevent spread of infection
Provide toys, games for quiet play	Promotes diversionary activity to detract from pain
Inform child that palpation will cause some pain and inform of any other procedures that cause pain	Warns child of discomfort to expect and promotes trust of caretaker

Information, Instruction, Demonstration

Interventions	Rationales
Explain cause of pain to parent(s) and child and measures that are taken to relieve pain	Promotes understanding of condition and reasons for treatments and medication
Inform parent(s) of behavioral responses to pain that child is manifesting and that as pain subsides, child will return to usual behavior patterns	Promotes understanding of behavior changes common to an age group in presence of pain

Discharge or Maintenance Evaluation

- Preoperative or postoperative pain relieved and/or controlled
- Limits movement or procedures that increase pain
- Child rests comfortably with absence of behavioral responses to pain
- Analgesic therapy administration based on severity of pain and age with desired results

Risk for infection

Related to: Inadequate primary defenses (ruptured appendix), invasive procedure (surgery)

Defining characteristics: Spread of infection in peritoneal cavity, absent bowel sounds, diffuse abdominal pain followed by an absence of pain, abdominal distention, vomiting, increased pulse and respirations, fever, redness, swelling, drainage at incision site whether closed by primary intension (appendectomy) or open and draining (ruptured appendix)

Outcome Criteria

Incision site free of infectious process
Infection maintained at lower right abdomen
Absence of spread of peritonitis

Interventions	Rationales
Assess closed incision site for redness, swelling, pain, drainage, approximation of edges, healing	Provides information indicating incision infection
Assess open incision site for drainage and characteristics, drain placement and patency, need for dressing change	Provides information about effectiveness of wound drainage to prevent abscess formation and spread of peritonitis
Administer antibiotic therapy IV as ordered	Destroys infectious agent with selection of medications based on culture and sensitivities of wound drainage
Position in sidelying or semi-Fowler's	Facilitates drainage through wound drain and prevents spread of infection upward in abdomen
Redress incision wound using sterile technique	Promotes cleanliness of wound and prevents introduction of pathogens

Interventions	Rationales
Change dressings on open wound or reinforce as needed, use Montgomery straps to hold dressings in place	Maintains clean, dry dressings and allows for frequent changes without removing tape
Apply warm, wet pack to open incision as ordered	Promotes circulation to the area and reduces inflammation
Irrigate open wound with antibiotic solution as ordered	Cleanses wound and destroys pathogens
Initiate wound isolation precautions	Prevents transmission of infectious agents to or from the child

Information, Instruction, Demonstration

Interventions	Rationales
Inform parent(s) and child of reason for infection and risk of spread of infection	Promotes understanding and cooperation in treatments to prevent spread of existing infection or risk of infection of appendectomy incision
Inform parent(s) of incision care, dressing change, removal of drainage, healing process	Promotes understanding of wound healing and progression to infection resolution
Inform parent(s) and child that isolation is needed to prevent spread of infection and length of time isolation is carried out	Promotes compliance with isolation techniques

Discharge or Maintenance Evaluation

- Infection confined to lower right abdomen
- Administration of antibiotic therapy
- Appendectomy incision free of infectious process and healing
- Open incision area draining and healing
- Dry and clean wound dressings maintained with changes as needed
- Wound isolation precautions maintained until culture is negative for infectious fast agent

Anxiety

Related to: Change in health status of child, hospitalization of child, possible surgery of child

Defining characteristics: Increased apprehension that condition might worsen and appendix rupture, expressed concern and worry about impending surgery, need for IV, NPO and N/G tube and other treatments and procedures while hospitalized, lack of information about postoperative care

Outcome Criteria

Reduced parental and child anxiety verbalized as illness and surgery resolved
Verbalizes understanding of cause of fear and anxiety and positive effect of surgical treatment

Interventions	Rationales
Assess source and level of anxiety and how anxiety is manifested; need for information that will relieve anxiety	Provides information about anxiety level and need for interventions to relieve it; sources for the parent(s) include fear and uncertainty about treatment and recovery, guilt for presence of illness; sources for child include separation from parent(s), procedures, fear of mutilation or death, unfamiliar environment; anxiety in the child may be manifested by crying, inability to play or sleep or eat, clinging aggression
Allow expression of concerns and ask questions about condition, procedures, recovery surgery by parent(s) and child	Provides opportunity to vent feelings and fears and secure information to reduce anxiety
Communicate with parent(s) and answer questions calmly and honestly; use pictures, drawings, and models for explanations to child	Promotes calm and supportive trusting environment
Allow parent(s) to stay with child and encourage to assist in care or open visitation	Allows parent(s) to care for and support child and continue parental role

Interventions	Rationales
Give parent(s) and child as much input in decisions about care and routines as possible	Allows for more control over situation

Information, Instruction, Demonstration

Interventions	Rationales
Inform parent(s) and child of disease process, physical effects and symptoms of illness	Provides information to relieve anxiety by knowledge of what to expect
Explain reason for each pre and postoperative procedure or type of therapy, diagnostic tests, surgical procedure and rationales including IV, N/G tube and dressings to parent(s) and child as appropriate for age	Reduces fear which decreases anxiety
Inform parent(s) of child's condition and difficulty in diagnosing and interpreting symptoms of illness in children	Promotes understanding and reduces anxiety caused by diagnosis process
Inform parent(s) and child that hospitalization for an appendectomy is 4-7 days and for an appendectomy for a ruptured appendix is about 2 weeks	Reduces anxiety and allows for postoperative planning
Demonstrate and instruct in wound care and dressing changes; allow for return demonstration; inform to protect dressing from diaper	Ensures wound healing without complication of infection or recurrence of infection
Inform parent(s) and child of activity restrictions and length of time before returning to school (usually 1 week following discharge)	Ensures wound healing without complication of infection or recurrence of infection
Instruct to report changes in wound indicating infection (redness, swelling, pain, drainage)	Allows for immediate treatment in presence of infectious process

Interventions	Rationales
Instruct parent(s) of dietary progression following removal of N/G tube	Promotes return to nutritional baseline and bowel elimination

Discharge or Maintenance Evaluation

- Expresses reduction in anxiety about illness, preoperative and postoperative care and procedures
- Parent(s) verbalize that anxiety decreases as acute phase is resolved
- Verbalizes positive effect of caring for and supporting ill child
- Participates in care and decision making regarding child
- Demonstrates wound care and dressing changes postoperatively and other procedures to enhance wellness and verbalizes comfort with knowledge and performance of postoperative care with reduced anxiety
- States signs and symptoms to report postoperatively

Appendicitis

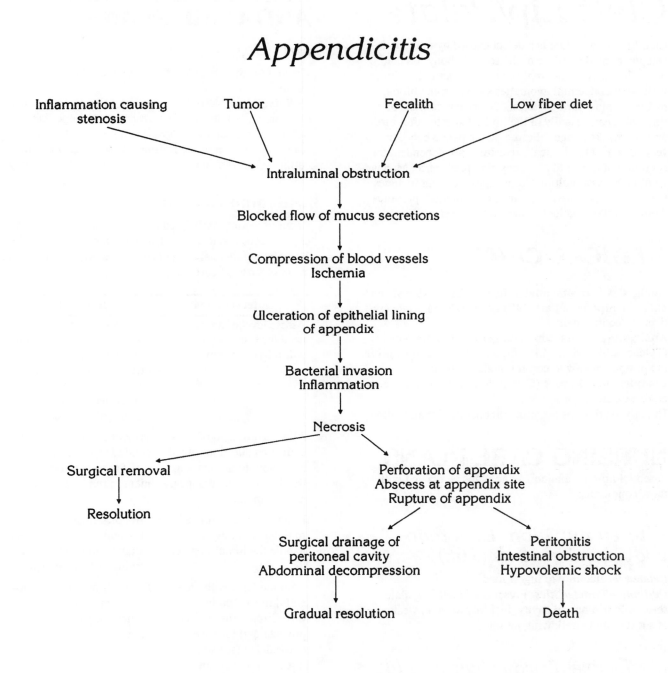

Cleft Lip/Palate

Cleft lip and/or palate is a defect caused by in utero development by the failure of the soft and bony tissue to fuse. They may occur singly or together and often occur with other congenital anomalies such as spina bifida, hydrocephalus, cardiac defect. Treatment consists of surgical repair, usually of the lip first shortly after birth or at 10 weeks of age followed by the palate between 1-3 years of age. The surgical procedures are dependent on condition of the child and physician preference. Management involves a multidiscipline approach that includes the surgeon, pediatrician, nurse, orthodontist, propthodontist, otolaryingologist, speech therapist.

MEDICAL CARE

Analgesics (narcotic analgesics): codeine (Methyl-morphine), morphine sulfate (MS) given SC, IM postoperatively to control pain.
Analgesics (non-narcotic analgesics): acetaminophen (Tylenol tablet, elixir, Liquiprin solution or drops) given PO postoperatively to control moderate pain.
Complete blood count (CBC): done as a routine preoperative examination.
Urinalysis: done as a routine preoperative examination.

NURSING CARE PLANS

Essential nursing diagnoses and plans associated with these conditions:

Altered nutrition: Less than body requirements (168)

Related to: Inability to ingest food
Defining characteristics: Presence of cleft lip/palate, sore, inflamed buccal cavity, inability to suck, weakness of sucking and swallowing muscles

Ineffective airway clearance (42)

Related to: Tracheobronchial aspiration of feedings, trauma of surgery
Defining characteristics: Abnormal breath sounds, dyspnea, tachypnea, cyanosis, changes in rate or depth of respirations, cough with or without sputum, postoperative edema

SPECIFIC DIAGNOSES AND CARE PLANS

Anxiety

Related to: Situational crisis of congenital defect of infant
Defining characteristics: Severe reaction to appearance of infant with a facial defect, responses to imperfect infant (shock, denial and grief), expression of guilt, blame and helplessness, feelings of inadequacy and uncertainty, worried and anxious about impending surgery

Outcome Criteria

Reduced anxiety verbalized and optimism increased as explanations about care and correction of the defect given Verbalizes understanding of cause of anxiety and positive effect of surgical correction

Interventions	Rationales
Assess level of anxiety and need for information that will relieve anxiety	Provides information to ally anxiety manifested by the infant's appearance at birth with level increased with the location and extent of the defect (lip and/or palate defect)
Allow expression of concerns and questions about condition, to discuss negative feelings about appearance of infant	Provides an environment conducive to venting of feelings to facilitate adjustment to the infant's defect
Provide an accepting environment and attitude and handle the infant in a gentle, caring way	Promotes trust and conveys to parent(s) that infant is a valuable human baby deserving of love and caring
Communicate with parent(s) in a calm, honest, way, discuss the surgical procedure(s) for correction of the defect(s) using pictures and models and allow to view pictures of children with successful defect repair	Promotes a calm and supportive environment to reduce anxiety and instill hope
Allow parent(s) to stay with infant and encourage to assist in care as appropriate	Reduces anxiety and promotes bonding that may be blocked by infant's appearance

Interventions	Rationales
Emphasize the infant's positive features when providing information	Promotes positive feelings for infant

Information, Instruction, Demonstration

Interventions	Rationales
Suggest visits with parent(s) who have a child with a similar defect	Provides support and information to reduce anxiety
Inform parent(s) of usual ages for cleft lip repair and/or cleft palate, stages of surgery and type of procedure performed	Provides information to reduce fear and anxiety and to know what to expect

Discharge or Maintenance Evaluation

- Express reduction in anxiety as feelings about defect(s), correction and prognosis are discussed
- Verbalizes positive effect of caring for and supporting infant
- Demonstrates accepting attitude towards infant with progressive adjustment to appearance of defect(s)

Knowledge deficit of parent(s), caretaker

Related to: Lack of information about preoperative care
Defining characteristics: Request for information about cause of defect(s), feeding techniques, prevention of complications caused by defect(s) preoperatively

Outcome Criteria

Absence of aspiration, upper respiratory infection, otitis media resulting from feeding
Feeding techniques modified to maintain nutritional status preoperative
Adequate knowledge acquired regarding cause and type of defect and preoperative preparation

Interventions	Rationales
Assess parent(s) ability to feed infant with a defect and acceptance of methods used, knowledge, cause and type of defect(s), preoperative needs and care, ability of infant to swallow	Provides information about defect which may be inherited or congenital, partial or complete, unilateral or bilateral cleft of lip and/or palate; adequate nutritional status and freedom from infection before surgery done
Instruct parent(s) to hold infant while feeding with the head in an upright position, use a nipple or feeding device for feeding, allow feeder to control the flow or the infant to express the formula, apply gentle, steady pressure on the bottom of the bottle and avoid removing the nipple frequently: instruct in feeding method that will be used postoperatively	Holding head upright reduces possibility of aspiration, pressure at the base of the bottle prevents choking or coughing, special nipples or devices are used because the cleft interferes with the ability to suck and liquid often flows into the nose when taken into the mouth, use of a nipple encourages development of sucking muscles
Instruct to feed slowly and in small amounts, burping frequently (tends to swallow air), and extend nipple or feeding device well back into the mouth	Prevents choking, abdominal distention, possible flow of liquid into nose or aspirated into lungs causing pneumonia or otitis media or upper respiratory infections
Inform parent(s) that feeding should not last any longer than 20-30 minutes	Prolonged feedings may deplete an infant's energy and cause fatigue
Instruct in use and care of preoperative orthodontic device (plastic palate mold) for infant with cleft palate including removing and cleaning daily, replacing, preventing infant from removing palate	Promotes the alignment of maxilla and more normal speech sounds and prevents food from entering nasal cavity
Instruct parent(s) to cleanse lip, oral cavity and nose with water before and after feeding; apply mineral oil to lips	Prevents infection or skin breakdown with cleft lip or palate

Interventions	Rationales
Instruct parent(s) about need to avoid prone position and place child on back or side, use arm restraints, use cup for feeding if palate repair to be done, feed upright if lip repair is to be done for the period preoperatively	Accustoms the child to treatments that will be done postoperatively
Inform parent(s) of procedure for correction of defect(s), medications and procedures done to prepare infant for surgery, what to expect postoperatively	Prepares parent(s) for surgical correction of defect(s) and what to expect during convalescence

Discharge or Maintenance Evaluation

- Verbalizes understanding of defect(s) and preoperative requirements before surgical correction
- Performs safe, effective feeding techniques and maintains nutritional status and weight gains
- Absence of infection or aspiration (upper respiratory, otitis media)
- Maintains clean cleft lip and/or palate
- Verbalizes understanding of need to carry out care and procedures that will be utilized postoperatively

Risk for injury

Related to: Internal physical factor of surgery (broken skin)
Defining characteristics: Trauma to suture line, use of protective device, formula or drainage at suture site, improper mouth care and teeth brushing, hands or other objects in mouth, redness, swelling and drainage from incision site, crying caused by pain of incision, improper feeding method

Outcome Criteria

Suture line free of trauma, accumulation of substances, infection
Sutures intact and healing with protective device in place

Interventions	Rationales
Assess suture line for cleanliness, redness, swelling or drainage	Provides information indicating possible infection and need for cleansing away formula or drainage

Interventions	Rationales
Assess for respiratory distress following palate surgery	Monitors breathing through a smaller airway caused by edema and breathing through nose
Cleanse suture site of lip repair with gauze or cotton tipped applicator with saline, apply medicated ointment after cleansing as prescribed; rinse mouth with water before and after each feeding	Removes material to prevent inflammation or sloughing and final cosmetic result expected
Place in sidelying position, gently aspirate mouth of any secretions; maintain suture at end of tongue if present	Facilitates breathing and prevents aspiration; suture at end of tongue extends tongue to prevent obstruction of airway
Apply warm compresses to suture site on lip if prescribed	Reduces swelling
Provide air humidification or place in mist tent for a short time following surgery	Decreases dry mouth and nose mucous membranes
Monitor lip protective device taped on operative site	Relaxes the site and prevents tension on sutures caused by facial movement or crying
Provide analgesic therapy for pain, hold, cuddle or rock child, anticipate needs to prevent crying	Promotes comfort and prevents crying caused by pain which creates tension on suture line
Apply soft elbow restraints and remove periodically to perform ROM on arms and allow for some movement and holding; a child may need a jacket restraint to prevent rolling over	Prevents child from touching or injuring operative site
Remove sharp objects or toys, avoid use of forks, straws or other pointed objects	Prevents trauma to mouth and suture line
Feed with a cup or spoon if palate repair done; avoid placing spoon in mouth	Prevents damage to suture line
Accompany child when playing or ambulating	Prevents trauma caused by accidental falls

Information, Instruction, Demonstration

Interventions	Rationales
Instruct, parent(s) in cleansing suture site and apply antibiotic ointment	Prevents infection and enhances comfort and healing
Instruct parent(s) in feeding method of infant and allow to practice appropriate technique using a syringe soft tube in mouth away from any suture line or using a cup for older child	Promotes nutrition following surgery without sucking on a nipple
Instruct parent(s) in soft diet inclusions and avoidance of toast, hard cookies or foods	Provides nutritional needs until incision heals completely
Explain to parent(s) and child to keep hands and objects away from mouth or to maintain use of restraints with removal until incision is healed	Prevents trauma to suture line
Advise parent(s) not to allow child to play with small toys or those that are sharp or require sucking or blowing; suggest soft, stuffed toys for infant	Removes possibility of placing toy in mouth or damage incision
Explain to parent(s) that usual feeding patterns may be resumed in 2 weeks for lip repair or in 4-6 weeks for palate repair	Provides estimated times based on suture removal and healing to resume regular bottle feeding or return to baseline dietary status

Discharge or Maintenance Evaluation

- Absence of trauma to incision site
- Surgical incision healing without infection or injury
- Facilitates feeding without trauma to suture line
- Provides comfort measures and pain control
- Verbalizes and demonstrates dietary inclusions and restrictions
- Demonstrates proper positioning and restraining procedures

- Cleanses suture site properly before and after feeding and when needed

Ineffective family coping: Compromised

Related to: Inadequate information and temporary family disorganization caused by defect(s) and future correction
Defining characteristics: Expression of concern about defect(s), long-term care required for successful outcome, confirmation of worry about normal growth and development, limited family support and assistance

Outcome Criteria

Development of family coping skills and support for long-term care of child with a defect correction
Adaptation of family members to child's condition and possible stigma and effect on child body image
Adequate knowledge regarding interdisciplinary approach to therapy

Interventions	Rationales
Assess family coping methods used and their effectiveness, family ability to cope with child that needs long-term care and guidance, stress on family relationships, developmental level of family, perception of crisis situation by family, response of siblings	Provides information identifying coping methods that work and need to develop new coping skills, family attitudes directly affect child's feeling of self-worth, child with special needs may strengthen or strain family relationships
Assess knowledge of long-term treatment of defect(s)	Provides a basis for information needed about therapy
Encourage family members to express problem areas and explore solutions responsibly	Reduces anxiety and enhances understanding; provides opportunity to identify problems and problem solving strategies
Assist family to establish short- and long-term goals for child and importance of integrating child into family activities	Promotes involvement and control over situations and maintains parental role
Encourage to follow home routines and meet child's needs with participation of family members	Increases child's sense of security and sense of belonging

Interventions	Rationales
Give positive feedback to family and praise family efforts in development of coping and problem solving techniques in caring for child	Encourages family to continue involvement in long-term care

Information, Instruction, Demonstration

Interventions	Rationales
Inform parent(s) and family that overprotective behavior may hinder growth and development and to treat the child as normally as it is possible	Enhances family understanding of importance of making child one of the family and adverse affects of overprotection of child
Discuss the long-term treatment of speech therapy, hearing impairment preventions, dental corrections for crossbite or malocclusion or other therapies	Promotes a positive outcome when family collaborates with the health team
Inform parent(s) to observe for hearing deficits and to schedule hearing tests as prescribed	Provides preventative therapy for permanent changes in ear caused by frequent otitis media
Inform parent(s) of importance of care and placement of any device or appliance and instruct in mouth care and teeth brushing to teach child	Provides support to defect area to prevent complications of mouth or dentition development
Inform parent(s) to stimulate speech after sutures removed by playing games, encourage use of words beginning with F, P, S, T, encourage chewing and swallowing of foods	Promotes speech development
Inform family of community agencies, March of Dimes, American Cleft Palate Association	Provides information and support services for families of children with cleft defect

Discharge or Maintenance Evaluation

- Verbalizes and clarifies child's and family's knowledge about long-term needs and rehabilitation following surgery
- Develops and uses coping skills and problem solving techniques effectively
- Supports and cares for child by family members while meeting own needs
- Preserves family relationships and minimizes family stressors with differences resolved
- Implements preventative measures to ensure optimal hearing, speech outcomes
- Progressive adaption and acceptance of long-term disorder and therapy by family
- Contacts community resources for assistance and support

Cleft Lip/Palate

In utero failure of maxillary
processes to fuse with nasal
elevations

↓

Cleft lip malformation

Unilateral   Bilateral

May be associated
with cleft palate

↓

Surgical correction early
in life or delayed for further
facial development
Surgery done before palate
closure

In utero failure of palatine or
processes to fuse with each
other and the primary palate
to form the roof of the mouth

↓

Cleft palate malformation

Isolated defect   Associated with
cleft lip

Midline involvement
of uvula only or
extend through soft
and hard palate

Midline of soft
palate and
extends to
hard palate on
side of cleft lip

Surgical correction later
in life (6 months-5 years)

Gastroenteritis

Gastroenteritis is an acute infectious process affecting the gastrointestinal tract caused by bacteria or viruses. Younger children are most commonly affected with specific organisms found in different age groups. At highest risk are those in daycare centers and schools with immune system abnormalities. The disease is transmitted by ingestion of contaminated food, water, contaminated hands, linens, equipment and supplies. Its most serious complication is dehydration and electrolyte losses which may lead to metabolic acidosis and death.

MEDICAL CARE

Antibiotics: selection depends on identification and sensitivity to organism revealed by culture, whether therapy is prophylactic and term of treatment with use of doxycycline (Vibramycin) in children over 8 years of age.
Stool examination: reveals toxins, culture reveals ova and parasites, specific pathogen for treatment mode.
Electrolyte panel: reveals decreases in electrolyte levels (K) in persistent diarrhea.
Complete blood count: reveals decreased RBC, Act, Hgb with blood loss in persistent diarrhea and inflammation of bowel mucosa; increased WBC in severe infectious process of tract.

NURSING CARE PLANS

Essential nursing diagnoses and plans associated with this condition:

Risk for fluid volume deficit (222)

Related to: Excessive losses through normal routes, NPO status
Defining characteristics: Vomiting, diarrhea, decreased skin turgor, dry skin and mucous membranes, weakness, fever, decreased urinary output, decreased pulse volume, increased pulse rate

Risk for impaired skin integrity (397)

Related to: External factor of excretions and secretions
Defining characteristics: Redness, excoriation at anal site and perineum, presence of persistent diarrhea

Altered nutrition: Less than body requirements (168)

Related to: Inability to ingest and digest foods
Defining characteristics: NPO status, nausea, vomiting, diarrhea, weight loss, anorexia, abdominal cramps

Hyperthermia (112)

Related to: Illness (infectious process)
Defining characteristics: Increase in body temperature above normal range, warm to touch, increased pulse and respirations

Diarrhea (171)

Related to: Dietary intake, contaminants, toxins, inflammation and irritation of bowel
Defining characteristics: Abdominal pain, cramping, increased frequency of bowel sounds, increased frequency, loose, liquid stools, changes in color, urgency

SPECIFIC DIAGNOSES AND CARE PLANS

Knowledge deficiency of parent(s), child

Related to: Lack of information about disease and treatment
Defining characteristics: Request for information about effect and treatment of the disease and preventions of transmission of disease

Outcome Criteria

Evidence of adequate knowledge about disease, transmission and compliance with treatment regimen

Interventions	Rationales
Assess knowledge of causes of types of enteritis, methods to treat and control disease, willingness and interest to implement treatment preventative measures	Promotes effective plan of instruction that is realistic to ensure compliance of medical regimen, prevents repetition of information

Interventions	Rationales
Provide parent(s) and child with information and clear explanations in understandable language, include teaching aids and encourage questions	Ensures understanding based on interest and need to know to promote compliance
Inform to avoid food and fluid (NPO) until diarrhea subsides and when allowed begin with rice cereal, bread, weak tea and progress as tolerated	Allows bowel to rest until foods allowed
Inform that abdominal cramping may occur, that diarrhea may occur after eating or if a new food is offered	Reveals symptom at associated entiritis
Instruct to offer fluids (Pedialyte) and avoid those fluids high in Na (milk, broth)	Provides and replaces fluids and electrolytes lost in frequent diarrheal stools, Na increases removal of fluid from cells by osmosis
Instruct in collection of stool specimen(s) for culture and procedure for stool Guaiac: collect stool specimens from other family members and inform to take to laboratory for examination	Reveals identification of specific organism responsible for enteritis as a basis for treatment and Guaiac test reveals occult blood in stool in severe inflammation of bowel
Instruct in enteric precautions and effective handwashing	Prevents transmission of organisms
Inform to take temperature by axillary method	Prevents additional irritation to rectum
Instruct to avoid over-the-counter drugs to treat diarrhea or vomiting	Prevents use of medications that may exacerbate condition
Demonstrate and instruct to insert antiemetic or sedative suppository	Treats vomiting and additional fluid loss and promotes rest
Instruct to measure I&O and determine imbalance to report	Prevents possible fluid imbalance complication which leads to dehydration
Instruct in antibiotic or other medication administration	Treats disease by organism-specific therapy

Discharge or Maintenance Evaluation

- Stool elimination decreases with return to baseline characteristics
- Disease transmission prevented with effective preventative measures
- Stools free from blood, mucus, infectious organisms
- Absence of fluid and electrolyte imbalance
- Nutritional status returned and maintained

Gastroenteritis

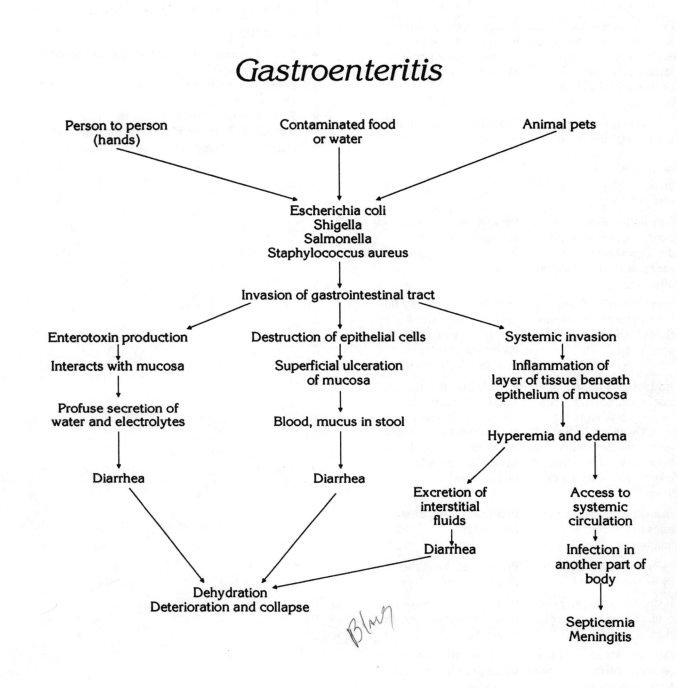

Person to person
(hands)

Contaminated food
or water

Animal pets

Escherichia coli
Shigella
Salmonella
Staphylococcus aureus

Invasion of gastrointestinal tract

Enterotoxin production

Interacts with mucosa

Profuse secretion of
water and electrolytes

Diarrhea

Destruction of epithelial cells

Superficial ulceration
of mucosa

Blood, mucus in stool

Diarrhea

Systemic invasion

Inflammation of
layer of tissue beneath
epithelium of mucosa

Hyperemia and edema

Excretion of
interstitial
fluids

Diarrhea

Access to
systemic
circulation

Infection in
another part of
body

Dehydration
Deterioration and collapse

Septicemia
Meningitis

Gastroesophageal Reflux (GER)

Gastroesophageal reflux (chalasia, cardiochalasia) is the return of gastric contents into the esophagus and possibly the pharynx. It is caused by an incompetent cardiac sphincter at the esophagus-stomach juncture. Reasons for this incompetence include an increase of pressure on the lower esophageal sphincter, following esophageal surgery, impaired local hormonal control mechanisms or immature lower esophageal neuromuscular function. The result of the persistent reflux is inflammation, esophagitis and bleeding causing possible anemia and damage to the structure of the esophagus as scarring occurs. It is also predisposing to aspiration of stomach contents causing aspiration pneumonia and chronic pulmonary conditions. Most commonly affected are infants and young children. As the condition becomes more severe or does not respond to medical treatment and experiences failure to thrive, surgical fundoplication to create a valve mechanism or other procedures may be done to correct the condition.

MEDICAL CARE

Analgesics: acetaminophen (Tylenol) to control reflux pain.
Cholinergics: bethanechol (Urecholine) given PO or SC to increase tone and peristaltic activity of esophagus and promotes gastric emptying: metoclopramide (reglan) given PO to increase tone of esophageal sphincter and lowers esophageal sphincter pressure, cisapride (Propulsid) increases tone and esophagus motility.
H₂ receptor antagonists: cimetidine (Tagumet) given PO to reduce gastric acidity and pepsin secretion.
Antacids: magaldrate (Riopan), aluminum hydroxide (Amphojel) given PO to neutralize gastric acid.
Antiflatulents: simethicone (Mylicon), given PO to break up gas bubbles for easier removal by belching or passing flatus to relieve gastric bloating.
Barium esophagram: reveals reflux of barium into the esophagus under fluoroscopy if done at time reflux occurs.
Manometry: reveals esophageal sphincter pressure of less than 6 mm Hg.

Intraesophageal pH monitoring: reveals pH measurements of the distal esophagus reflux contents.
Gastroesophageal scintigraphy: reveals reflux or aspiration following ingestion of a radioactive compound and scanning the esophagus.
Gastroscopy: endoscopic examination that reveals view of esophagus to not esophagitis or to remove tissue for biopsy.
Complete blood count: reveals decreased RBC, Hgb, Hct in persistent blood loss.

NURSING CARE PLANS

Essential nursing diagnoses and plans associated with this condition:

Altered nutrition: Less than body requirements (168)

Related to: Inability to ingest or digest food because of biological factors
Defining characteristics: Weight loss, vomiting, increased appetite, heartburn (older child), failure to thrive, gastric bloating

Risk for fluid volume deficit (222)

Related to: Excessive losses through normal route
Defining characteristics: Vomiting, diarrhea (postoperatively), decreased urine output, dehydration

Ineffective airway clearance (42)

Related to: Tracheobronchial aspiration and infection
Defining characteristics: Abnormal breath sounds, dyspnea, changes in rate or depth of respirations, fever, cough that is effective or ineffective and with or without sputum

SPECIFIC DIAGNOSES AND CARE PLANS

Risk for aspiration

Related to: Increased intragastric pressure with an incompetent cardiac sphincter
Defining characteristics: Laryngospasm, choking, coughing, apnea, cyanosis, wheezing, pneumonitis

Outcome Criteria

Absence of aspiration with breathing pattern maintained at baseline parameters

Absence of recurrent pulmonary infection

Interventions	Rationales
Assess respiratory status for rate, depth and ease, breath sounds before and after feedings	Provides information about respiratory pattern changes caused by aspiration
Assess vomiting, activity and position before and after feeding	Predisposes to aspiration of contents of reflux which is precipitated by factors associated with feeding
Place in prone position (30 degrees) or in an infant seat or on a reflux board	Maintains upright position to prevent reflux and risk of reflux
Offer frequent, small feedings of thickened formula, maintain upright position (60 degrees) for 1 hour following feedings	Prevents reflux and minimizes symptoms
Administer cholinergics as ordered	Promotes gastric emptying and lowers esophageal sphincter pressure
Have suctioning and O$_2$ equipment at hand	Removes aspirate and promotes airway patency and tissue oxygenation

Information, Instruction, Demonstration

Interventions	Rationales
Inform parent(s) of risk for aspiration and consequences of recurring aspiration associated with the condition	Provides information about potential for complications
Instruct parent(s) in feeding modifications, positions before and after feedings; burp as often as possible	Minimizes risk for reflux and aspiration
Instruct parent(s) in construction of an antireflux saddle, bed elevation or modification, use of foam rubber wedge, sling or in-	Provides optimal positioning to prevent reflux

Interventions	Rationales
fant seat; inform to maintain sitting position when feeding, bathing, diaper change; to carry infant upright with head resting on shoulder	
Inform parent(s) that sucking on pacifier reduces reflux episodes	Clears reflux contents from esophagus
Inform parent(s) to gradually change position from upright to flat when asymptomatic for 2 months	Provides safe return to normal positions without return of symptoms

Discharge or Maintenance Evaluation

- Aspiration absent or minimized with reflux or vomiting episodes
- Absence of recurring pulmonary infection
- Optimal positioning maintained for feeding, rest, bathing, diapering
- Formula modification with cereal added and rescheduling to reduce reflux episode and aspiration risk
- Medication administration with desired effects to control reflux

Risk for injury

Related to: Internal factors (malnutrition, abnormal blood profile)

Defining characteristics: Decreased Hgb with esophageal bleeding leading to anemia, severe reflux disorder leading to failure to thrive

Outcome Criteria

Absence of or minimized occurrence of complications of reflux disorder

Absence of frank or occult blood in vomits or stool

Interventions	Rationales
Assess for severity of reflux, weight loss or gain, failure to thrive, stool and vomit for occult blood	Provides information about complication of esophagitis or esophageal structure, anemia or failure to thrive

Interventions	Rationales
Prepare parent(s) and infant for diagnostic procedures and possible surgical procedure	Reveals severity of reflux and need for surgical interventions
Promote positioning and feeding actions to minimize symptoms	Allows for medical regimen to be tried before surgical interventions

Information, Instruction, Demonstration

Interventions	Rationales
Inform parent(s) that infant usually outgrows the disorder and achieves normal function by 6 weeks of age and those with a continuing problem of reflux usually improve by 6 months of age	Provides reassurance to parent(s) that medical regimen may be successful and complication may not occur
Instruct in performing Guaiac test on stool and vomitus and allow to return demonstration	Reveals presence of occult blood in esophagitis
Inform that severe reflux may require NPO status and nasogastric tube insertion with suction	Prevents distention and continuing reflux activity of stomach contents

Discharge or Maintenance Evaluation

- Absence of complications caused by severe reflux disorder
- Reflux activity minimized by preventative measures
- Diagnostic procedures performed without incident

Anxiety

Related to: Change in health status of infant, possible surgery of infant

Defining characteristics: Increased apprehension that condition might worsen and that surgery be required, expressed concern and worry about impending surgery, pre and postoperative care, gastrostomy and treatments while hospitalized and complications following surgery

Outcome Criteria

Reduced parental anxiety verbalized as disorder resolved by surgery
Verbalizes need of surgery with positive outcome of treatments

Interventions	Rationales
Assess source of level of anxiety and how anxiety is manifested: need for information that will relieve anxiety	Provides information about anxiety level and need for interventions to relieve it; sources for the parent(s) include fear and uncertainty about treatment and recovery, guilt for presence of illness
Allow expression of concerns and ask questions about condition, procedures, recovery surgery by parent(s)	Provides opportunity to vent feelings and fears and secure information to reduce anxiety
Communicate with parent(s) and answer questions calmly and honestly; use pictures, drawings, and models for explanations	Promotes calm and supportive trusting environment
Allow parent(s) to stay with child and encourage to assist in care or open visitation	Allows parent(s) to care for and support child and continue parental role
Give parent(s) as much input in decisions about care and routines as possible	Allows for more control over situation
Provide consistent care of infant with familiar staff assigned for care	Promotes trust and reduces anxiety

Information, Instruction, Demonstration

Interventions	Rationales
Inform parent(s) of disease process, physical effects and symptoms of illness	Provides information to relieve anxiety by knowledge of what to expect
Explain reason for each pre and postoperative procedure or type of therapy,	Reduces fear which decreases anxiety

Interventions	Rationales
apy, diagnostic test, surgical procedure and rationales including IV, N/G tube, dressings and gastrostomy tube	
Inform parent(s) that N/G tube is removed when postoperative ileus is resolved and gastrostomy tube is removed 2 or more weeks after surgery	Reduces anxiety that the tube placements and care evokes
Instruct in care of and feeding via gastrostomy tube and inform of complications of choking, delayed gastric emptying, inability to vomit, gas bloating that may occur following surgery	Information of what to expect will reduce anxiety
Demonstrate and instruct in wound care and dressing changes; allow for return demonstration, inform to protect dressing from diaper	Ensures wound healing without complication of infection or recurrence of infection
Instruct parent(s) in feeding techniques, allowing infant to take a long time to feed and to report any feeding problems	Familiarizes parent(s) with changes in feeding patterns to prevent complications of choking, aspiration
Instruct to report changes in wound indicating infection (redness, swelling, pain, drainage)	Allows for immediate treatment in presence of infectious procedure

Discharge or Maintenance Evaluation

- Expresses reduction in anxiety about illness, preoperative and postoperative care and procedures
- Parent(s) verbalize that anxiety decreases as acute phase is resolved
- Verbalizes positive effect of caring for and supporting ill child
- Participates in care and decision making regarding child
- Demonstrates wound care and dressing changes postoperatively and other procedures to enhance wellness and verbalizes comfort with knowledge and performance of postoperative care with reduced anxiety
- States signs and symptoms to report postoperatively

Gastroesophageal Reflux

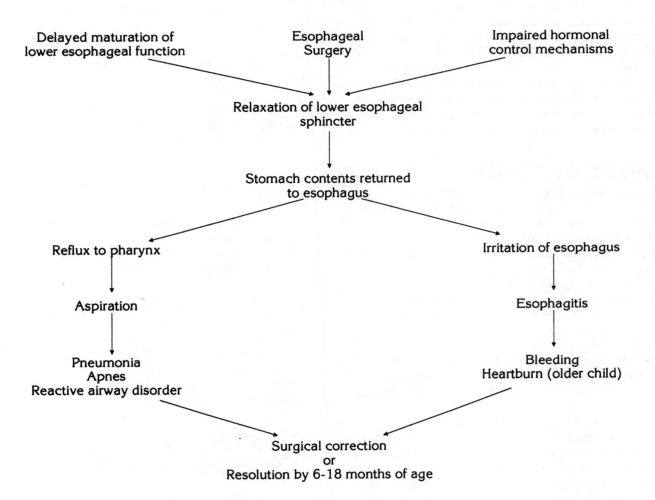

Hepatitis

Hepatitis is the inflammation of the liver caused by a virus. It includes four different types of viruses; namely, hepatitis A (HAV), hepatitis B (HBV), hepatitis D (HDV) and hepatitis non-A, non-B (NANB). Most common of the types found in children is the hepatitis A which is transmitted by the fecal-oral route. The incidence in children is increased in those living in crowded housing or attending daycare centers. The disorder is usually self-limiting with resolution within 2-3 months or may develop into chronic hepatitis. Symptomology varies with severity of the disease.

MEDICAL CARE

Immunizing agents: immune globulin (Gamma globulin) given IM primarily Ig as prophylaxis to provide passive immunity or modify severity of hepatitis A; hepatitis B immune globulin (H-BIG) given IM as prophylaxis after exposure to hepatitis B or to provide passive immunity if exposed to contaminated materials (blood serum); hepatitis B vaccine (Heptavax-B) given IM to immunize against hepatitis B in high risk children (hemodialysis, Down's dyndrome, immunodeficiency diseases, hemophilia).

Metabolic enzymes: alanine aminotransferase (ALT), aspartate aminotranferase (AST), lactic dehydrogenase (LDH) reveals increases as liver damage occurs and cells release enzymes; alkaline phosphatase reveals increase in liver disease.

Immunoglobulins: reveals IgM antibodies indicating hepatitis A virus antibodies for diagnosis of hepatitis A, IgG indicates susceptibility or past exposure to hepatitis A. Hepatitis B suface antigen (HBsAg); titer that reveals antibodies or antigens that are produced in response to hepatitis B and indicates chronic hepatitis B if present longer than 6 months or improvement as the antigen is decreased or disappears.

Bilirubin: reveals increases in indirect bilirubin if liver damaged.

Ammonia: reveals increases in poorly functioning liver.

Protein: reveals increased globulins and decreased albunin.

Prothrombin time: reveals increases in severe liver disease.

Urine urobilinogen: reveals increases in liver disease whether the serum bilirubin level changes or not.

Stool: reveals changes in color if bile is not produced as a result of liver disease.

Bromsulphalein excretion (BSP): reveals the dye in the bloodstream indicating that liver function is impaired and filtration and excretion of the dye is affected.

NURSING CARE PLANS

Essential nursing diagnoses and plans associated with this condition:

Altered nutrition: Less than body requirements (168)

Related to: Inability to ingest, digest food
Defining characteristics: Anorexia, nausea, vomiting, weight loss, fatigue, abdominal discomfort

Risk for fluid volume deficit (222)

Related to: Excessive losses through normal routes
Defining characteristics: Vomiting, diarrhea, reduced intake of fluids, reduced urinary output, signs and symptoms of dehydration, gastrointestinal bleeding

Risk for impaired skin integrity (397)

Related to: External factors of excretions and secretions, internal factor of altered pigmentation
Defining characteristics: Redness, irritation of perianal area with diarrhea, jaundice with pruritis

SPECIFIC DIAGNOSES AND CARE PLANS

Risk for activity intolerance

Related to: Generalized weakness, bed rest
Defining characteristics: Easy fatigue, malaise, preference for inactivity, deconditioning with bedrest

Outcome Criteria

Absence of fatigue with return to baseline activity

Interventions	Rationales
Assess intolerance to activity and manifestations	Provides information about extent of fatigue

Interventions	Rationales
Maintain bed rest while illness is in acute stage but allow for quiet play and progress as condition allows	Allows for time for liver to heal and prevents any further damage
Provide access to needed articles within reach, aids to assist in performing ADL	Preserves energy which improves endurance
Provide increasing activity participation as tolerated on a daily basis	Promotes recovery without compromising energy or causing fatigue

Information, Instruction, Demonstration

Interventions	Rationales
Instruct in a rest and activity schedule which can be adjusted to child's tolerance and allow child to regulate activity at own pace	Provides information to improve activity tolerance without causing fatigue or remission or disease
Inform parent(s) and child of level of activity necessary to return to school	Permits return to normal activity when possible

Discharge or Maintenance Evaluation

- Progresses in activities until baseline achieved
- Complies with activity and rest schedule
- Absence of fatigue and weakness

Knowledge deficit of parent(s), child

Related to: Lack of information about transmission of disease
Defining characteristics: Request for information about spread of disease, measures to take to prevent spread of disease and possible relapse of condition

Outcome Criteria

Spread of disease prevented or controlled
Secondary infection or relapse prevented

Interventions	Rationales
Assess knowledge of disease and isolation precautions to take to prevent transmission	Promotes knowledge and understanding of disease
Instruct parent(s) and child in proper handwash and inform to perform before meals, after using bathroom	Prevents transmission of microorganisms for type A which is carried via the oral-fecal route
Inform parent(s) and child that toys may become contaminated and that they should not be shared	Prevents transmission to others via handling of toys
Inform of need to use disposable gloves when handling blood, excrete any other body fluids	Prevents transmission of microorganisms
Instruct parent(s) to use disposable dishes, wash linens in hot soapy water and rinse well and dry, separate child's personal hygiene articles from other members of household	Prevents transmission of microorganisms to others
Inform parent(s) and child of signs and symptoms of disease, how disease is transmitted, dietary inclusions of protein and carbohydrate, activity program and signs, symptoms of disease recurrence (pain, anorexic fever, nausea and vomiting, jaundice) to report	Provides information about disease and treatments to prevent transmission or relapse
Inform parent(s) of immune globulin available for hepatitis A if given before exposure or after exposure if during early incubation period, or hyperimmune gamma globulin for hepatitis B if given after exposure but reserved for those at risk	Provides information about prophylactic measures available
Inform parent(s) and child to avoid over-the-counter drugs without physician advice	Prevents potential for toxicity if liver is unable to detoxify drugs

Discharge or Maintenance Evaluation

- Verbalizes understanding of disease process and transmission to others
- Performs precautions to prevent transmission of disease to others
- Acquires passive immunization if at risk
- Absence of reinfection or relapse of disease
- Maintains enteric precautions of strict isolation as indicated by type of hepatitis

Hepatitis

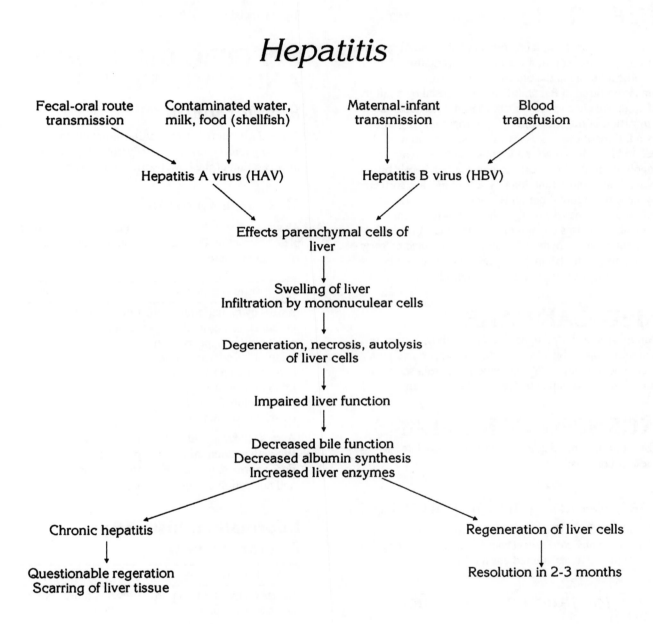

Hernia

A hernia results from a protrusion of abdominal contents through an opening in a weakened musculature. An umbilical hernia is the protrusion of intestine and omentum through the umbilical ring caused by a failure of complete closure after birth. Inguinal hernia is the protrusion of intestine through the inguinal ring caused by a failure of the processus vaginalis to atrophy to close before birth allowing for a hernial sac to form along the inguinal canal. Umbilical hernia usually resolves by 4 years of age; those that don't by school age are corrected by surgery. Inguinal hernia becomes apparent in the infant by 2-3 months of age when intra-abdominal pressure increases enough to open the sac. It is usually associated with a hydrocele. Both are corrected by surgical repair (herniorrhaphy) to prevent obstruction and eventual incarceration of a loop of bowel.

MEDICAL CARE

Analgesics: acetaminophen (Tylenol elixir, Liquiprin solution drops) given PO to reduce postoperative pain.
Herniogram: reveals visualization of hernia sac after injection of a radiopaque dye into the abdomen.

NURSING CARE PLANS

Essential nursing diagnoses and plans associated with these conditions:

Ineffective breathing pattern (45)

Related to: Pain, decreased lung expansion
Defining characteristics: Dyspnea, tachypnea, respiratory depth changes, altered chest excursion

Risk for fluid volume deficit (222)

Related to: Deviations affecting intake of fluids (postoperative status)
Defining characteristics: NPO status, altered intake, signs and symptoms of dehydration, I&O imbalance

Risk for impaired skin integrity (397)

Related to: Surgical incision

Defining characteristics: Disruption of skin surface, invasion of body structures, excreta in diaper contaminating the incision area

SPECIFIC DIAGNOSES AND CARE PLANS

Risk for injury

Related to: Internal factor of intestinal obstruction
Defining characteristics: Irreducible loop of bowel, incarceration of the bowel with complete obstruction

Outcome Criteria

Absence of complication associated with partial or complete obstruction by prompt evaluation and reporting of signs and symptoms

Interventions	Rationales
Assess by palpation for umbilical or inguinal swelling that appears when infant cries or when child strains or coughs, and ability to reduce swelling with gentle compression if bowel forced into sac	Reveals hernia that is reducible
Assess tenderness at hernia site with abdominal distention, anorexia, irritability and defecation changes	Indicates partial or complete obstruction caused by incarceration and strangulation

Information, Instruction, Demonstration

Interventions	Rationales
Instruct parent(s) to report signs and symptoms to physician; inform of reason for disorder and what signs are expected and those that indicate obstruction	Prevents more severe complication of eventual gangrene of bowel
Inform parent(s) of surgical procedure to repair hernia and possible hydrocele and course of progress to expect	Corrects and repairs hernia and hydrocele if present before complication arises

Interventions	Rationales
Inform parent(s) to prevent infant from crying as much as possible; hold and feed when hungry as preventative measures	Prevents bowel from being forced into sac
Instruct in dietary inclusions and restrictions to prevent straining	Modification of diet to prevent constipation, decreased straining and increased intra-abdominal pressure that forces bowel into sac
Inform parent(s) that hernia usually resolves itself and if not, surgery may be required to repair	Provides information regarding prognosis of disorder

Discharge or Maintenance Evaluation

- Bowel contents easily reduced from sac with compression
- Absence of signs and symptoms of partial or complete obstruction
- Preventative measures taken to reduce straining and intra-abdominal pressure
- Verbalizes signs and symptoms to report to physician

Pain

Related to: Biological injuring agent (surgical repair)
Defining characteristics: Irritability in infant, crying, moaning, guarding behavior, verbal descriptor of pain, refusal to move, change in facial expression in child

Outcome Criteria

Postoperative pain relieved or absent

Interventions	Rationales
Assess incision pain and associated symptoms	Provides information about need for analgesic therapy
Administer analgesic appropriate for severity of pain and age	Relieves pain and discomfort caused by incision
Maintain position of comfort	Promotes comfort and reduces pain caused by strain on incision
Support buttocks when lifting or changing position	Prevents strain and pull on incision site

Interventions	Rationales
Apply ice bag to scrotal area if hydrocele corrected and apply scrotal support if applicable	Promotes comfort by decreasing edema
Provide toys, games for quiet play	Promotes diversionary activity to detract from pain

Information, Instruction, Demonstration

Interventions	Rationales
Inform parent(s) to hold infant when feeding or when irritable, burp frequently to remove swallowed air	Reduces strain on incision and promotes comfort
Inform parent(s) to change diapers frequently	Prevents irritation and pain at incision area caused by damp diapers
Explain cause of pain to parent(s) and child and measures taken to relieve it	Promotes understanding of treatments for pain postoperatively

Discharge or Maintenance Evaluation

- Postoperative pain relieved or controlled
- Takes measures to prevent pain postoperatively
- Infant/child rests comfortably with absence of behavioral responses to pain
- Analgesic therapy administered based on severity and age with desired results

Knowledge deficit of parent(s), caretaker

Related to: Lack of knowledge about postoperative care
Defining characteristics: Request for information about activity allowed, wound care, diet, bathing and comfort measures

Outcome Criteria

Evidence of adequate knowledge about compliance with postoperative medical regimen

Interventions	Rationales
Assess knowledge of causes of hernia, surgical procedure performed, willingness and interest to implement treatment regimen	Promotes effective plan of instruction to ensure compliance
Provide parent(s) and child as appropriate with information and clear explanations in understandable language, include teaching aids and encourage questions	Ensures understanding based on learning ability and age
Inform to maintain incision site design until it peels off and to apply diaper so that it does not cover incision or to change it frequently	Maintains dry and clean incision site
Inform to give sponge baths until incision heals	Maintains incision integrity
Hold infant when crying and to feed, activity is not usually restricted; advise child to refrain from lifting, pushing or engaging in strenuous play or gym classes at school	Reduces strain on incision and possible recurrence of hernia
Advise parent(s) to increase and progress diet and fluids baseline achieved	Promotes return to nutritional status without causing gastrointestinal strain on incision
Inform parent(s) that infant usually tolerates surgery well and progresses to wellness without incident and that this condition is one of the most common surgeries in infancy	Provides assurance and comfort to parent(s) in giving care

- Verbalizes comfort in caring for infant/child postoperatively
- Absence of postoperative complications or recurrence of hernia

Discharge or Maintenance Evaluation

- Verbalizes and demonstrates postoperative care including restrictions and progressive return to baselines
- Incision healing, fluid and dietary status maintained, activity monitored according to age

Hernia

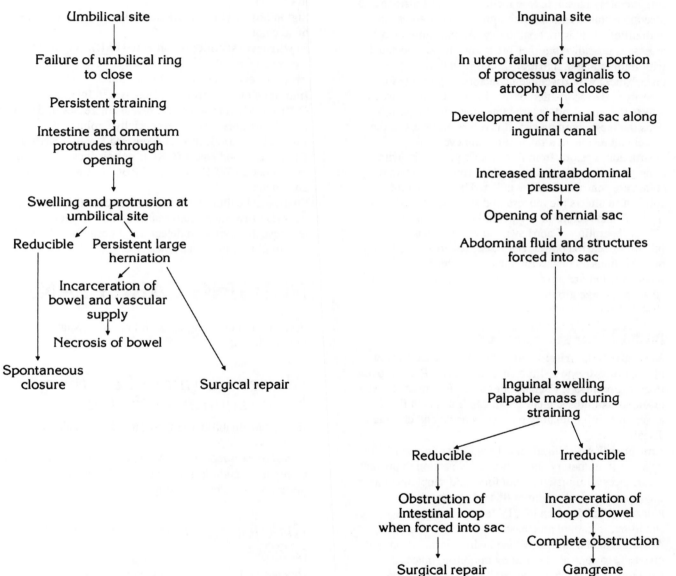

Umbilical site

↓

Failure of umbilical ring
to close

↓

Persistent straining

↓

Intestine and omentum
protrudes through
opening

↓

Swelling and protrusion at
umbilical site

Reducible   Persistent large
herniation

Incarceration of
bowel and vascular
supply

↓

Necrosis of bowel

Spontaneous
closure

Surgical repair

Inguinal site

↓

In utero failure of upper portion
of processus vaginalis to
atrophy and close

↓

Development of hernial sac along
inguinal canal

↓

Increased intraabdominal
pressure

↓

Opening of hernial sac

↓

Abdominal fluid and structures
forced into sac

↓

Inguinal swelling
Palpable mass during
straining

Reducible   Irreducible

Obstruction of
Intestinal loop
when forced into sac

Incarceration of
loop of bowel

↓

Complete obstruction

↓

Surgical repair   Gangrene

Inflammatory Bowel Disease

Inflammatory bowel disease includes Crohn's disease and ulcerative colitis with similar signs and symptoms but with different intestinal pathology. Actual cause of either disease is unknown but they are known to be associated with immunologic, nutritional, and infectious disturbances with psychogenic factors responsible for severity and exacerbation of the disease. Crohn's disease affects the small and/or large intestine with the terminal ileus the most common site. It involves all layers of the bowel and results in a thickening and eventual obstruction. Lesions from this disease are patchy with areas of normal tissue while lesions from ulcerative colitis are continuous in the affected bowel. Ulcerative colitis also affects the mucosa and submucosa of the large intestine and rectum in a hyperemia and edema of which effects absorption of nutrients and eventually a narrowed, inflexible, scarred bowel. Both diseases are characterized by remissions and exacerbations and occur in children of school age but are most commonly found in the adolescence age group.

MEDICAL CARE

Anti-inflammatories: hydrocortisone (Cortisol) given PO; hydrocortisone sodium succinate (Solu-Cortef) given IM, IV; prednisone (Delatasone) given PO: methylprednisolone sodium succinate (Solu-Medrol) given IM, IV, to suppress inflammatory process in acute and chronic disease.

Anti-infectives: sulfasalazine (Azulfidine) given PO for its anti-inflammatory and anti-infective action to prevent recurrences administered with folic acid supplement as it interferes with utilization of this substance; metronidazole (Flagyl) given PO, IV to treat perianal condition, intestinal amebiasis.

Antidiarrheals: diphenoxylate hydrochloride (Lomotil) given PO to control diarrhea by inhibiting mucosal receptors responsible for peristaltic reflex to reduce motility.

Anticholinergics: propantheline bromide (Pro-Banthine) given PO to control diarrhea by reducing smooth muscle contraction in the intestinal tract.

Analgesics: codeine (Methylmorphine) given PO to control pain.

Gastrointestinal x-ray (Barium enema): reveals colon abnormalities.

Gastrointestinal x-ray (Barium swallow): reveals small intestine abnormalities.

Colonoscopy: reveals view of colon abnormalities such as intermittent mucosa involvement, mucusal erosion, cobblestoning, granularity.

Bowel biopsy: taken during colonoscopy or sigmoidoscopy at different sites reveals bowel pathology especially in Crohn's.

Sigmoidoscopy: reveals abnormalities in rectum, sigmoid colon.

Erythrocyte sedimentation rate (ESR): reveals increases in Crohn's.

Protein: reveals decreases in albumin.

Immunoglobulins: reveals decreases in IgG, IgA.

C-Reactive protein (CRP): reveals increases in presence of inflammatory disorder, especially Crohn's.

Electrolyte panel: reveals decreased K with diarrhea.

Complete blood count (CBC): reveals increased with inflammation WBC, decreased RBC, Hct with blood loss and anemia.

Stool: fecal culture reveals presence of pathologic organisms that may cause diarrhea; fecal analysis for fat content reveals absorption defect; fecal occult blood reveals bleeding from intestinal tract.

NURSING CARE PLANS

Essential nursing diagnoses and plans associated with this condition:

Altered nutrition: Less than body requirements (168)

Related to: Inability to ingest and digest food, absorb nutrients

Defining characteristics: Anorexia, diarrhea, abdominal cramping, weight loss, growth retardation, abdominal distention, possible vomiting

Risk for fluid volume deficit (222)

Related to: Excessible losses through normal routes

Defining characteristics: Diarrhea, output greater than intake, signs and symptoms of dehydration, electrolyte imbalance (K)

Diarrhea (171)

Related to: Irritation, or malabsorption of bowel, dietary intake

Defining characteristics: Abdominal pain, cramping, increased frequency, increased frequency of bowel sounds, loose, liquid, watery stools, urgency, changes in color and constituents (blood, mucus), ingestion of high fiber foods

Risk for impaired skin integrity (397)

Related to: External factor of secretions and excretions, internal factor of extra-intestinal skin lesions

Defining characteristics: Irritation, redness, pain at perianal area, disruption of skin surfaces, chronic and excessive diarrhea

Altered growth and development (419)

Related to: Effects of physical disability

Defining characteristics: Altered physical growth, delay in sexual maturation, delay in bone age, weight loss, school absences during exacerbations

SPECIFIC DIAGNOSES AND CARE PLANS

Pain

Related to: Biological injuring agents, inflammation and irritation of the bowel

Defining characteristics: Abdominal cramping, abdominal distention, intermittent pain aggravated by eating or pain that is constant and aching, verbalization of other pain descriptors, guarding and protective behavior towards abdomen

Outcome Criteria

Relief and control of severe pain symptoms with treatment

Interventions	Rationales
Assess severity of pain, onset and precipitating factors, location, duration, remissions and exacerbations	Provides information symptomatic of inflammatory bowel disease with pain common in Crohn's disease and less frequent in ulcerative colitis; pain is associated with dietary intake in both diseases
Administer analgesics, antispasmodics and anti-inflammatories and assess effect of medications in relieving discomfort	Relieves pain, bowel activity and the inflammatory process associated with pain
Allow to assume position of comfort	Promotes comfort to reduce pain
Provide toys, TV, book, games for quiet play during painful episodes	Promotes diversionary activity to detract from pain

Information, Instruction, Demonstration

Interventions	Rationales
Instruct child in relaxation exercises and guided imagery, use of music for relaxation	Provides child with methods to control discomfort by diversion
Explain cause of pain to child and measures taken to relieve pain	Provides information for understanding of condition and reasons for treatments and medication
Inform child of factors that exacerbate pain episodes and to express presence of pain at onset	Promotes opportunity to avoid those foods or stressful situations that contribute to pain and provides for immediate relief

Discharge or Maintenance Evaluation

- Pain relieved or controlled
- Limits or avoids factors that initiate or increase pain
- Analgesic therapy administration based on severity of pain and age with desired result
- Participates in self-concept (body image), change in health status

Anxiety of child

Related to: Threat to self-concept (body image), change in health status

Defining characteristics: Expressed fear and uncertainty, feelings of inadequacy among peer group, feeling of helplessness about consequences, delayed growth and sexual maturation, feeling of being different or frequency of being ill, school absences, ongoing dietary restrictions, presence of a colostomy if colectomy performed

Outcome Criteria

Verbalized reduction in anxiety
Acceptance by family and child of a more positive attitude about the chronicity, long-term nature of disease process and treatments

Interventions	Rationales
Assess level of anxiety of child and how it is manifested; the need for information that will relieve anxiety	Provides information about source and level of anxiety and need for interventions to relieve it; sources for the child may be procedures, fear of mutilation or death, unfamiliar environment of hospital and may be manifested by restlessness, inability to play or sleep or eat, clinging, aggression, withdrawal
Assess possible need for special counseling services for child	Reduces anxiety and supports child dealing with a long-term illness and promotes adjustment to lifestyle changes
Allow expression of concerns about illness and procedures and treatments	Provides opportunity to vent feelings and fears to reduce anxiety
Communicate with child at appropriate age level and answer questions calmly and honestly; use pictures, models and drawings for explanations	Promotes understanding and trust
Allow child as much input in decisions about care and routines as possible	Allows for more control and independence in situations

Information, Instruction, Demonstration

Interventions	Rationales
Inform child of disease process, physical effects, signs and symptoms of disease	Provides information to promote understanding and relieve anxiety

Interventions	Rationales
Explain reason for each procedure or type of therapy, diagnostic tests and what to expect	Reduces fear of unknown which evokes anxiety

Discharge or Maintenance Evaluation

- Expresses reduction in anxiety as a result of information
- Participates in self-care and decision-making regarding care
- States reason for anxiety and behavior

Impaired adjustment

Related to: Disability requiring change in lifestyle, inadequate support systems
Defining characteristics: Verbalization of nonacceptance of health status change, unsuccessful in ability to be involved in problem solving, lack of movement towards independence

Outcome Criteria

Progressive adaptation to change in lifestyle
Utilization of support systems for assistance with changed health status

Interventions	Rationales
Assess for ability of child and family to adapt, willingness of family and child to support medical regimen and need to change lifestyle, ability to problem solve and utilize coping mechanisms	Provides information about ability of family and child to modify lifestyle, make plans for a constructive lifestyle within limits imposed by change in health status
Encourage to identify strengths and roles of family and child, coping mechanisms that have been successful in the past, resources and support groups available	Allows for support needed to manage long-term illness of child
Assist child and family to develop a health care regimen by making decisions regarding care, sharing goals and progress, accepting accountability for specific aspects of care	Promotes independence and control over care and situations

Interventions	Rationales
Assist child and family to deal with denial behavior and to differentiate between denial of change in health status and denial of limits imposed by change in health status	Permits realistic lifestyle changes that are congruent with health status changes
Maintain a positive, hopeful attitude about lifestyle changes accomplished to promote health	Promotes maximal use of personal resources and acceptance of support systems

Information, Instruction, Demonstration

Interventions	Rationales
Provide information about disease process, treatment, potential disability, prognosis	Promotes understanding of disease and effect on lifestyle
Inform family and child of importance of adhering to medical regimen including medication administration, dietary restrictions and inclusions, rest requirements over an extended period of time even if symptoms have decreased or been eliminated	Promotes compliance to prevent exacerbation of episodes
Inform and prepare child and family for colostomy or ileostomy surgery if indicated and emphasize the positive aspects of such a surgery and possibility of fairly normal life regardless of bowel diversion (permanent recovery, normal growth and sexual development)	Provides information that may begin to lead to acceptance of change in bowel elimination
Inform of resources such as insurance assistance (government and private, support groups, social services, colitis and Ileitis Foundation, United Ostomy Association	Assists family and child to seek out support and information over long period of time for current treatment development and research and economic and psychological assistance

Discharge or Maintenance Evaluation

- Modifies lifestyle within limitations
- Maximizes strengths and resources towards acceptance and adjustment of lifestyle changes
- Demonstrates self-care and independence in health care
- Accepts responsibility and need for involvement and cooperation by family and child
- Verbalizes progress towards acceptance of health status (including ostomy if present)
- Utilizes social services, dietary consult, community agencies and resources if appropriate
- Complies with medication and dietary regimen

Knowledge deficit of parent(s), child

Related to: Lack of information about long-term medical regimen
Defining characteristics: Request for information about medication, dietary regimen, care of colostomy or ileostomy

Outcome Criteria

Knowledge of continuing care to control disease process that will result in reduction or elimination of signs and symptoms
Adequate knowledge of care required for bowel diversion

Interventions	Rationales
Assess parent(s) and child for knowledge of prescribed medical regimen and postoperative care if applicable	Provides information of learning needs of parent(s) and/or child
Instruct in special nutritional needs including diet that is high in protein and calories and low in fat and fiber	Provides replacement of nutritional losses caused by the disease and to promote metabolic function and energy levels
Inform that mouth care before meals and bland foods should be encouraged if mouth pain is present	Promotes comfort if stomatitis present

Interventions	Rationales
Instruct in long-term administration of anti-inflammatories, anti-spasmodics, folic acid supplement including actions, dosages during acute and chronic stages, frequency, times, side effects, effect of discontinuing a steroid without tapering, signs and symptoms to report	Ensures compliance with medication regimen to reduce exacerbations
Instruct and demonstrate and allow for return demonstration for ostomy care including, application and removal of appliance peristomal skin care, emptying and cleansing of ostomy bag, odor control; continent ileostomy care and catheterization of the pouch	Promotes independence in ostomy care with as normal a return to activities as possible; procedure done if child does not respond to medical treatment
Inform of nasogastric tube feedings or total parenteral nutrition if required	Provides information about alternate methods of nutritional support during acute state of disease

Discharge or Maintenance Evaluation

- Complies with medication and dietary regimen
- Demonstrates safe, effective ostomy care
- Maintains long-term remission

Inflammatory Bowel Disease

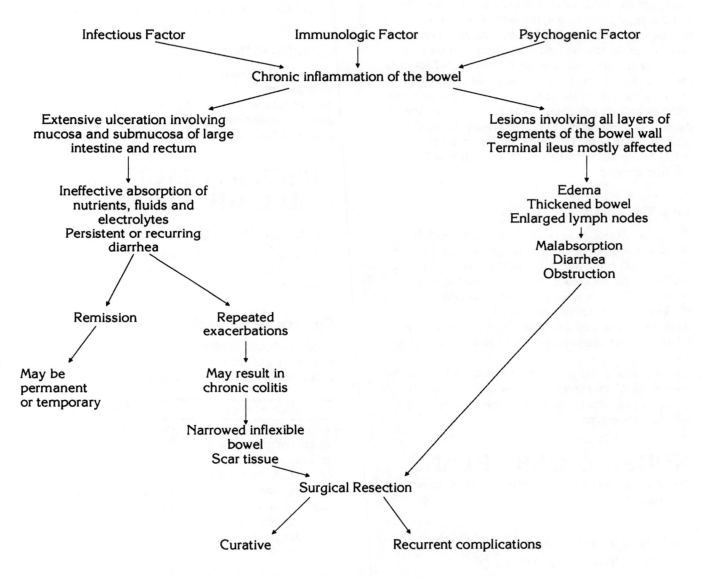

Infectious Factor   Immunologic Factor   Psychogenic Factor

Chronic inflammation of the bowel

Extensive ulceration involving mucosa and submucosa of large intestine and rectum

Lesions involving all layers of segments of the bowel wall
Terminal ileus mostly affected

Ineffective absorption of nutrients, fluids and electrolytes
Persistent or recurring diarrhea

Edema
Thickened bowel
Enlarged lymph nodes

Malabsorption
Diarrhea
Obstruction

Remission

Repeated exacerbations

May be permanent or temporary

May result in chronic colitis

Narrowed inflexible bowel
Scar tissue

Surgical Resection

Curative   Recurrent complications

Intussusception

Intussusception is a telescoping of one section of the bowel into another section resulting in obstruction to passage of the intestinal contents and in inflammation and decreased blood flow to the parts of the walls that are pressing against one another. If left untreated, eventual necrosis, perforation and peritonitis occurs. It occurs in infants most commonly between 3-12 months of age or in children 12-24 months of age. The actual cause is unknown but risk for the condition increased in children with Meckel's diverticulum, celiac disease, cystic fibrosis, diarrhea or constipation. Surgical correction is done if the obstruction of the involved segment cannot be reduced manually or by barium enema or if bowel becomes necrotic.

MEDICAL CARE

Analgesics (narcotic analgesics): codeine (Methylmorphine), morphine sulfate (MS) given SC, IN preoperatively before diagnostic test or postoperatively for pain.
Analgesics (non-narcotic analgesics): acetaminophen (Tylenol tablets, elixir, Liquiprin solution or drops) given PO for moderate pain postoperatively.
Antibiotics: ampicillin sodium (SK-Ampicillin-N) given IV, IM or other anti-infectives to prevent or treat peritonitis.
Lower gastrointestinal x-ray: barium enema reveals an obstruction which prevents the flow of barium into the colon; may be done to reduce the telescoping bowel by hydrostatic pressure.

NURSING CARE PLANS

Essential nursing diagnoses and plans associated with this condition:

Altered nutrition: Less than body requirements (168)

Related to: Inability to ingest and digest foods
Defining characteristics: Vomiting, abdominal pain, NPO status, N/G tube pre and postoperatively

Risk for fluid volume deficit (222)

Related to: Excessive losses through normal routes
Defining characteristics: Vomiting, decreased urine output, altered intake with NPO status, signs and symptoms of dehydration or electrolyte imbalance

Constipation (173)

Related to: Medications, diagnostic procedure using barium enema
Defining characteristics: Hard formed, barium colored stools, decreased bowel sounds, less frequent passage of stools and flatus, abdominal discomfort

SPECIFIC DIAGNOSES AND CARE PLANS

Risk for injury

Related to: Internal factor of bowel function
Defining characteristics: Severe abdominal pain, bowel obstruction

Outcome Criteria

Absence of complication associated with obstruction by reporting signs and symptoms to allow correction by hydrostatic reduction of bowel invagination

Interventions	Rationales
Assess presence of acute abdominal pain with loud crying and drawing knees up to chest which may be episodic, vomiting, passage of a brown stool followed by red, currant jelly-like stool, pallor, irritability	Provides information that indicates that intussusception is present which may lead to obstruction and signs of peritonitis if not treated
Assess presence of diarrhea, constipation, episodes of vomiting and colic in older child	Indicates presence of intussusception and need for further evaluation
Provide N/G tube attached to suction, IV fluids to decompress bowel and maintain hydration status and maintain patency of therapy	Prevents vomiting and dehydration and prepares child for barium enema procedure to diagnose and reduce the invagination

Interventions	Rationales
Note bowel elimination and stool characteristics and ability to eliminate barium following the procedure	Indicates success of the procedure in reducing the affected bowel as the condition may recur within 36 hours
Provide reassurance to parent(s) and allow to accompany child during procedure	Promotes trust and reduces anxiety
Provide information about all care given and allow for opportunity to ask questions about procedures	Reduces anxiety

Information, Instruction, Demonstration

Interventions	Rationales
Inform parent(s) of reasons for IV and N/G tube, NPO status	Provides information about treatments for understanding and reduction of anxiety
Inform parent(s) that surgical reduction may be necessary if barium enema does not reduce the invagination	Prepares parent(s) for possibility of surgical correction
Inform parent(s) that child will be hospitalized for 3 days for the reduction	Provides opportunity to observe child following procedure for recurrence of problem
Inform parent(s) of surgical reduction by reinforcing information given by physician and possibility of temporary colostomy if resection of a portion of bowel is indicated	Provides information about surgery intervention if barium enema reduction not successful or if bowel obstruction and gangrene is present

Discharge or Maintenance Evaluation

- Invagination reduced by barium enema procedure
- Bowel pattern returned to normal with passage of brown stools
- Absence of signs and symptoms of bowel obstruction
- Monitoring of chronic intussusception and reporting signs and symptoms as they occur

Knowledge deficit of parent(s), caretaker

Related to: Lack of information about condition
Defining characteristics: Request for information about causes of condition, postoperative or postprocedural care

Outcome Criteria

Evidence of adequate knowledge about compliance with postoperative or postprocedural care
Complications prevented and reported if present

Interventions	Rationales
Assess knowledge of condition, causes, treatment regimen following procedure(s), willingness and interest in providing care and comply with treatment regimen	Promotes development of effective plan of instruction to ensure compliance and wellness
Provide parent(s) with information and clear explanation in understandable language, include aids in teaching and encourage questions	Ensures understanding of care needs based on ability to learn
Inform parent(s) of signs and symptoms of incision infection and demonstrate and allow for return demonstration of dressing change	Promotes awareness of signs and symptoms to report to treat complication of wound infection
Inform to report any blood in stool, change in stool characteristics or diarrhea or constipation or absence of stools	Indicates gastrointestinal bleeding and possible recurrence or chronicity of condition
Inform parent(s) of reason for preparation procedures for reduction by barium enema or surgery and antibiotic and postoperative care given to child	Provides information regarding care to expect during hospitalization
Inform parent(s) that child will be NPO and when advisable, will be offered clear fluids and slowly progress to usual diet	Prevents vomiting or abdominal distention until condition resolved

Interventions	Rationales
Inform parent(s) of activity restrictions	Allows condition and/or wound to heal and resolve itself without complications
Inform parent(s) that bowel elimination of brown stools indicate that condition has been corrected	Provides parent(s) with baseline expected with successful resolution of problem

Discharge or Maintenance Evaluation

- Verbalizes and demonstrates competence in postoperative or postprocedural care
- Verbalizes baselines that are expected with the appropriate care
- Return of fluid, dietary, activity within limitations progressively as instructed
- Absence of complications or recurrence of invagination of bowel
- Compliance with monitoring of sign and symptoms indicating a complication that should be reported

Intussusception

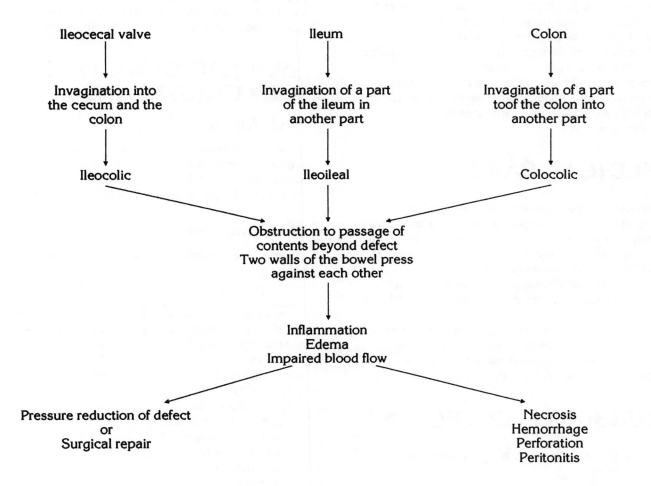

Ileocecal valve

Invagination into
the cecum and the
colon

Ileocolic

Ileum

Invagination of a part
of the ileum in
another part

Ileoileal

Colon

Invagination of a part
toof the colon into
another part

Colocolic

Obstruction to passage of
contents beyond defect
Two walls of the bowel press
against each other

Inflammation
Edema
Impaired blood flow

Pressure reduction of defect
or
Surgical repair

Necrosis
Hemorrhage
Perforation
Peritonitis

Pyloric Stenosis

Pyloric stenosis is a hypertrophic disorder of the circular muscle of the pylorus in which the pylorus is greatly enlarged and hyperplasic causing progressive narrowing of the canal between the stomach and duodenum. As the canal becomes obstructed over time, associated inflammation and edema results in complete obstruction. The exact cause is unknown although heredity is suspected. The abnormality is most common in young children between 1-6 months of age. Pyloric obstruction is treated successfully with surgical correction (pyloromyotomy).

MEDICAL CARE

Analgesics (narcotic analgesics): codeine (Methylmorphine) given SC, IM postoperatively for pain control.
Analgesics (non-narcotic analgesics): acetaminophen (Tylenol elixir, liquiprin solution and drops) given PO postoperatively for moderate pain.
Upper gastrointestinal x-ray: reveals delayed gastric emptying with an elongated canal between stomach and duodenum.
Ultrasound: reveals narrowed canal between stomach and duodenum without the use of barium swallow.
Electrolyte panel: reveals increased Hgb, Hct as hemoconcentration occurs with fluid depletion.

NURSING CARE PLANS

Essential nursing diagnoses and plans associated with this condition:

Risk for fluid volume deficit (222)

Related to: Excessive losses through normal routes, NPO status pre and postoperatively
Defining characteristics: Vomiting with an eventual projectile character, electrolyte losses, signs and symptoms of dehydration, hemoconcentration, decreased urine output

Altered nutrition: Less than body requirements (168)

Related to: Inability to ingest, digest food
Defining characteristics: Excessive vomiting especially after eating, chronic hunger, weight loss, failure to gain weight, diminished stools, abdominal distention, N/G tube pre and postoperatively for stomach decompression

SPECIFIC DIAGNOSES AND CARE PLANS

Risk for injury

Related to: Internal factor of pyloric obstruction
Defining characteristics: Vomiting that increases in severity leading to dehydration, hunger, weight loss and reduction in frequency and amount of bowel elimination

Outcome Criteria

Absence of or correction of fluid and nutritional deficits before surgery

Interventions	Rationales
Assess pattern of vomiting, development of projectile vomiting, vomiting that occurs after feeding or hours after feeding, weight loss, diminished stools, palpable mass in the epigastrium to the right of the umbilicus, presence of visible gastric peristaltic waves across the epigastrium	Provides information about presence of hypertrophic pyloric stenosis causing obstruction as the canal to the duodenum narrows
Maintain NPO status and N/G tube connected to suction, position with head slightly elevated	Decompresses stomach for 24-36 hours in preparation for surgery
Assess skin for decreased turgor, elasticity, loss of subcutaneous tissue, sunken eyeballs, urinary output	Provides information about the presence of dehydration caused by excessive vomiting
Maintain IV fluids and electrolytes (Na, K, Ca, Cl), glucose for nutritional support	Provides hydration and replaces lost glycogen stores and electrolytes for 24-36 hours in preparation for surgery or when needed

Interventions	Rationales
Weigh daily at same time on same scale	Reveals losses or gains related to fluid and nutritional

Information, Instruction, Demonstration

Interventions	Rationales
Inform parent(s) of diagnostic tests and procedures done and reason for them	Provides information needed to reduce anxiety
Inform parent(s) of importance of emphasis on fluid and nutritional replacements to decrease surgical risk	Promotes understanding of all preoperative care

Discharge or Maintenance Evaluation

- Absence of dehydration, electrolyte imbalance
- Adequate nutritional support maintained with vomiting controlled
- N/G and IV tubes patent
- Preoperative preparation complete with restoration of hydration, electrolytes, depleted protein stores

Anxiety

Related to: Change in health status of infant, surgical correction of condition

Defining characteristics: Increased apprehension and expressed concern and worry about impending surgery, pre and postoperative care, treatments while hospitalized and complications following surgery

Outcome Criteria

Reduced parental anxiety verbalized as disorder resolved by surgery and infant improves
Verbalizes understanding of need for surgery with an expected positive outcome

Interventions	Rationales
Assess source and level of anxiety and how anxiety is manifested; need for information that will relieve anxiety	Provides information about anxiety level and need for interventions to relieve it; sources for the parent(s) include fear and uncertainty about treatment and recovery, guilt for presence of illness
Allow expression of concerns and ask questions about condition, procedures, recovery surgery by parent(s)	Provides opportunity to vent feelings and fears and secure information to reduce anxiety
Communicate with parent(s) and answer questions calmly and honestly; use pictures, drawings, and models for explanations	Promotes calm and supportive trusting environment
Allow parent(s) to stay with child and encourage to assist in care and feeding or open visitation	Allows parent(s) to care for and support child and continue parental role
Give parent(s) as much input in decisions about care and routines as possible	Allows for more control over situation
Provide consistent care of infant with familiar staff assigned for care	Promotes trust and reduces anxiety

Information, Instruction, Demonstration

Interventions	Rationales
Inform parent(s) of disease process, physical effects and symptoms of illness	Provides information to relieve anxiety by knowledge of what to expect
Explain reason for each pre and postoperative procedure or type of therapy, diagnostic tests, surgical procedure and rationales including IV, N/G tube, dressings that will be in place	Reduces fear which decreases anxiety
Inform parent(s) surgical procedure done (pyloromyotomy) and that this is standard treatment to correct the disorder and is usually safe and effective	Reduces anxiety and concern about surgery and outcome
Demonstrate and instruct parent(s) in wound care and dressing changes and allow for return demon-	Ensures wound healing without complication of infection

Interventions	Rationales
stration; apply and pin diaper low or use a urine collecting system to maintain dry dressing and wound	
Instruct parent(s) in reporting redness, swelling, drainage at wound site	Indication that infectious process is present
Instruct parent(s) in feeding after N/G tube removed and allow to feed clear liquids slowly and frequently and progress to formula or breast milk expressed by mother or to limit nursing to 5 minutes and gradually increase until previous pattern established	Promotes comfort and bonding with infant with continuation of parenting role until feeding pattern returns; prevents overdistention of stomach and vomiting
Instruct parent(s) to hold infant upright and use nipple that does not flow too rapidly, burp frequently and place on right side or abdomen after feeding	Facilitates feeding postoperatively and prevents vomiting and possible aspiration
Inform parent(s) to sponge bathe infant until incision heals	Promotes comfort and cleanliness of infant

Discharge or Maintenance Evaluation

- Expresses reduction in anxiety about illness, preoperative and postoperative care and procedures
- Parent(s) verbalize that anxiety decreases as acute phase is resolved
- Verbalizes positive effect of caring for and supporting ill child
- Participates in care and decision making regarding child care
- Demonstrates wound care and dressing changes postoperatively and other procedures to enhance wellness and verbalizes comfort with knowledge and performance of postoperative care with reduced anxiety
- State signs and symptoms to report postoperatively
- Complies with a progressive postoperative feeding regimen successfully with weight gain and absence of vomiting

Pyloric Stenosis

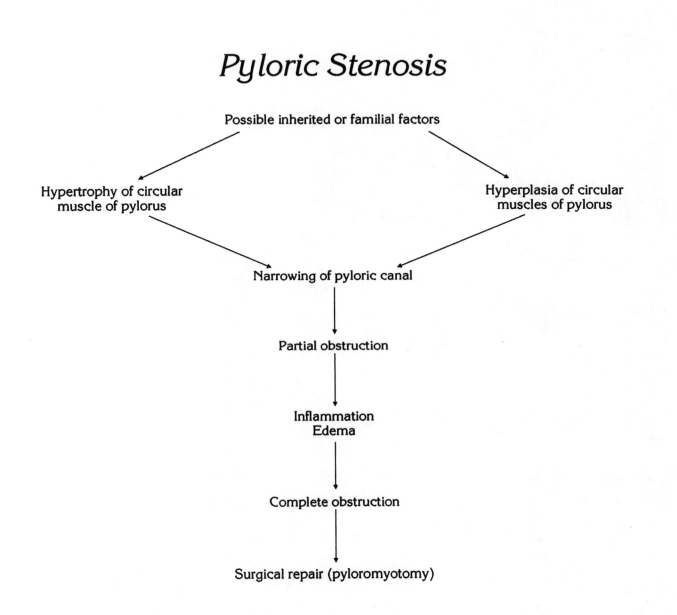

Possible inherited or familial factors

Hypertrophy of circular
muscle of pylorus

Hyperplasia of circular
muscles of pylorus

Narrowing of pyloric canal

Partial obstruction

Inflammation
Edema

Complete obstruction

Surgical repair (pyloromyotomy)

Renal/Urinary System

Renal/Urinary System

The urinary system comprises the kidneys, ureters, urinary bladder and urethra. The urinary system is categorized into two tracts: the upper tract (kidneys and ureters) and the lower tract (urinary bladder and urethra). The kidneys regulate fluid and electrolytes, body pH, and excretion of the end products of protein metabolism (urea). This is accomplished by urine formation, and tubular reabsorption and secretion in response to body's requirements for water and electrolyte balance. Another kidney function is the production of enzymes (erythropoietin stimulating factor and renin) which acts to stimulate red blood cell production in the bone marrow and produce angiotensin to increase blood pressure and stimulate aldosterone production. The urinary bladder and urethra provide for the storage and drainage of urine after passage from the kidneys via the ureters. Disease involving the upper and lower urinary tract are common in children and affect urinary excretion by causing inflammation, damage and scarring of tissue and dysfunction of the organs or structures of the organs. These structural or functional abnormalities may obstruct urine flow and cause renal disorders although obstruction in children may also be a result of a congenital malformation and lead to chronic renal damage and failure. Although the system functions the same as in an adult, the functional deficiency in the infant/child's kidney ability to concentrate urine affects its handling of fluid and electrolyte fluctuations, and increases proneness to dehydration states when the body is stressed by disease. With growth and maturity of the system, the renal/urinary organs progressively function within adult parameters.

GENERAL RENAL/URINARY CHANGES ASSOCIATED WITH PHYSICAL GROWTH AND DEVELOPMENT

Renal and urinary organ structure/anatomy

- Kidney size of infant is three times proportionately larger than adult size

- Number of nephrons increase until one year of age with continued maturation of the nephrons throughout development of the young child
- Tubules and glomeruli continue to form and enlarge after birth; tubular length of nephrons is highly variable but glomeruli size is less variable; tubular length increases until 3 months of age
- The loop of Henle is short in the infant which affects ability to reabsorb water and sodium causing urine to be dilute
- The length of the urethra in children is proportionately shorter according to their growth and age
- The urinary bladder increases in size with growth and development and is considered an abdominal organ in infancy; it becomes a pelvic organ with growth
- Urinary output and bladder capacity increases with growth:

Infant:	350-550 ml/24 hr
Child:	500-1000 ml/24 hr
Adolescent:	700-1400 ml/24 hr

Growth and developmental changes to structure and function of the renal system

- Glomerular filtration and absorption values are reached between 1-2 years of age
- Kidneys' ability to concentrate urine at 3 months of age with urea synthesis and excretion reaching adult levels by this time; by age 2, urine is concentrated at the adult level
- Excretion of water and hydrogen ion is reduced during infancy and excretion of sodium is also reduced during the first month of life with an inefficient reabsorption of sodium
- Volume of urinary output varies with age:

Infant:	5-10 ml/hr
10 yr old:	10-25 ml/hr

- Number of voidings/day vary but decrease with age as urine becomes more concentrated
- Voluntary control of urethral sphincter achieved between 18-24 months of age with night control of bladder usually achieved by 3 years of age; by 4 years of age, bladder capacity reaches 250 ml which allows child to remain dry at night
- The amount of total body water varies with age, growth, sex and decreases as the child grows and develops

Birth:	75-80% of weight
3 yr old:	63% of weight
12 yr old:	58% of weight

- The amount of extracellular fluid changes with age, growth and development with decreases of 45% to 27% in the first year of life, and with the gradual change in water distribution as cells will increase intracellular fluid volume with increased muscle growth, organ size and decrease of secretions into the gastrointestinal tract
- The infant and young child have greater intake and output relative to size than older children, and water loss or decreased intake are more likely to cause dehydration as this age group are more vulnerable to fluid and electrolyte alterations
- The increased amount of extracellular fluid results in a high water turnover (50% of the extracellular fluid is exchanged daily) and higher tendency to develop dehydration
- Water loss through respirations, increased metabolism is greater in children; the greater surface area increases water loss through the skin
- Acid-base balance is maintained by a buffer system that is less mature in children
- The newborn is at risk of developing severe metabolic acidosis due: hydrogen ion excretion is reduced, acid secretion is lower for the first year of life, plasma bicarbonate levels are low, and the inability to excrete a water load at rates similar to the adult
- Sodium excretion is reduced in the immediate newborn period, and the kidneys are less able to adapt to deficiencies and excesses of sodium
- Infants have a diminished capacity to reabsorb glucose and during the first few days of life, to produce ammonium ions

ESSENTIAL NURSING DIAGNOSES AND CARE PLANS

Risk for fluid volume deficit

Related to: Excessive losses through normal routes
Defining characteristics: Vomiting, diarrhea, excessive renal excretion, dry skin and mucous membranes, weight loss, decreased urinary output, altered intake, sunken fontanels in infant, decrease of tears and saliva, sunken soft eyeballs
Related to: Loss of fluid through abnormal routes
Defining characteristics: Nasogastric suction, fistula
Related to: Factors influencing fluid needs
Defining characteristics: Hypermetabolic states, temperature elevation (diaphoresis), increased insensible loss (respirations, perspirations), failure to absorb or reabsorb

water, excessive renal excretion, extremes of age, water output exceeds intake
Related to: Medications
Defining characteristics: Use of diuretics, improper administration of IV fluids containing NaCl

Outcome Criteria

Fluid I&O and electrolytes in balance with absence of dehydration
Absence of fluid deficit

Interventions	Rationales
Assess fluid losses, sources, amounts, and effects; urinary output (should be 1-2 ml/kg/hr; weigh diapers for infant and calculate as 1 ml/Gm); vomiting (include spitting up); diarrhea (include watery or bloody); stoma drainage (liquid); nasogastric aspirate (suctioning); insensible losses (respirations, diaphoresis from body temperature or ambient temperature); wound damage hemorrhage (fluid volume reduced); injury (burns)	Provides information about body fluid losses and depletion which can lead to serious consequences in the infant/child; include output analysis when comparing to intake; causes include failure to absorb or reabsorb water, reduced intake or NPO status, excessive renal excretion, inappropriate ADH secretion, increased temperature or respirations, over-use of diuretic therapy, improper fluid replacement
Assess intake and accurately compare to losses q2-8h for I&O determination and balance; oral intake (liquids, fluid content of foods/formula, foods that become liquid at body temperature, fluids given with medications); parenteral (IV, IM, TPN); enteral (N/G, gastrostomy tube feedings)	Provides strict I&O to determine positive or negative balance and potential for fluid deficit/dehydration; mild dehydration: less than 50 ml/kg fluid loss; moderate dehydration: 50-90 ml/kg; severe dehydration: about 100ml/kg
Assess infant's weight (undressed without diaper) on the same scale; weights are usually ordered BID (at 6 a.m. and 6 p.m., before meals)	Determines losses related to fluid deficit and potential for dehydration; mild dehydration: loss of 5% in infant, 3% in older child; moderate: loss of 10% in infant, 6% in older child; severe: loss of 15% in infant, 9% in older child

Interventions	Rationales
Assess for presence of dehydration q2-8h including decreased urinary output, poor skin turgor testing, dry skin and mucous membranes, gray or mottled color to skin, reduced or absent tears and saliva, sunken, soft eyeballs, sunken fontanels in infants, increased Sp.Gr. and serum osmolality, blood urea nitrogen (BUN), creatinine, hemoglobin, creatinine hematocrit, thirst in the older child, vital signs changes (tachycardia, lowered blood pressure, postural changes in blood pressure)	Reveals signs and symptoms of dehydration and hydration status; dehydration occurs when output exceeds intake and is classified as isotonic dehydration (water and electrolyte deficits equal); hypertonic dehydration (water loss is greater than sodium loss); hypotonic dehydration (sodium loss is greater than water loss)
Assess for presence of electrolyte depletion and possible etiology	Reveals signs and symptoms of electrolyte imbalance which are related to specific diseases; provides information regarding fluid/electrolyte imbalances, kidney function and risk for acidosis or alkalosis
Potassium (K): muscle weakness and cramping, irritability, fatigue, hypotension, arrhythmias	K: excessive urinary output, diuretic therapy, vomiting, diarrhea, N/G aspirate (functions in neural transmission in smooth, skeletal and cardiac muscle)
Sodium (Na): nausea, abdominal cramps, weakness, dizziness, apathy	Na: excessive water loss via any route, fever, diaphoresis, vomiting, diarrhea, N/G aspirate, fistula or wounds (functions to control movement of fluid between fluid compartments)
Calcium (Ca): tingling of fingertips, toes, hypotension, muscle irritability, tetany	Ca: renal insufficiency, loss through gastrointestinal route, inadequate Ca intake or vitamin D deficiency (functions to prevent metabolic acidosis)

Interventions	Rationales
Assess urinalysis, electrolyte panel, serum and urine osmolality, blood urea nitrogen, creatinine, arterial blood gases, as indicated	Provides information regarding fluid/electrolyte imbalances, kidney function and risk for acidosis or alkalosis
Encourage increased oral fluid intake in proportion to losses; provide a varied selection of beverages; if the fluid volume deficit is due to diarrhea, the following recommendation is: diarrhea is not managed by encouraging intake of clear fluids by mouth, such as fruit juices, carbonated soft drinks, gelatin, chicken broth or beef broth; allow child to request oral fluid preferences (sweet tea, diluted juice, decarbonated soda); start with rapid replacement for 4-6 hours and continue over 24 hours for maintenance therapy as tolerated: Infant: 150 ml/kg/day Toddler: 120 ml/kg/day Preschool: 100 ml/kg/day Schoolage: 75 ml/kg/day	Provides replacement of lost fluids if able to retain PO; child requires 750-2000 ml/day fluids depending on age and weight and calculation of losses; fluids with a high carbonation content, usually have a low electrolyte content; the caffeine in caffeinated soft drinks acts as a mild diuretic and may lead to increased loss of water and sodium; chicken or beef broth contains excessive sodium and inadequate carbohydrates
Provide oral rehydraton therapy (i.e., Pedialyte, Rehydralyte, Infalyte) for infant, alternate formula feedings with water feedings, if appropriate	Promotes fluid and electrolyte replacement and prevents risk of dehydration and electrolyte deficits
Maintain NPO status, prepare child and initiate IV fluid therapy with solution selection, rate and amount based on type and cause of dehydration	Provides immediate replacement and ongoing prevention of losses for those who are unable to ingest fluids PO, are dehydrated or who suffer from gastric distention
Use infusion pump or volume control chamber for IV with a pediatric infusion set with long tubing and restrain body parts as needed	Provides regulated and accurate fluid rate and volume with a microdrip IV infusion set (60 gtt/ml); long tubing allows for movement in bed, and proper restraining and monitoring provides safe IV administration

Interventions	Rationales
Monitor IV hourly for amount, site infiltration, tube patency or displacement; change fluid bag and tubing q24h, use a transparent occlusive dressing over IV site (i.e., IV House)	Ensures safe fluid administration; allows for ROM of restrained parts, prevents complication of IV therapy
Provide non-nutritive sucking for infant, hold and cuddle child, mouth care (spray water into mouth) for oral dryness, Vaseline to lips	Provides support and comfort to infant/child
During IV therapy, note presence of headache, cramps, vomiting, crackles, muscle twitching, lethargy, decreased urine output	Indicates overhydration
Discontinue IV when fluids are tolerated orally; begin with small amounts of clear fluids, gradually increase in amounts and frequency as tolerated including Jell-o, popsicles, low salt soup, baby food for infants	Resumes oral fluid intake when condition improves; oral intake may be resumed as soon as 5-10 hours after surgery
Employ play at developmental level including games, use of straws, small cup (medicine or animal image cup)	Promotes oral intake of fluids when child is ill and doesn't fulfill fluid goals
Place water and cup in room and allow to take frequent sips; praise child for drinking fluids	Promotes adequate intake of fluids and promotes independence
Allow child to participate in the fluid selection and scheduling, to record intake using symbols or checks with colors	Promotes independence and control over the situations and enhances compliance

Information, Instruction, Demonstration

Interventions	Rationales
Explain to parent(s) and child the amount of fluid needed by the infant/child daily and therapeutic need based on disorder or illness	Provides information about fluid needs as a basic need and increase of fluid need as treatment for deficit
Instruct and demonstrate measurement of I&O to parent(s) and allow for return demonstration by calculating and measuring for 24 hours	Permits accurate monitoring of I&O to determine risk for dehydration
Inform parent(s) of signs and symptoms of K, Na, Ca depletion based on reason for fluid deficit	Prevents electrolyte imbalance which may lead to serious complications
Inform parent(s) and child of reasons for fluid loss; types of fluid to give for replacement of fluid loss and amount of fluid needed/day depending on output	Prevents future fluid and electrolyte loss and dehydration
Inform parent(s) and child of IV method, reasons and effect; inform child that it is not a punishment	Promotes cooperation and reduces anxiety; children are fearful of "shots"
Develop list of preferred fluids; inform parent(s) which are clear liquids and how to progress to full liquids PO	Prevents offering liquids or foods that may exacerbate disorder that caused deficit
Suggest referral to a nutritionist for administration of electrolyte formula, dilution of fluids, caloric and sodium content of commercial fluids	Provides information and instruction and support to parents for safe fluid administration PO

Discharge or Maintenance Evaluation

- Absence of fluid and electrolyte imbalance, adequate circulating fluid volume
- Absence of presence of or risk for dehydration, assesses I&O ratio

- Correct calculation and administration of fluids in proportion to losses
- Progressive return to baseline fluid intake PO
- Maintains NPO status when needed
- Administers IV fluids, electrolytes as prescribed safely and accurately without complications
- Encourages compliance and independence in adequate fluid intake
- Verbalizes reason and treatment for increased fluid loss and the prevention of recurrence

Chronic Renal Failure

Chronic renal failure (CRF) is the progressive deterioration of kidney function that reaches 50% or more loss or a creatinine level of less than 2 mg/dl. Causes include congenital kidney and urinary tract abnormalities in children less than 5 years of age, glomerular and hereditary kidney disorders in children 5-15 years of age. The disease involves all body systems as abnormalities include water, Na, Ca losses, K, P, Mg increases, reduced Hgb, Hct that result in metabolic acidosis, anemia, growth retardation, hypertension, bone demineralization. Eventually, if untreated, uremic syndrome develops as the kidneys are not able to maintain fluid and electrolyte balance. End stage renal disease (ESRD) is defined as loss of kidney function at 90% or greater. ESRD is the term applied when the kidneys are no longer able to clear wastes from the body. Eventually the disease terminates in death unless kidney transplantation or dialysis is performed.

MEDICAL CARE

Electrolyte panel: at diagnosis lab results will reveal decreased Ca, CL, Co2; and <u>increased</u> K, phosphorus, Na, Hydrogen ions. With diuretic therapy and increased K intake, lab results may display decreased K and Na.

Diuretics: furosemide (Lasix) given PO or IV, chlorothiazide (Diuril) given PO, hydrochlorothiazide (Hydrodiuril tablet or Intenso solution) given PO to promote excretion of water and electrolytes to reduce edema associated with renal failure.

Antihypertensives: severe hypertension is treated with a combination of a beta blocker and a vasodilator (Proprolol and hydralazine); others may include: nifedipine, atenolol, minoxidil, prazosin, captopril or labetal (these may be used singly or in combination).

Alkalizing agents: metabolic acidosis is treated with alkalizing agents (PO), such as sodium bicarbonate or a combination of sodium and potassium citrate (Bicitra, Polycitra, or Shohl solution).

Antibiotics: specific to identified microorganisms and sensitivity to specific antimicrobials to prevent or treat infection with dosage adjusted to renal function to prevent toxicity.

Vitamins/Minerals: fat-soluble vitamins (A, E, and K) are not supplemented. Water-soluble vitamins may be prescribed (B, C, folic acid, niacin) and Vitamin D is prescribed. Folic acid (and sometimes ferrous sulfate) is prescribed to enhance iron absorption. To increase calcium and phosphorus absorption: (PO) dehydrotachysterol (Hytakerol); or (PO) 1,25 dihydroxyvitamin D3 (Rocaltrol); or ergocalciferol (Calciferol).

Renal scan/Renal ultrasound: reveals renal abnormality diagnosis.

Blood urea nitrogen (BUN): reveals increases as renal failure progresses and protein catabolism increases.

Serum creatinine: reveals increases as renal failure progresses and glomerular filtration rate is reduced.

Electrolyte panel: reveals decreased Na, Ca, Cl and increased K, CO_2.

Complete blood count: reveals decreased RBC, Hct, Hgb, WBC, reticulocyte count.

Prothrombin time (PT): activated partial thromboplastin time (APPT): reveals prolonged time as erythropoeitin production is reduced.

Calcium carbonate preparations (used as phosphate binders): calcium acetate, also act as a calcium supplement and as an alkalizing agent.

Aluminum hydroxide gels: are effective phosphorus binders. Only used for severe or unresponsive hyperphosphatemia due to risk of aluminum toxicity.

Epogen {Epoeitin alpha, (subcutaneous or IV)}: recombinant Human Erythropoletin (rHuEPO) is prescribed to treat anemia. It also has decreased the need for blood transfusions.

Growth hormone: recombinant human growth hormone is used to treat growth retardation secondary to CRF and following renal transplant.

NURSING CARE PLANS

Essential nursing diagnoses and plans associated with this condition:

Fluid volume excess (5)

Related to: Compromised regulatory mechanism
Defining characteristics: Edema, water and Na retention, weight gain, clothes begin to feel tight, decreased urine output, facial puffiness, altered electrolyte, shortness of breath, crackles, hypertension, vascular congestion

Altered nutrition: Less than body requirements (168)

Related to: Loss of appetite
Defining characteristics: Anorexia, nausea, fatigue, weight loss, limited K, P and protein food intake, poor

absorption of Ca, iron by intestines, growth retardation; may observe weight gain (due to fluid retention and oliguria) or weight loss (due to anorexia and electrolyte disturbances)

Hyperthermia (112)

Related to: Illness (renal failure)
Defining characteristics: Frequent infections, increase in body temperature above normal range that is recurrent, malaise

Risk for impaired skin integrity (397)

Related to: Internal effects of chronic renal failure
Defining characteristics: Dryness, pruritis, uremic frost, sallow color, disruption of skin surfaces from scratching secondary skin breakdown (due to edema)

Altered growth and development (419)

Related to: Loss of appetite, depletion of body protein, decreased erythropoietin production, and related metabolic disturbances
Defining characteristics: Altered physical growth, delay in sexual maturation, frequent absences from school and disruptions in socialization, inability to participate in activities, frequent hospitalizations

SPECIFIC DIAGNOSES AND CARE PLANS

Activity intolerance

Related to: General weakness
Defining characteristics: Complaints of fatigue on exertion, preference for quiet play, lack of energy

Outcome Criteria

Participation in activities within limitations imposed by disease
Optimal energy level preserved

Interventions	Rationales
Provide information, instruction and support to assess degree of weakness, fatigue, ability to participate in activities (active and passive)	Provides information about effect of activities on fatigue and energy reserves

Interventions	Rationales
Schedule care and provide rest periods following an activity; encourage child to set own limits in amount of exertion tolerated	Promotes independence and control of situations as the presence of a chronic disease may encourage independence
Provide for quiet play, reading, TV, games during times of fatigue	Provides diversion, stimulation and requires minimal energy expenditure

Information, Instruction, Demonstration

Interventions	Rationales
Explain to child reason for restrictions; explain when to stop activity and rest to child	Promotes understanding of the need to conserve energy and rest
Inform parent(s) and child that full participation in activities is important and should be encouraged for as long as possible (within capabilities and disease restriction)	Promotes an active and normal life for the child with a chronic illness

Discharge or Maintenance Evaluation

- Conserves energy and minimizes fatigue
- Participation in activities within capabilities and disease restrictions
- Balances activity with rest periods

Risk for infection

Related to: Pulmonary edema, metabolic acidosis, uremia, loss of appetite
Defining characteristics: Changes in respiratory pattern, productive cough with yellow or other abnormal color, adventitious sounds, elevated temperature, cloudy, foul smelling urine, dysuria, urgency, frequency

Outcome Criteria

Absence of pulmonary or urinary infection

Interventions	Rationales
Assess lab results for infection (elevated WBC and positive blood cultures)	To prevent and treat infection

Interventions	Rationales
Assess temperature, respiratory and urinary system changes as disease progresses	Provides information about presence of infection caused by progressive chronic disease and its deteriorating effect on all systems
Administer antibiotic therapy as ordered in doses related to decreased renal function	Prevents or treats infection
Perform handwashing, medical or surgical asepsis during procedures or care as appropriate	Prevents transmission of pathogens to child
Secure urine or sputum cultures for analysis	Identifies presence and type of microorganism responsible for infection and specific sensitivities to antibiotic therapy

Information, Instruction, Demonstration

Interventions	Rationales
Instruct child and parent(s) in handwashing technique, proper disposal of tissues and used articles	Prevents transmission of infectious agents to child
Inform parent(s) and child of importance of daily bathing, cleansing after toileting, wearing of loose undergarments	Promotes comfort and measures to prevent urinary infection
Inform child to avoid contact with persons with upper respiratory infections	Prevents transmission of infectious agents that may lead to pneumonia

Discharge or Maintenance Evaluation

- Absence of infections
- Controls transmission of pathogens to child
- Participates in measures to prevent infections

Body image disturbance

Related to: Biophysical and psychosocial factors

Defining characteristics: Verbal and nonverbal responses to change in body appearance, disruptions in school attendance and participation in school activities and socialization, negative feelings about body, multiple stressors and change in daily living, severe growth retardation (in height and weight); dry skin, facial puffiness

Outcome Criteria

Body image improved, preserved and maintained
Accommodations made for special needs of child with long-term illness:
- Verbalization of positive feelings about limitations
- Progressive social acceptance and adjustment to special help when needed

Interventions	Rationales
Assess child for feelings about abilities, chronic illness, difficulty in school and social situations, short stature, inability to keep up with peers	Provides information about status of self-concept and special needs
Encourage expression of feelings and concerns and support communication with parent(s), teachers, and peers	Provides opportunity to vent feelings and reduce negative feelings about change in appearance
Stress positive activities and accomplishments, avoid negative comments	Enhances sense of positive body image, confidence, self-esteem

Information, Instruction, Demonstration

Interventions	Rationales
Inform parent(s) of importance of maintaining support for child regardless of their needs	Encourages acceptance of the child with special needs (dialysis, dietary requirements, urinary device, medications)
Instruct parent(s) of need for flexibility in care of child and need to integral care and routines into family routines	Promotes well-being of child and sense of belonging
Inform child and parent(s) about food selections which can be tolerated when eating out with friends	Promotes social interactions with peers within limitations imposed by disease

Discharge or Maintenance Evaluation

- Verbalizes improved body image, sense of well-being, and self-confidence
- Participates in school and social activities as appropriate
- Verbalizes feelings about special needs in positive terms
- Supports positive body image and promotes adjustment to chronic illness

Anticipatory grieving

Related to: Perceived potential loss of child by parent(s); perceived potential loss of physiopsychosocial well-being by child

Defining characteristics: Expression of distress of potential loss, inevitable kidney failure, kidney dialysis, premature death of child

Outcome Criteria

Progressive grief resolution over prolonged time of illness by parent(s)
Management of stages of grieving process

Interventions	Rationales
Assess stage of grief process, problems encountered, feelings regarding long-term illness and potential loss of child	Provides information about stage of grieving as time to work through the process varies with individuals; the longer the illness, the better able the parent(s) and family will be able to move towards acceptance
Provide emotional and spiritual comfort in an accepting environment and avoid conversations that will cause guilt or anger	Provides for emotional needs of parent(s) and assist them to cope with ill child without adding stressors that are difficult to resolve
Allow for parental and child responses and expression of feelings	Allows for reactions necessary to work through grieving
Assist to identify and use effective coping mechanisms and to understand situations over which they have no control	Promotes use of coping mechanisms over long period of time of illness; chronic disease causes physical and emotional stress on family members which may be positive or negative

Interventions	Rationales
Refer to social worker and/or counseling as appropriate	Offers information and support to parent(s) and family in need of psychologic, economic assistance

Information, Instruction, Demonstration

Interventions	Rationales
Inform parent(s) of stage of grieving and behaviors that are acceptable in resolving grief	Promotes understanding of feelings and behaviors that are manifested by grief
Instruct parent(s) and child in coping skill, problem solving skills and approaches that may be used	Promotes coping ability over prolonged period of illness and assists in resolution of family stress
Refer to clergy, local support groups for kidney diseases, National Kidney Foundation	Provides support and assistance in adapting and accepting chronic illness and services and information for care

Discharge or Maintenance Evaluation

- Verbalizes understanding of grief process and responses
- Shares feelings with professionals and other members of family
- Secures assistance from support persons and/or groups
- Identifies and uses coping skills that assist in adaptation and acceptance of chronic illness and deterioration
- Performs normal parental tasks/interventions with child
- Verbalizes hope after diagnosis is made and prospect of dialysis and kidney transplant is explained

Risk for injury

Related to: Internal factor of regulatory mechanism (renal failure)

Defining characteristics: Complications of impaired renal function, hypertension, anemia, metabolic acidosis, osteodystrophy, neurologic manifestations, uremic syndrome if disorder untreated

Outcome Criteria

Complications of disease prevented with compliance of medical regimen

Interventions	Rationales
Assess blood pressure for alterations; administer antihypertensives and directs as ordered singly or in combination	Provides data regarding hypertension evident in advanced renal disease
Assess I&O, electrolyte panel, and creatinine; administer diuretics as ordered (for excessive water retention)	Provides indication of renal function affecting output with water and electrolyte retention as disease progresses and nephrons are destroyed
Assess RBC, Hct, Hgb and administer iron and transfusion of packed red blood cells, as ordered	Provides indication of anemia caused by the reduced production of erythropoietin by the failing kidneys and inadequate intake of iron in a restricted diet
Assess bone pain and deformities affecting ambulation and activities; administer supplemental vitamin D, calcium and alkalizing agents, as ordered	Provides indication of osteodystrophy caused by a calcium phosphorus imbalance resulting in bone demineralization and growth retardation; kidney disease results in the inability to synthesize vitamin D needed to absorb Ca, acidosis causes dissolution of alkaline salts of bone and phosphate is increased and calcium decreased as glomerular filtration is reduced
Assess presence of acidosis by pH, bicarbonate losses and administer alkalizing agents	Provides indication of impending metabolic acidosis caused by the inability of the failing kidneys to excrete metabolic acids that are byproducts of metabolism the hydrogen ion is retained and bicarbonate is lost as the tubules are unable to reabsorb it
Assess for sensory loss, confusion and changes in consciousness	Reveals possible changes in neurologic status as kidney function deteriorates and uremic syndrome appears

Information, Instruction, Demonstration

Interventions	Rationales
Instruct in accurate medication administration including actions, dosage, frequency, side effects to report	Ensures compliance of correct medication administration; long-term of many medications are given for disease to prevent complications and uremic syndrome
Inform parent(s) of importance of long-term treatments, follow up care	Promotes effective management of renal function and treatment of systemic signs and symptoms present with this disease
Instruct parent(s) and child in dietary regimen, to restrict Na, K, P and include Ca, iron in diet, to restrict protein and water intake if appropriate and amounts allowed; offer lists of foods and sample menus for planning	Promotes compliance with dietary inclusions or restrictions depending on degree of renal failure
Inform parent(s) and child of dialysis procedure and frequency if appropriate; include biological, psychological and social effects	Provides information if renal dialysis is needed; usually based on creatinine level which indicated the ability of the kidneys to excrete waste materials and the degree of renal failure

Discharge or Maintenance Evaluation

- Controls systemic complications with medical regimen
- Complies with follow-up supervision of renal function
- Administers medications accurately and reports adverse effects if present
- Verbalizes and promotes therapy to prevent uremic syndrome

Chronic Renal Failure

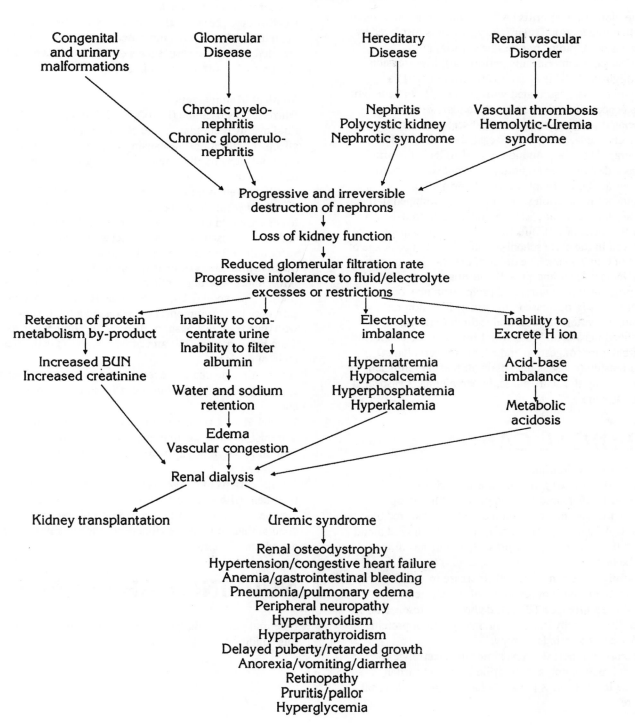

Congenital and urinary malformations

Glomerular Disease → Chronic pyelo-nephritis / Chronic glomerulo-nephritis

Hereditary Disease → Nephritis / Polycystic kidney / Nephrotic syndrome

Renal vascular Disorder → Vascular thrombosis / Hemolytic-Uremia syndrome

→ Progressive and irreversible destruction of nephrons
→ Loss of kidney function
→ Reduced glomerular filtration rate / Progressive intolerance to fluid/electrolyte excesses or restrictions

Retention of protein metabolism by-product → Increased BUN / Increased creatinine

Inability to concentrate urine / Inability to filter albumin → Water and sodium retention → Edema / Vascular congestion

Electrolyte imbalance → Hypernatremia / Hypocalcemia / Hyperphosphatemia / Hyperkalemia

Inability to Excrete H ion → Acid-base imbalance → Metabolic acidosis

→ Renal dialysis → Kidney transplantation / Uremic syndrome

Renal osteodystrophy
Hypertension/congestive heart failure
Anemia/gastrointestinal bleeding
Pneumonia/pulmonary edema
Peripheral neuropathy
Hyperthyroidism
Hyperparathyroidism
Delayed puberty/retarded growth
Anorexia/vomiting/diarrhea
Retinopathy
Pruritis/pallor
Hyperglycemia

Glomerulonephritis (Acute)

Acute glomerulonephritis (AGN) is an alteration in renal function due to glomerular injury, which is displayed by the classic symptoms of gross hematuria, mild proteinuria, edema (usually periorbital), hypertension and oliguria. AGN is also classified as either: 1) a primary disease, associated with group A, Beta hemolytic streptococcal infection; or 2) a secondary disease, associated with various systemic diseases (ie., systemic lupus erythema, sickle cell disease, henochschonlein purpura). The most common type of AGN is the primary disease, described as an immune-complex disease (or an antigen-antibody complex formed during the streptococcal infection which becomes entrapped in the glomerular membrane, causing inflammation 8-14 days after the onset of this infection). AGN is primarily observed in the early school-age child, with a peak age of onset of 6 to 7 years. The onset of the classic symptoms of AGN is usually abrupt, self-limiting (unpredictable) and prolonged hematuria and proteinuria may occur. AGN results in decreased glomerular filtration rate causing retention of water and sodium (edema); expanded plasma and interstitial fluid volumes than lead to circulatory congestion and edema (hypervolemia); hypertension (cause is unexplained; plasma renin activity is low during the acute phase, hypervolemia is suspected to be the cause).

MEDICAL CARE

Diagnostic Evaluation
Urinalysis: reveals gross hematuria, and some proteinuria, increased specific gravity. Microscopic examination of the urine sediment will reveal: red blood cells, leukocytes, epithelial cells, granular and red blood cast cells. Bacteria are not present, and urine cultures will be negative.
Creatinine clearance: reveals increase in AGN. It will determine presence of severe renal impairment.
Blood urea nitrogen (BUN): determines presence of renal disease, dehydration, hemorrhage, high protein intake, corticosteriods therapy.
Electrolyte panel: will reveal normal electrolytes (sodium, potassium, and chloride ions) and carbon dioxide levels (unless the AGN has progressed to renal failure).

Complete blood count: reveals decreased RBC, Hct, Hgb and increased WBC.
Throat culture: positive cultures of the pharynx (occur in only a few cases).
Antistreptolysin O (ASO): an ASO titer of 250 Todd units or higher is diagnostic for AGN, as is a rising titer in 2 samples taken a week apart.
Erythrocyte sedimentation rate (ESR), C-reactive protein (CRP), and Serum mucoprotein test: are all elevated during the early stages of AGN and then gradually return to normal as healing occurs.

Medical Management
Diuretics: furosemide (Lasix) PO, IV to treat edema and fluid overload but may not be effective since the disease affects the filtration rate causing limited Na reaching the distal tubules and the action of the drug is to inhibit reabsorption of water and Na.
Antihypertensives: hydralazine (Apresoline) PO with a diuretic, hydrochlorothiazide (HydroDiuril) PO for mild hypertension to increase excretion of water and Na, Cl and acts on vascular smooth muscles to cause vasodilation. In the absence of encephalopathy complications, hydralazine (IV or IM) may be given with furosemide. Alternate antihypertensives include prazosin (PO), propranolol (PO), or reserpine (IM). If hypertension is causing symptoms of encephalopathy, treatment with diazoxide (IV push, or drip for 30 minutes) or sodium nitroprusside (IV) and furosemide (IV) is the treatment of choice.
Antibiotics: no change, except is indicated only if persistent streptococcal infections exist (usually are not present).
Hyperkalemia treatment: if hyperkalemia is present, administration of calcium, glucose and insulin, or a sodium polystyrene sulfonate (Kayexalate) enema may be required.
Complications of congestive heart failure: will require treatment with fluid restrictions and diuretics. Also, it may be treated with intravenous inotropic agents, such as dobutamine, or with vasodilatation, such as nitroglycerin or sodium nitroprusside.

NURSING CARE PLANS

Essential nursing diagnoses and plans associated with this condition:

Fluid volume excess (5)

Related to: Compromised regulatory mechanism
Defining characteristics: Dependent edema, periorbital edema, pleural effusion, puffiness in the face, moderate blood pressure increases, intake greater than output, weight gain, azotemia, crackles and pleural effusion (occasionally is seen if pulmonary congestion occurs), decreased Hgb and Hct, altered electrolytes, decreased urinary output

Altered nutrition: Less than body requirements (168)

Related to: Loss of appetite
Defining characteristics: Anorexia, fatigue, nausea, vomiting, malaise, no added-salt diet, lethargy, abdominal discomfort

Altered tissue perfusion: Cerebral (6)

Related to: Hypervolemia, hypertensive encephalopathy, cerebral ischemia
Defining characteristics: Early signs of hypertensive encephalopathy: headache, dizziness, abdominal discomfort, and vomiting; if hypertensive encephalopathy worsens: transient loss of vision and/or hemiparesis, disorientation, generalized convulsions (tonic/clonic type), coma

Risk for impaired skin integrity (397)

Related to: Internal factor of edema, altered circulation
Defining characteristics: Bedrest, impaired tissue perfusion, pressure on skin and bony prominences, pink or redness of skin, disruption of skin from IV infusions

SPECIFIC DIAGNOSES AND CARE PLANS

Activity intolerance

Related to: Generalized weakness, bedrest
Defining characteristics: Expressed weakness and fatigue, anemia, lethargy

Outcome Criteria

Interventions	Rationales
Assess weakness, fatigue, ability to move about in bed and participate in play activities	Provides information about energy reserves during the acute phase of the disease and acceptance of bedrest status
Schedule care and provide rest periods following any activity in a quiet environment	Provides adequate rest and reduces stimuli and fatigue
Maintain bedrest during the acute stage, disturb only when necessary	Conserves energy and decreases production of waste materials which increases work of the kidneys
Provide for quiet play, reading, TV, games as symptoms subside	Provides diversion, stimulation and requires minimal energy expenditures

Information, Instruction, Demonstration

Interventions	Rationales
Explain reason for activity restriction to parent(s) and child	Promotes understanding of the need to conserve energy and rest to promote recovery
Inform parent(s) and child to rest following ambulation or any activity	Prevents fatigue and conserves energy during recovery
Instruct parent(s) and child to rest when feeling tired	Prevents fatigue and promotes recovery

Discharge or Maintenance Evaluation

- Conserves energy and minimizes fatigue and weakness
- Engages in activities progressively within capabilities and disease restrictions
- Provides rest and activity balance

Risk for infection

Related to: Chronic disease
Defining characteristics: Persistent streptococcal infections

Outcome Criteria

Absence of presence of infection or transmission to other

Interventions	Rationales
Assess temperature, chills, sore throat, cough (presence or recurrence)	Indicates persistence of streptococcal infection
Obtain throat culture for analysis and sensitivities	Identifies streptococcal microorganism and sensitivity to specific antibiotic therapy
Administer antibiotic therapy to child and to family members if ordered	Destroys microbial agents by preventing cell wall synthesis and prevents transmission to family members
Provide for disposal of used tissues and articles properly	Prevents transmission of microorganisms to others or reinfection

Information, Instruction, Demonstration

Interventions	Rationales
Instruct child and family to wash hands after sneezing/coughing and to dispose of used articles	Prevents spread of disease
Instruct parent(s) about antibiotic therapy and to administer full course of medication	Promotes compliance with medication regimen
Instruct parent(s) to avoid exposure of child to others with upper respiratory infection	Prevents respiratory infections in the susceptible child
Inform parent(s) to report fever, cough, sore throat	Indicates infection and provides for early intervention

Discharge or Maintenance Evaluation

- Absence of streptococcal infection (nephritogenic)
- Controls transmission of the streptococcal microorganism
- Complies with medication regimen

Risk for injury

Related to: Internal factor of regulatory mechanism (renal function)
Defining characteristics: Complications of impaired renal function, hypertension, cardiac failure, renal failure; risk of complications (i.e., encephalopathy, congestive heart failure, acute renal failure)

Outcome Criteria

Complications of disease prevented

Interventions	Rationales
Assess BP, pulse, respirations q4h; monitor BP q1h if diastolic is more than 90, pulse and respirations q1h if tachycardia, tachypnea of dyspnea present	Provides information about complication of hypertension which may lead to encephalopathy, pulse and respirations which change with heart failure and pulmonary edema
Assess changes in I&O, extent of edema, decreased urinary output, headache, pallor, electrolyte balance	Indicates signs and symptoms of possible renal failure
Administer anti-hypertensives, diuretic therapy, cardiac glycoside and monitor for expected results	Provides therapy for complications if a more severe renal impairment is present
Limit fluids if output is reduced; allow intake of the amount lost via urine and insensible losses	Prevents further fluid retention and edema in the presence of renal damage
Limit foods high in Na, K and protein during the acute phase of AGN; encourage a diet with the increased carbohydrates and fats (only during acute phase of AGN)	Provides nutrition during the acute period with limitation of K during oliguria, Na with presence of edema, protein limitation if oliguria is prolonged
Note behavior changes including lethargy, irritability, restlessness associated with hypertension and administer anticonvulsives if ordered	Indicates need for safety precautions associated with seizure activity as a result of cerebral changes

Information, Instruction
Demonstration

Interventions	Rationales
Inform parent(s) of potential for complications and signs and symptoms to report (increased weight, blood in urine with decreased amount of output, complaints of headache and anorexia)	Provides for early intervention to prevent severe renal impairment
Instruct in dietary inclusions and restrictions; offer a list of foods to include and avoid that comply with Na, K, protein allowances	Provides nutrition while disease is being resolved
Instruct to allow activity/rest periods as energy and fatigue requires; progressively increase as condition warrants	Prevents fatigue and conserves energy during acute stage and convalescence
Inform parent(s) of importance of compliance with follow-up care and supervision	Ensures ongoing monitoring of child for chronic renal disease or persistent streptococcal infection

Discharge or Maintenance
Evaluation

- Absence of complications of acute disease
- Complies with medication, activity, dietary regimen
- Complies with follow-up supervision of renal function

Glomerulonephritis

Post streptococcal infection
(group A, Beta hemolytic)

↓

Release of material from the organism into the
circulation (antigen)

↓

Formation of antibody

↓

Immune-complex reaction in the
glomerular capillary

↓

Inflammatory response

↓

Proliferation of endothelial cells lining
glomerulus and cells between endothelium and
epithelium of capillary membrane

↓

Swelling of capillary membrane and infiltration
with leukocytes
Increased permeability of base membrane

↓

Occlusion of the capillaries of glomeruli
Vasospasm of afferent arterioles

↓

Decreased glomeruli filtration rate

↓

Decreased ability to form filtrate from
glomeruli plasma flow

↓

Retention of water and sodium
Reduced circulatory volume (hypovolemia)
Circulatory congestion

↓

Edema (peripheral and perorbital)
Hypertension
decreased urinary output (hematuria, proteinuria)
Urine dark in color
Anorexia
Irritability, lethargy

↓

Acute glomerulonephritis

Hypospadias/ Epispadias

Hypospadias and epispadias are congenital defects of the penis resulting in incomplete development of the anterior urethra. The congenital defect results in an abnormal urethral opening at any place along the shaft of the penis and may open onto the scrotum or perineum. The incidence of this defect in the U. S. is approximately 3.2 in 1000 live male births or about 1 in every 300 male children. The etiology of this defect is unknown but is associated with a higher familial tendency and by race/ethnic background (more common in whites, Italians, and Jews). Chordee, an abnormal curvature of the penis, is frequently associated with hypospadias. Other associated anomalies/diseases include: undescended testes (9%-32%); inguinal hernia (9%-17%); and Wilm's tumor. The goal of treatment of this defect is to reconstruct a straight penis with a meatus close to the normal anatomical location. Age for repair is being performed at progressively younger ages to avoid emotional distress in the young child. Currently, the recommended age for repair is between 3 and 12 months (for hypospadias/epispadias or urethroplasty) versus 6 to 18 months of age; and during the first year (for chordee repair or orthoplasty). Three objectives of surgical correction of this defect include: 1) to ensure the child's ability to void in the standing position with a straight stream (will minimize child and parent anxiety); 2) to improve the child's physical appearance and ensure a positive body image; and 3) to preserve sexual function.

MEDICAL CARE

Analgesics: acetaminophen (Tylenol tablets or syrup, Liquiprin solution codeine (Methylmorphine) PO postoperatively to control pain.

Antibiotics: ampicillin (Amcill) PO, ampicillin sodium (SK-Ampicillin-N) IM to prevent infection or treat infection postoperatively; oral antimicrobials (Ceclor for 2 days followed by Bactrim for 8-12 days; anticholinergics (Ditropan) when urinary drainage is used.

Trimethoprim-sulfa (Septra or Bactrim); or Nitrofurantoin (PO): may be helpful in preventing postoperative cystitis complications.

Testosterone stimulation: enlargement of the penis (or artificial erection) is sometimes required to facilitate

surgical intervention, especially prior to orthoplasty (the release of chordee).

Artificial erection: can be accomplished by the following methods:

1) 5% testosterone cream: is rubbed on the genitals daily for 3 weeks.

2) Dihydrotestosterone (DHT): {25 mg Im once per week for 3 weeks} can also be used for this purpose.

Testosterone cypionate (Andronate) {PO} can also be used for this purpose.

Injectable saline/epinephrine: a tourniquet is placed at the base of the penis, and a corpus cavernosum is injected with injectable saline/epinephrine.

Tegaderm wrap: a postoperative dressing, which facilitates diffuse pressure to be applied by placing the penis onto the abdominal wall for compression (used primarily for distal hypospadias).

<u>In patients (without a urinary diversion):</u> the dressing can be removed at home in 24 to 48 hours.

<u>In patients (with a urinary diversion):</u> the dressing can be removed at home after 72 hours.

Dripping stent: is used postoperatively in patients age 6 to 18 months (to allow healing of the urethra). Today, most surgeons avoid foley catheters due to the increased risk of bladder spasms with their usage. Usage of stents also usually avoids postoperative complications of meatal edema, crusting, or synechia.

Sitz baths (twice a day): are recommended postoperatively to facilitate meatal patency (if a stent is not left in place).

Antispasmodics: flavoxate hydrochloride (Urispas) PO to relax smooth muscle of bladder and reduce discomfort caused by bladder irritation.

Methantheline bromide (Banthine) {1/3 of a suppository}: is used to treat bladder spasms.

Oxybutynin chloride (PO): is used to treat bladder spasms.

Hormones: testosterone cypionate (Andronate) PO preoperatively to increase size of penis which may facilitate surgery at an earlier age.

Complete blood count: reveals increased WBC if infection present.

Urinalysis/urine culture: reveals urinary tract infection.

Chromosome analysis: testosterone level reveals male hormone if ambiguous genitalia is present.

NURSING CARE PLANS

Essential nursing diagnoses and plans associated with this condition:

Risk for impaired skin integrity (397)

Related to: External factor of surgical incision
Defining characteristics: Disruption of skin surface, surgical correction of defect, catheter site irritation, poor wound healing or wound infection, edema within the urethra

Risk for fluid volume deficit (222)

Related to: Factors influencing fluid needs
Defining characteristics: NPO preoperatively, temperature elevation with infection, decreased urinary output, inadequate fluid replacement postoperatively, risk of intraoperative hemorrhage and postoperative bleeding

Hyperthermia (112)

Related to: Presence of postoperative wound infection or UTI
Defining characteristics: Increase in body temperature above normal range, warm to touch, increased pulse and respiratory rate, evidence of infection at surgical site, evidence of lower urinary tract infection

SPECIFIC DIAGNOSES AND CARE PLANS

Anxiety

Related to: Threat to self-concept, change in health status, change in environment (hospitalization)
Defining characteristics: Expressed apprehension and concern about correction of defect by surgery and the imperfect appearance of the penis following surgery, preoperative and postoperative care

Outcome Criteria

Reduced parental anxiety verbalized
Verbalizes positive effects of surgical correction
Acceptance of imperfect penis of child after surgery

Interventions	Rationales
Assess source and level of anxiety and need for information that will relieve anxiety	Provides information about anxiety level and need to relieve it; concerns include the type of procedure and appearance of penis after

Interventions	Rationales
	surgery; whether the penis will be sexually adequate; possibility that correction may need to be done in stages if child is old enough; fear of castration and change in body image
Allow expression of concerns and time for parent(s) and child to ask questions about condition, procedures, recovery	Provides opportunity to vent feelings and fears and secure environment
Answer questions calmly and honestly; use pictures, drawings, and models for information	Promotes trust and a calm, supportive environment
Allow parent(s) to stay with child during hospitalizations and encourage to assist in care	Allows parent(s) to care for and support child and continue parental role
Give parent(s) as much input into decisions about care and usual routines as possible	Allows for more control over situations and maintains familiar routines for care

Information, Instruction, Demonstration

Interventions	Rationales
Inform parent(s) of cause of defect, and extent of defect to be corrected, whether a mild defect or severe defect, that correction is best done between 3-9 months, placement of meatus on penis and possible number of procedures necessary to correct defect	Provides information that will enhance understanding of the defect to relieve anxiety
Inform parent(s) of reason for surgery (urethroplasty), type of procedure, appearance of penis following surgery and cosmetic results to expect; inform older child that penis will not be cut off and that procedure is not a form of punishment	Provides rationale for surgery which includes voiding in a standing position with ability to direct stream, improve appearance of penis and preserve self image, and to develop a sexually adequate penis

Interventions	Rationales
Inform parent(s) of post-operative care; indwelling meatal or suprapubic catheter or stents will be in place; restraints may be in place; medications will be administered to control pain and promote sedation	Provides information about postoperative care and what to expect following surgery
Instruct parent(s) in relaxation techniques and how to deal with child's anxiety and irritability	Reduces anxiety and promotes ability to provide calm and supportive care
Inform parent(s) and child (if appropriate) that defect or surgery will not affect sexual activity or orientation and will not affect reproductive ability	Relieves anxiety produced by fear caused by misinformation

Discharge or Maintenance Evaluation

- Verbalizes reduction in anxiety about defect and surgical correction
- Verbalizes positive effects of surgical correction
- Parents participate in care and support of child and decision making during postoperative experience

Pain

Related to: Physical injuring agent (surgery)
Defining characteristics: Communication of pain descriptors, crying, irritability, restlessness, withdrawal, increased P, increased R, increased BP

Outcome Criteria

Absence or control of incision pain

Interventions	Rationales
Assess verbal and nonverbal behavior; type, location and severity of pain depending on child's age	Provides information about pain as basis for analgesic therapy
Administer analgesic and sedative, as ordered	Reduces pain and promotes rest which reduces stimuli and pain
Place in position of comfort; position catheter to avoid tension and kinking	Promotes comfort and prevents pain from pulling on or manipulating catheter
Apply ice pack if ordered	Reduces edema and pain

Information, Instruction, Demonstration

Interventions	Rationales
Inform parent(s) that medications will prevent pain and restlessness and allow for healing	Provides information about need for pain medications for child's comfort

Discharge or Maintenance Evaluation

- Absence of pain and associated responses
- Administers correct medication to prevent and/or control pain
- Controls pain provoking actions when giving care or positioning child

Risk for infection

Related to: Inadequate primary defenses (surgical incision); invasive procedure (catheter)
Defining characteristics: Redness, swelling, drainage at incision site; cloudy, foul smelling urine, elevated temperature, positive urine or wound culture

Outcome Criteria

Absence of infection at any site
Wound intact and healing
Urinary catheter and drainage system sterility and patency maintained

Interventions	Rationales
Assess wound for redness, swelling, drainage on dressing, healing	Provides information indicating presence of infection or poor healing
Assess catheter insertion site for redness, irritation, swelling; assess urine collected in drainage system for cloudiness, foul odor, sediment	Indicates infectious process at catheter site or in urinary bladder
Collect urine specimen for culture and sensitivities	Provides information about specific organism and sensitivity to antibiotic
Administer anti-infective if culture results are 100,000 ml/mm or more as ordered	Treats specific organism causing urinary infection or prevents infection when catheter is in place

Interventions	Rationales
Use sterile technique when changing dressings or giving catheter care or emptying drainage bag	Prevents contamination by introducing organisms into sterile wound or cavity
Encourage to increase fluid intake according to age needs	Promotes dilution of urine to prevent urinary infection and after catheter removed will encourage voiding
Maintain catheter and collection bag below level of bladder and a closed drainage system free of kinks in the tubing (if a drainage device is used: then maintain catheter and collection bag — marked in red	Provides information that will enhance understanding of the defect to relieve anxiety
Immobilize arms and legs with restraints, remove periodically; use a bed cradle following surgery	Prevents accidental removal or disturbance of catheter or contamination of wound if surgical correction done for a more severe defect
Avoid change of dressing, reinforce as needed, and secure catheter to penis with dressing and tape, and to leg or abdomen with tape	Promotes comfort and prevents infection and catheter displacement
Note urinary output of at least 1 ml/kg/hr and report if less	Indicates that catheter obstruction may be present with urinary retention which leads to infection

Information, Instruction, Demonstration

Interventions	Rationales
Instruct and demonstrate to parent(s) catheter care, irrigation, emptying of drainage bag or use of diaper for urine drainage, how to tape catheter and bag to leg; allow for return demonstration	Provides information and skill in caring and maintaining patency for catheter as child may be discharged with a catheter or stent in place
Inform parent(s) to avoid allowing child to straddle toys, play in a sandbox, swim or engage in rough activities until advised by physician	Prevents trauma to or dislodging of catheter or infection

Interventions	Rationales
Inform parent(s) to sponge bathe the child and use loose fitting clothing, avoiding contact of feces with wound and instruct in cleansing after each bowel elimination	Promotes cleanliness and comfort without constriction
Instruct parent(s) in signs and symptoms of infection to report	Provides information about need for reporting to allow for early treatment

Discharge or Maintenance Evaluation

- Absence of urinary tract infection
- Patency and placement of catheter maintained
- Wound healing without infection or complications
- Complies with preventative measures and anti-infective therapy

Altered urinary elimination pattern

Related to: Mechanical trauma (urethroplasty), mental stenosis
Defining characteristics: Dysuria, frequency, urgency, retention, bladder spasms, inadequate output, edema of the urethra

Outcome Criteria

Voiding resumed after removal of catheter

Interventions	Rationales
Assess I&O ratio, voiding stream, color and amount of urine on first voiding and each subsequent voiding	Provides information about voiding pattern after clamping or removal of catheter
Assess for pain, abdominal distention, inability to void for 8 hours after catheter	Indicates urinary dysfunction and possible obstruction or continuing edema of meatus
Support child after catheter is removed and provide privacy for voiding	Prevents embarrassment which is common in an older child
Encourage increased fluid intake after catheter removed, offer preferred liquids qlh	Promotes micturition

Information, Instruction, Demonstration

Interventions	Rationales
Inform parent(s) to notify physician if urinary pattern changes or if child is unable to void	Allows for early intervention to prevent complications

Discharge or Maintenance Evaluation

- Return of urinary elimination pattern through new or corrected meatus after catheter removed
- Absence of signs and symptoms of urinary retention or dysfunction

Hypospadias/Epispadias

In utero development

Failure of fusion of the folds
that close the urethra in
the penis

Urethral orifice on
ventral surface of
penis

Urethral orifice on
dorsal surface of
penis

Hypospadias

Epispadias

Surgical repair to normalize
urethra and penis by
6-18 months of age

Nephrotic Syndrome

Nephrotic syndrome is an alteration to renal function due to increased glomerular basement membrane permeability to plasma protein (albumin). Alterations to the glomerulus result in classic symptoms of gross proteinuria, hypoalbuminemia, generalized edema (anasarca), oliguria, and hyperlipidemia. Nephrotic syndrome is classified as either by etiology or the histologic changes in the glomerulus. Nephrotic syndrome is also classified into 3 types: primary minimal change nephrotic syndrome (MCNS), secondary nephrotic syndrome, and congenital nephrotic syndrome. The most common type of nephrotic syndrome is MCNS (idiopathic type) and it accounts for 80% of cases of nephrotic syndrome. MCNS can occur at any age but usually the age of onset is during the preschool years. MCNS is also seen more in male children versus female children. Secondary nephrotic syndrome is frequently associated with secondary renal involvement or with systemic diseases. Congenital nephrotic syndrome (CNS) is caused by a rare autosomal recessive gene which is localized on the long arm of chromosome 19. Currently, CNS has a better prognosis due to early treatment of protein deficiency, nutritional support, continuous cycling peritoneal dialysis (CCPD) and renal transplantation. The prognosis for MCNS is usually good, but relapses are common, and most children respond to treatment.

MEDICAL CARE

Diagnostic Evaluation: is based on the history and the presence of classic clinical manifestations of MCNS.
Urinalysis: reveals great increases of protein (proteinuria) of 3+ to 4+ or 300-1000 mg/dl; increased Sp. Gr.; hyaline casts and few RBC.
Renal biopsy: provides information regarding the glomerulus status, type of nephrotic syndrome, expected response to steroids and prognosis.
Creatinine clearance: reveals increase in MCNS. It will determine presence of severe renal impairment.
Blood Urea Nitrogen (BUN): determines presence of renal disease, dehydration, hemorrhage, high protein intake, corticosteriods therapy.
Serum protein: reveals decreases in total proteins (albumin and globulin) with electrophoresis revealing a great decrease in albumin.

Serum Lipids: reveals increases with a great increase in cholesterol to 450-1500 mg/dl.
Electrolyte panel: reveals decreased Na and Ca and K at normal level.
Complete blood count: reveals normal Hct and Hgb and increased platelet count of 500,000-1,000,000 cu/mm resulting from hemoconcentration.
Medical Management:
Corticosteroid therapy: choice drug is Prednisone (Deltasone) PO given until the urine is free from protein and remains normal for 10 days to 2 weeks. The daily dosage for Prednisone is 2 mg/kg and given in 3 to 4 divided doses. A positive response to therapy usually occurs in 6 to 14 days.
Immunosuppressant therapy: is used for patients who experience a relapse of symptoms. The drug of choice is cyclophosphamide (Cytoxan), an oral alkylating agent. It is given for 2 to 3 months, alternating it with Prednisone. An alternate drug, Chlorambucil (PO), is effective when given with Prednisone.
Plasma expanders: human albumin (Albuminar) IV is recommended for severe edema to increase plasma protein level and promote diuresis.
Diuretics: diuretics are typically not used. Diuretics are used for edema which interferes with respirations or which results in secondary skin breakdown. Loop diuretics (furosemide) will be administered in combination with Metolazone.
Salt-poor human albumin (0.5 to 1.0g/kg, given IV over 60 minutes): is used for severely edematous children. It is given IV, to be followed within 30 minutes by IV furosemide.
Diet: salt is restricted by a no-added salt diet and a diet generous in protein. A high-protein diet is a contraindication with the presence of azotemia and renal failure.

NURSING CARE PLANS

Essential nursing diagnoses and plans associated with this condition:

Fluid volume excess (5)

Related to: Compromised regulatory mechanism
Defining characteristics: Edema (pitting), periorbital and facial puffiness in morning and dependent in the evening, abdominal ascites, scrotal or labial edema, edema of mucous membranes of intestines, anasarca, slow weight gain, decreased urine output, altered electrolytes, Sp. Gr., BP, R

Altered nutrition: Less than body requirements (168)

Related to: Inability to ingest and digest foods and absorb nutrients
Defining characteristics: Anorexia, edema of intestinal tract affecting absorption, weight loss, loss of protein (negative nitrogen balance), rejection of low salt diet

Risk for impaired skin integrity (397)

Related to: Internal factor of edema
Defining characteristics: Disruption of skin surface, waxy pallor, stretched and shiny appearance, muscle wasting, decreased tissue perfusion, pressure on edematous area, irritation of anal area with diarrhea

Diarrhea (171)

Related to: Inflammation, edema, malabsorption of bowel
Defining characteristics: Increased frequency, loose, liquid stools, abdominal discomfort

Risk for fluid volume deficit (222)

Related to: Change in appearance (severe fluid overload, edema)
Defining characteristics: Puffiness in face, severe generalized edema (anasarca) ascites, labial or scrotal swelling, obesity and Cushing syndrome (due to long-term corticosteriod therapy side effects)

Risk for fluid volume deficit (222)

Related to: Medications, intravascular fluid loss
Defining characteristics: Diuretic therapy, increased fluid output, urinary frequency, rapid weight loss, hypotension, hypovolemia, protein and fluid loss, edema

SPECIFIC DIAGNOSES AND CARE PLANS

Fatigue

Related to: States of discomfort
Defining characteristics: Extreme edema, lethargy, easily fatigued with any activity

Outcome Criteria

Progressive return to activities within disease limitations as edema subsides

Interventions	Rationales
Assess degree of weakness, fatigue, extent of edema and difficult movement or activity in bed	Provides information about fatigue and tendency of lying in prone position and not moving or changing position
Maintain bedrest during most acute stage	Prevents energy expenditure when edema is severe
Provide selected play activities as tolerated and adjust schedule to allow for rest periods and after activity	Provides stimulation and activity within endurance level as edema is relieved
Plan activities with discretion and observe for behavior changes after activity	Prevents fatigue while improving endurance; inactivity and steroid therapy and disease results in mood swings and irritability in the child
Allow for quiet play followed by unrestricted activity and encourage child to set own limits when feasible	Promotes independence and control of situations

Information, Instruction, Demonstration

Interventions	Rationales
Inform child to rest when feeling tired	Reduces fatigue and conserves energy
Inform parent(s) and child that full participation in activities will be allowed as the disease is resolved	Promotes return to active life for child

Discharge or Maintenance Evaluation

- Conserves energy and minimizes fatigue
- Participates in play and activities within capabilities in a progressive fashion
- Balances activity with rest periods

Risk for infection

Related to: Inadequate secondary defenses
Defining characteristics: Fluid overload, edema, elevated temperature, immunosuppression, suppressed inflammatory response, leukopenia

Outcome Criteria

Absence of infectious process, upper respiratory cellulitis, cystitis, or other sites

Interventions	Rationales
Assess temperature elevation, respiratory changes (dyspnea, productive cough with yellow sputum), urinary changes (cloudy, foul smelling urine), skin changes (redness, swelling, pain in an area)	Indicates presence of infectious process resulting from steroid and immunosuppressant therapy given to enhance body defenses and reduce relapse rate
Prevent visits from those with illnesses or infectious processes	Protects child from infected persons that may transmit pathogen to immunosuppressed child
Provide private room or share room with children who are free from infections	Protects child from pathogen transmission
Maintain medical aseptic techniques and handwash when giving care	Promotes measures to prevent infection
Maintain warmth for child, regulate room environmental temperature and humidity	Prevents chilling and predisposition to upper respiratory infection
Administer antibiotic therapy if ordered	Prevents or treats infection based on culture and sensitivities

Information, Instruction, Demonstration

Interventions	Rationales
Instruct parent(s) and child of need to avoid exposure to those with infections	Provides understanding of susceptibility to infections
Inform parent(s) and child of importance of handwash and other techniques to maintain a healthy environment	Prevents transmission of infectious agents to the child
Inform parent(s) that an infection may initiate a relapse of the disease	Provides rationale for preventative measures
Instruct parent(s) to report any sign or symptom of infection to physician immediately	Allows for immediate medical intervention to prevent relapse

Discharge or Maintenance Evaluation

- Absence of infections
- Controls transmission of pathogens to child
- Participates in measures to prevent infections

Knowledge deficit

Related to: Lack of exposure to information about disease
Defining characteristics: Expressed need for information about disease, medication administration, follow-up care and procedures, anxiety associated with relapse of disease

Outcome Criteria

Verbalization of knowledge and demonstration of follow-up care

Interventions	Rationales
Assess knowledge of disease, signs and symptoms of relapse, dietary and activity aspects of care, medication administration and side effects, monitoring urine and VS	Provides information about teaching needs for follow-up care
Assess level of anxiety and need for support in care of ill child and possible relapse	Anxiety will interfere with learning process

Information, Instruction, Demonstration

Interventions	Rationales
Instruct in medications administration including side effects of steroids and immunosuppressives; that these are reversible when discontinued and must be discontinued gradually	Promotes compliance of accurate medication administration and what can be expected from drug therapy
Inform parent(s) that immunizations may be postponed	Provides safety measure to prevent complications in a child that is immunosuppressive
Inform parent(s) and child of potential for relapse and support social isolation as needed	Prevent risk of infection that may precipitate a relapse
Instruct and demonstrate and allow for parent(s) to return demonstration of urine testing by dipstick for albumin, monitor for edema, taking daily weights and BP and to report changes of increased weight or presence of albumin in urine to physician immediately	Allows for monitoring of possible relapse of disease
Reinforce physician instructions about Na restriction, activity progression and pacing	Promotes return to usual patterns of living
Provide information about disease, its causes, need for frequent hospitalizations if disease becomes prolonged or is a relapsing type with remissions and exacerbations	Promotes understanding of disease process and importance of compliance with therapy to prevent exacerbation

Discharge or Maintenance Evaluation

- Verbalizes signs and symptoms of disease and importance of immediate reporting
- Complies appropriately with an administration of medications with knowledge of side effects to expect
- Complies with follow-up care requirements in diet and activity
- Collects specimen and tests for albumin
- Monitors for edema, daily weights for increases, BP for increases
- Minimizes potential for relapse of disease
- Verbalizes comfort with implementation of follow-up care
- Encourages return to school and socialization for child within limitations imposed by the disease

Nephrotic Syndrome (Nephrosis)

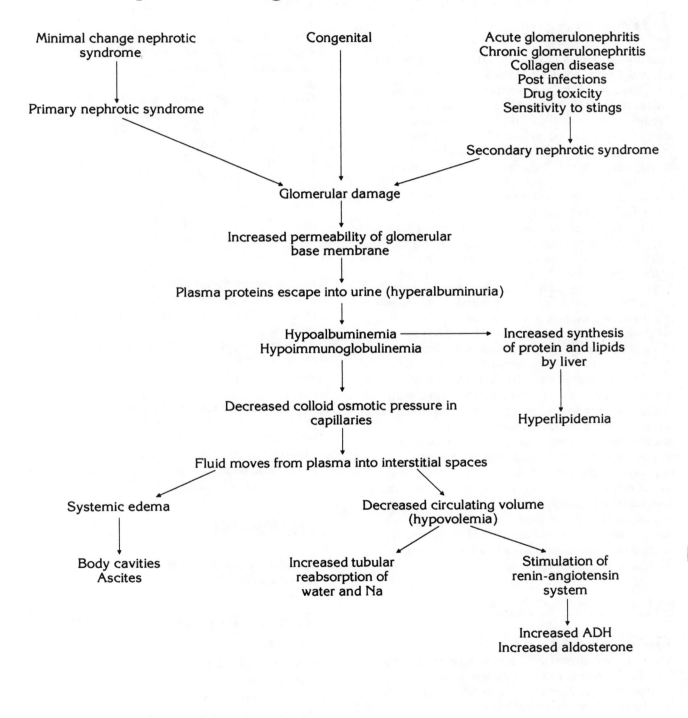

Sexually-Transmitted Diseases

Sexually transmitted diseases (STD), previously termed venereal disease, are described as a diverse group of viral, bacterial, protozoa and ectoparasitic infections which are due to a common route of transmission through sexual intercourse. Infectious organisms associated with STD(s) include: Chlamydia tractor (urethritis and cervicitis); Neisseria gonorrhea; epididymitis (due to C. trachomatis or N. gonorrhea); Pelvic Inflammatory Disease (PID) (due to C. trachomatis, N. gonorrhea, or Mycoplasma hominis); vaginal infections (bacterial vaginosis, vulvovaginal candidiasis, or trichomoniasis); syphilis (during SO pregnancy, or congenital syphilis, or syphilis with AIDS); Haemophilus ducreyi (chancroid); herpes simplex; papillomavirus (genital warts); and genital herpes. Infection by each of the above organisms has its own pattern of clinical patterns; medications/treatments; prognosis; transmission dynamics/host response to infection; and patterns of sexual contact. STDs are identified as one of the major causes of morbidity during adolescence. Three factors, unique to the adolescent, predispose this age group to STDs: developmental maturity, biology, and environment. Developmentally: evolving identity and emerging sexuality; reproductive capabilities but insufficient maturity to make safe decisions and to communicate effectively with their partner. Biologically: the adolescent female is at increased risk due to thin layer of columnar cells in the area of the endocervix; the unchallenged immune system does not provide adequate antibody response to exposure to these organisms; and during anovulatory cycles estrogen may facilitate the transport of pathogens. Environmentally: include barriers to the adolescent's direct access to contraceptive usage.

MEDICAL CARE

Diagnostic Evaluation
Diagnosis is completed by identification of the organism from direct smear or culture techniques.
Asymptomatic males: screening by detection of pyuria in the urine (positive for Neisseria gonorrhea).

Homosexual males: should receive pharyngeal, urethral, and rectal cultures.
Acute or asymptomatic females: cervical and urethral smears is required for all types of STDs.

Medical Management
Antibiotic therapy: (is specific to the infecting organism and the age of patient)
Chlamydia: Adults: Doxycycline (PO- 100 mg) or Azithromycin (PO- 1 gm., once). For the neonate: Erthromycin (12.5 mg/kg can be given PO or IV for 14 days).
Gonorrhea: Adults: Ceftrizxone (IM- 125 mg, once or IV- 1 gm., 7-10 days). For the neonate: Ceftriaxone (IM- 125 mg, once or 25 mg/kg/ IV, 7-10 days; or 25mg/kg/IM, 10-14 days).
Epididymitis: Adults: Ceftrioxone (IM- 200 mg, once) followed by Doxycycline (PO- 100 mg BID, 10 days).
Vaginal infection: Adults: Metronidazole (PO 2 grams once or 500/mg BID for 10 days).
Syphilis: Adults: Penicillin G (IM once, or IM weekly for 3 weeks, or IV for 10-14 days)
Chancroid: Adults: Erythromycin (PO- 500 mg, for 7 days; or IM- 250 mg, once; or PO- 1 gram, once).
Herpes simplex: Acycloir (PO- 400 mg, 7-10 days; or PO- 800, 7-10 days; or PO- 400 mg, 5 days for recurrent infection; or PO - 400 mg, BID, for prevention of reoccurrence).
Antibiotics: (is specific to the infecting organism and the age of patient).
Keratolytics: podophyllum resin (Podofin) TOP to treat warts.
Venereal disease research laboratory (VDRL): reveals presence of the Treponema pallidum (syphilis) by antibody tests (FTA-ABS and TPI).
Cultures: Urethral and/or cervical smears for microorganism identification in gonorrhea, Chlamydia, urethritis; lesion smear to detect herpes, syphilis.

NURSING CARE PLANS

Essential nursing diagnoses and plans associated with these conditions:

Risk for impaired skin integrity (397)

Related to: External factor of excretions and secretions, internal factor of infectious agent invasion
Defining characteristics: Disruption of skin surface, invasion of body structures, pus from urethra or cervix, vesicles on genitalia, buttocks, thighs, penile or vaginal

discharge, chancre lesion on penis or female genitalia, skin rash, popupapules on skin, blisters and ulcerations on genitalia, itching and burning of lesions or sores, conjunctivitis, pharyngitis, dermatitis

Hyperthermia (112)

Related to: Illness (pelvic inflammatory disease)
Defining characteristics: Increase in body temperature above normal range, warm to touch, increased pulse and respiratory rate, evidence of infectious process

SPECIFIC DIAGNOSES AND CARE PLANS

Knowledge deficit

Related to: Lack of information about disease
Defining characteristics: Expressed need for information about treatment and prevention of recurrence of sexually transmitted disease

Outcome Criteria

Knowledge of care and treatment of specific disease
Knowledge and implementation of measures to prevent

Interventions	Rationales
Assess knowledge of diagnostic and reporting methods, signs and symptoms of specific diseases, risk factors in acquiring or transmitting disease and potential complications	Provides information about the disease causes, treatment and preventative measures
Inform of type of culture and blood testing done for diagnosis of disease	Provides information about need to identify specific organisms by culture of discharge from lesions, urethra, vagina, and cervix
Instruct to note pain, tingling, burning, dysuria, frequency, purulent discharge or leukorrhea, itching of genitalia	Indicates active disease caused by lesion, inflammation
Instruct in administration of antibiotics, analgesics, topical agents as ordered; emphasize need to take full course of ordered antibiotic	Provides treatment of choice for specific disease and instructions for administration

Interventions	Rationales
and follow-up exam for syphilis, gonorrhea, pelvic inflammation, chlamydial infection; application of topical chemical agent and removing the drug by washing off in 4-6 hours to remove warts; topical application of topical antiviral to treat herpes	
Inform that disease is contracted and transmitted by sexual contact and to avoid sexual contact with an infected partner and during active phase of the disease; instruct to use male or female condom protection if sexually active	Prevents spread of the disease to others and recurrence in the infected person
Instruct in handwashing technique to be used following toileting and to avoid touching face with hands	Prevents transmission of infectious agents to genitalia or other body parts
Explain consequences of disease if left untreated or follow-up evaluation avoided, especially in gonorrhea and syphilis	Prevents progression or complications of the disease; may lead to infertility or second stage syphilis
Inform that information will be kept confidential according to state laws	Promotes environment conducive to instruction and that is nonjudgmental and accepting
Inform of causes of flare-ups of herpes and to avoid changes in environment extremes, tight clothing, colds, exposure to sun	Prevents recurrence of herpes lesions that commonly occur with illnesses, trauma, or changes that may lower resistance
Inform of importance of reporting the disease and contacts	Promotes control of disease by tracing and treating contacts as well as the infected person
Instruct on the recommended use of spermicide-coated latex condoms	Usage helps prevent transmission of infections
Communicate to the adolescent the best form of prevention is avoiding exposure (by sexual activity)	This information may decrease incidence and reoccurrence of STDs in the adolescent

Interventions	Rationales
Provide education to the adolescent that STDs are not contracted from toilet seats, drinking glasses or bath towels; also, that hormonal contraceptive methods do not provide protection against STDs	Adolescents are often uninformed or lack accurate information regarding how STDs are contracted

Discharge or Maintenance Evaluation

- Verbalizes signs and symptoms specific to disease present
- Administers oral and topical medications correctly with desired effect
- Complies with measures to prevent transmission or recurrence of the disease
- Complies with follow-up treatment
- Absence of signs and symptoms of spread of disease or complications
- Avoids factors that exacerbate disease and maintains nutrition, activity, rest needs for optimal health
- Verbalizes adequate knowledge about disease, treatment, transmission, prevention and follow-up care
- Participates in sex education classes

Sexually Transmitted Diseases

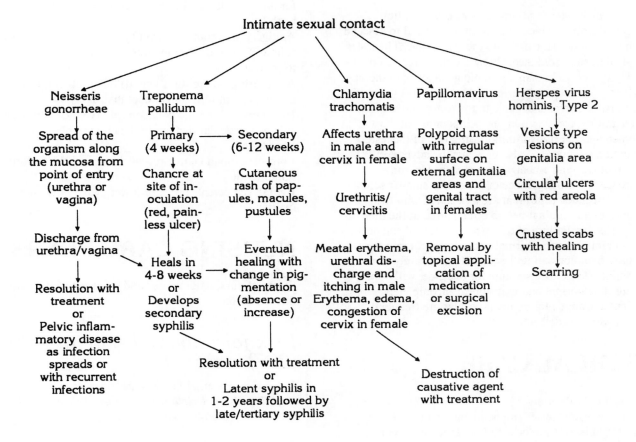

Intimate sexual contact

Neisseris gonorrheae
↓
Spread of the organism along the mucosa from point of entry (urethra or vagina)
↓
Discharge from urethra/vagina
↓
Resolution with treatment
or
Pelvic inflammatory disease as infection spreads or with recurrent infections

Treponema pallidum
↓
Primary (4 weeks) → Secondary (6-12 weeks)
↓
Chancre at site of inoculation (red, painless ulcer)
↓
Heals in 4-8 weeks or Develops secondary syphilis

Cutaneous rash of papules, macules, pustules
↓
Eventual healing with change in pigmentation (absence or increase)
↓
Resolution with treatment
or
Latent syphilis in 1-2 years followed by late/tertiary syphilis

Chlamydia trachomatis
↓
Affects urethra in male and cervix in female
↓
Urethritis/ cervicitis
↓
Meatal erythema, urethral discharge and itching in male Erythema, edema, congestion of cervix in female

Papillomavirus
↓
Polypoid mass with irregular surface on external genitalia areas and genital tract in females
↓
Removal by topical application of medication or surgical excision
↓
Destruction of causative agent with treatment

Herspes virus hominis, Type 2
↓
Vesicle type lesions on genitalia area
↓
Circular ulcers with red areola
↓
Crusted scabs with healing
↓
Scarring

Undescended Testes

Undescended testes (cryptorchidism) is a condition present at birth in which one or both testes fail to descend through the inguinal canal into the scrotal sac. The testes usually descend spontaneously by 1 year of age. If not, a child may receive human chorionic gonadotropin therapy or surgery (orchiopexy) performed between 1-2 years of age. Surgery prevents damage to the testes that are affected by exposure to a higher temperature in the abdomen and the risk for tumor formation of the testes. Repair at a younger age also prevents the adverse effect on body image and embarrassment caused by the difference in the appearance of the empty smaller scrotal sac. Undescended testes that are associated with the presence of an inguinal hernia are repaired at the time of herniorrhaphy. Failure of the testes to descend can occur at any point along the normal path of descent into the scrotum. Symptoms of undescended testes rarely causes discomfort. The entire scrotum, or one side, will appear smaller than normal and may appear incompletely developed. Congenital inguinal hernias are frequently present with this defect.

MEDICAL CARE

Diagnostic Evaluation
Retractile testes: testes can be manually pushed back down (or milked) into the scrotum. True undescended testes cannot be manually pushed back down into the scrotum.
Cremasteric reflex: (after 6 months of age and peaks by 4 to 5 years of age). Procedure: drawing up of the scrotum and testicle when the skin over the front and inside thigh is stimulated, will result in spontaneous retraction of testes back into the scrotum.
Diagnostic tests, may include: Testicular Ultrasonography, Computed Tomography, and Laparoscopy. All can be performed to confirm undescended testes prior to surgical intervention and to rule out masses, tumors, or cysts.

Medical Management
By 1 year of age, the undescended testes will spontaneously descend into the scrotum in 75% of cases. If testes do not descend, surgery (orchiopexy is recommended before the child's second birthday).

Trial Hormone Therapy: {with luteinizing hormone-releasing hormone (nasal spray) and human chorionic gonadotropin (injection)}; may be helpful to stimulate spontaneous descent of testes. The response to hormone therapy to facilitating or initiating the descent of the testes back into the scrotum is not clearly understood.
Surgical intervention (Orchiopexy): is recommended for undescended testes repair before the child's second birthday.
Analgesics: acetaminophen (Tylenol tablets, Liquiprin solution), codeine (Methylmorphine) PO postoperatively to control pain.
Antibiotics: ampicillin (Amcill) PO or other anti-infective to prevent infection at operative site.
Hormones: chorionic gonadotropin (Choron 10) IM to enhance testicular descent in the absence of an anamotic impediment.
Complete blood count: reveals increased WBC if infection present.
Urinalysis: reveals upper or lower urinary tract abnormalities.

NURSING CARE PLANS

Essential nursing diagnoses and plans associated with this condition:

Risk for impaired skin integrity (397)

Related to: External factor of surgical incision
Defining characteristics: Disruption of skin surface, surgical invasion of body structure(s)

Hyperthermia (112)

Related to: Risk of infection in postoperative period (infection is rare preoperatively)
Defining characteristics: Increase in body temperature above normal range, warm to touch, increased pulse and respiratory rate, evidence of infectious process at surgical site, temperature elevation (greater than 38.8°C)

SPECIFIC DIAGNOSES AND CARE PLANS

Anxiety

Related to: Threat to self-concept, change in health status of child, hospitalization and surgery of child

Defining characteristics: Increased apprehension and expressed concern about future infertility and effect on body image, presence of empty scrotum and smaller size, expressed concern about impending surgery or need for future surgery and procedure performed to correct abnormality

Outcome Criteria

Reduced parental and child anxiety verbalized
Verbalizes positive effects of surgical correction
Body image remains intact with placement of testes in scrotum

Interventions	Rationales
Assess source and level of anxiety and how it is manifested; need for information that will relieve anxiety	Provides information about anxiety level and need for interventions to relieve it; source for the parent(s) include fear and uncertainty about treatment and recovery; source for child include embarrassment by different shape and size of scrotum after school age
Allow expression of concerns and opportunity to ask questions about diagnosis, procedures, effect of abnormal placement on testes and future fertility	Provides opportunity to vent feelings and fears and secure information to reduce anxiety
Communicate with parent(s) and child and answer questions calmly and honestly; use pictures, models and drawings as aids where helpful in explanations	Promotes calm and supportive trusting environment
Give parent(s) and child as much input in decisions about care and routines as possible	Allows for more control over situation

Interventions	Rationales
Provide as much privacy to the child as possible during assessments	Promotes comfort and prevents embarrassment

Information, Instruction, Demonstration

Interventions	Rationales
Inform parent(s) that surgery is ideally performed after the age of one but may be done during the preschool years by the age of 5 if testes have not spontaneously descended on their own	Provides information about need for surgical correction before schoolage to prevent psychological and cosmetic embarrassment to the child and that exposure to the higher temperature in the abdomen may damage testes and predispose to formation of tumor and infertility
Inform the parent(s) and child that a suture secures the testes after it is brought down into the scrotum and is then attached to the thigh without tension applied to the scrotum; an overnight stay in the hospital may be necessary	Explains the surgical procedure to correct the deformity (orchiopexy); some procedures do not include a traction suture attached to the thigh
Inform child that his penis will remain in place and that the surgery will not affect the penis in any way	Alleviates any fear that the penis may be cut off
Inform parent(s) about the prognosis for sterility and concerns about changes in sexual orientation	Relieves fear about sterility and homosexuality
Instruct parent(s) and child of activity restrictions (3-7 days) and play appropriate to age and trauma of surgery	Provides information about return to normal activity without injury to operative area or disconnect the suture which may lead to testes again returning into inguinal canal
Instruct and demonstrate self-examination of testes and allow for return demonstration; inform to report any change felt	Allows for early detection of a neoplasm

Discharge or Maintenance Evaluation

- Verbalizes reduction in anxiety about abnormality, procedure to correct it, risk of complications
- Verbalizes positive effects of surgical correction
- Participates in decision making and postoperative care
- Complies with activity restrictions, self-examination of testes

Risk for infection

Related to: Inadequate primary defenses (broken skin)
Defining characteristics: Surgical incision proximity to urine and feces

Outcome Criteria

Absence of infectious process at surgical site

Interventions	Rationales
Assess wound for redness, warmth, swelling, discharge	Indicates infection at site
Apply ice to wound post-operatively	Reduces swelling
Carefully cleanse perineal area of any urine or stool as needed	Prevents contamination of wound and risk of infection
Administer antibiotic therapy as ordered	Prevents or treats infection by preventing synthesis of cell wall of microorganisms

Information, Instruction, Demonstration

Interventions	Rationales
Instruct parent(s) and demonstrate cleansing of perineum, wound cleansing and dressing	Prevents infection of suture line
Instruct to complete course of antibiotic therapy	Prevents recurrence of infection
Inform child to wear clean undergarments or parent(s) to change child's diaper frequently and not leave	Maintains cleanliness of surgical area and prevents contamination

child in soiled diaper

Discharge or Maintenance Evaluation

- Absence of infection of surgical area
- Maintains clean perineal and wound areas
- Complies with antibiotic regimen as instructed
- Protects surgical area from bathing and urine and/or feces

Undescended Testes (Cryptorchid)

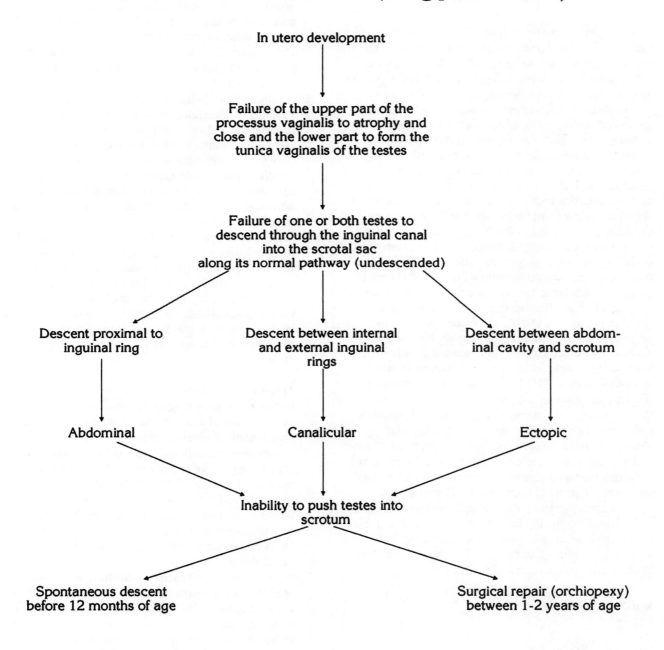

Urinary Tract Infection

Urinary tract infection (UTI) is defined as infection located in the lower tract (bladder or urethra) or in the upper tract (ureters or kidneys). The peak incidence of UTI observed in children occurs between 2 and 6 years of age, but can be observed at any age. The incidence of UTI in children also varies by gender: females have a 10% to 30% greater risk of developing a UTI; males have a 50% greater risk of developing a recurrent UTI; and during the newborn age range only, male infants are at a greater risk of developing a UTI. Etiologic factors associated with UTI in children include: 75% to 80% of bacterial infections are due to Escherichia coli; bacterial organisms occur more frequently than viral or fungal organisms; greater in low-birth weight and preterm infants; higher incidence in female children is attributed to the female child's anatomical differences from the male child (shorter urethra with an increased chance of contamination due to the close proximity to the anus); structural factors affecting complete urine drainage (resulting in urinary stasis); metabolic dysfunctions; hygeine practices (especially in younger girls and sexually active adolescents); and external factors (i.e., foley catheter, tight fitting diapers, exposure to bubble baths). Diagnosis of UTI can be made on a urine culture from a clean-catch or a catheterized specimen. However, there is a high risk for contamination with clean-catch specimens. Lab result criteria for a UTI diagnosis: Colony counts of 100,000 colonies in a clean-catch urine; and any urine culture greater than 5,000 colonies from urine obtained on a suprapubic puncture or catheterized specimen. Signs and symptoms of UTI in pediatric patients are age-related. For example, unique symptoms of UTI displayed by the infant: failure to thrive and fever; by the preschooler: anorexia and somonolence; by the school-ager: enuresis and personality changes; and those by the adolescent: fatigue and flank pain.

MEDICAL CARE

Diagnostic Evaluation
Diagnosis is dependent upon: age-related symptoms of UTI; an accurate and thorough history of UTI symptoms, patterns of voiding, health practices at home, recurrent treatment of UTI, physical growth and examination, and urine culture lab results.

Urine culture and sensitivity: the gold standard for the diagnosis of UTI, to determine the presence of bacteria in the urine and the drugs to which they are sensitive. UTI will have > 100,000 colony formation units/ml in the first urine specimen in the morning. Evidence of a contaminated urine sample will reveal a report of less than 10,000 colony formation. Low colony formation may also occur due to very dilute or acidic urine, frequent voiding, chronic infection, or antibacterial therapy.

Urinalysis: may show elevated protein, leukocytes, casts, pus cells. The urinalysis may be normal, with a positive urine culture.

Radiographic studies: (may be performed to identify any structural or functional renal abnormalities). These may include: renal ultrasound (RUS), voiding cystourethrogram (VCUG), intravenous pyelogram (IVP), and dimercaptosuccinic acid (DSMA).

Voiding cystourethrogram (VCUC): reveals anatomic abnormality of bladder and urethra and reflux of urine into ureters reflex which predisposes to recurrent infection.

Intravenous pyelogram (IVP): reveals abnormalities in renal or bladder function caused by recurrent infections.

Renal Ultrasound (RUS): radiologic test to determine renal obstructions and structural abnormalities; renal size; renal calculit; and polycystic kidney.

Dimercaptosuccinic Acid (DSMA): a renal scan which is very accurate in making a diagnosis of UTI, pyelonephritis, integrity of renal parenchyma and renal function.

Medical Management
Is directed at early diagnosis, elimination of infection, identification of causative factors to prevent infection and preservation of renal function.

Antibiotics: (usually use are broad-spectrum, against both gram positive and gram negative organisms). In children older than 12 months, a single oral antibiotic is recommended for a 14-day course, such as: trimethaprim/sulfamethoxazole, amoxicillin, ampicillin, nitrofurantoin or cephalosporin. If there is no improvement in 24-48 hours post onset of antibiotic therapy, the child should be hospitalized.

Nitrate tests with reactive reagent urine strips: may be used to identify reoccurrence of UTI symptoms in the home, if used on the first AM specimen. It is not 100% accurate, since all organisms do not produce nitrates and leukocytes. Recommended for home monitoring with children at risk for recurrence of UTI.

Follow-up management: urine cultures should be repeated monthly for 3 months, every 3 months for 6 months, and annually thereafter to ensure early detection of any recurrent symptoms. The relapse rate of UTI is high in children and tends to occur within 1-2 months after termination of antibiotic therapy.

Anti-infectives: penicillins and sulfonamides dependent on identification of the microorganism and sensitivity to specific anti-infectives; ampicillin (Amcill) or sulfisoxazole (Gantrisin) PO are possible choices.

Urine culture: reveals colonization of bacteria and identification of specific organism and sensitivity to antimicrobials.

NURSING CARE PLANS

Essential nursing diagnoses and plans associated with this condition:

Hyperthermia (112)

Related to: Illness (urinary tract infections)
Defining characteristics: Age-related symptoms of UTI in the pediatric patient, fever (temperature greater than 38.5°C), positive urine culture and sensitivity for bacterial in the urine

Risk for fluid volume deficit (222)

Related to: Abnormal loss of fluids and deviations affecting intake of fluids
Defining characteristics: Fever and chills; vomiting and diarrhea; anorexia, abdominal pain; reluctance of child to drink fluids; attempts to hold urine for long periods; enuresis; urgency and dysuria with voiding

SPECIFIC DIAGNOSES AND CARE PLANS

Knowledge deficit of parent(s), child

Related to: Diagnosis of new onset UTI or evidence of recurrence of UTI
Defining characteristics: Lacks accurate information related to diagnosis; treatment of current UTI and prevention or recurrent UTI; age-related signs and symptoms of UTI; home management and follow-up needs

Outcome Criteria

Adequate information for preventative measures to avoid recurrence
Absence of urinary tract infection

Interventions	Rationales
Assessment of parent(s) knowledge of age-related signs and symptoms of UTI, associated anatomy effects related to UTI (girls vs boys); assess history and past treatments for UTI, compliance of previous UTI management	Provides information needed to develop plan of instruction to ensure compliance of medical regimen; UTI commonly occur in females and are prone to recurrent episodes; vesicourethral reflux predisposes to UTI

Information, Instruction, Demonstration

Interventions	Rationales
Inform parent(s) of causes of the infection and predisposing factors; to be alert to dysuria, frequency, urgency, fever, foul odor to urine, cloudiness of urine, enuresis in the toilet trained child or flank pain, chills and fever, abdominal distention; and to report the presence of these signs and symptoms to physician	Provides information that indicates lower or upper urinary tract infection
Instruct parent(s) to collect a mid-stream urine specimen for laboratory analysis before and after antibiotic therapy	Reveals presence of infection and identifies organism responsible and if treatment is effective or needs changing
Instruct parent(s) and child in antibiotic therapy and to take full course of medication; stool softener if constipated	Ensures compliance with medication therapy for effective resolution of infection and prevention of relapse; prevent possible obstruction of urination by constipation
Inform parent(s) and child to avoid bubble baths and tub baths and take showers; to wipe female from front to back and instruct child to do same after toileting	Provides information about prevention of recurrence of infection and irritation to the urethra

Interventions	Rationales
Instruct child to void frequently and increase daily fluids according to age, include fluids that are acidic (citrus and cranberry juice)	Prevents retention and stasis of urine which predisposes to infection; fluids flush out bacteria and acidic fluids change pH of urine from alkaline to acid
Inform parent(s) and child to avoid wearing tight nonabsorbable undergarments	Predisposes to harboring of bacteria, entry and ascending into urinary tract
If diagnostic tests are to be performed, provide information about type of procedure, reason for procedure to be done, what to expect during procedure, after care following procedure	Prepares child and parent(s) for procedures to diagnosis anatomic abnormalities that may be the source of UTI
Instruct parents to obtain urine for analysis from the first morning void	The first morning void is considered the most accurate for assessing growth of organisms; urine specimens will show a decline in colonization throughout the day due to diuresis and frequent voiding
Instruct parents to avoid giving the child caffeine beverages and carbonated beverages	Caffeine and carbonated beverages may cause irritation to the bladder mucosa
Instruct sexually active adolescents to void immediately after sexual intercourse	This measure is associated with decreasing the risk of exposure to UTI; it may also help prevent recurrence of UTI; this measure will aid in flushing out bacteria
Instruct parents on associated signs of infections (i.e., scratching between legs and around anal area)	These behaviors are identified as signs of related intestinal parasites and should be evaluated
Instruct parents on proper technique of urine collection; urine culture should be as sterile as possible	Contamination during urine collection can alter results and affect treatment
Urine culture specimens can be kept in the refrigerator for up to 24 hours; urine culture specimens should be tested immediately	Proper storage of urine culture specimens will prevent false positive culture results

Discharge or Maintenance Evaluation

- Verbalizes signs and symptoms of UTI
- Minimizes recurrent UTI by carrying out preventative measures
- Urinary culture negative for infectious organisms following treatment
- Complies appropriately with administration of anti-infective therapy
- Collects mid-stream urine specimen and takes to laboratory when signs and symptoms of urinary infection are present
- Complies with follow-up care requirements
- Prevents spread of infection to upper urinary tract
- Absence of constipation causing bladder neck obstruction and urinary stasis

Urinary Tract Infection

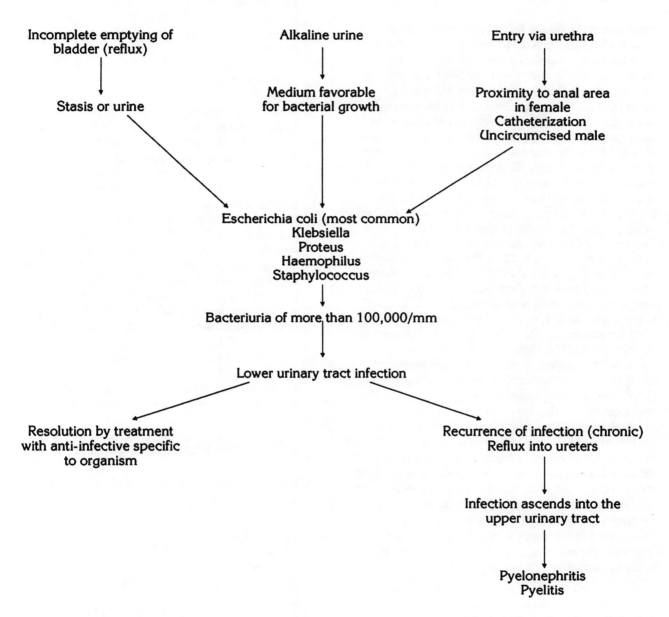

Incomplete emptying of
bladder (reflux)

Alkaline urine

Entry via urethra

Stasis or urine

Medium favorable
for bacterial growth

Proximity to anal area
in female
Catheterization
Uncircumcised male

Escherichia coli (most common)
Klebsiella
Proteus
Haemophilus
Staphylococcus

Bacteriuria of more than 100,000/mm

Lower urinary tract infection

Resolution by treatment
with anti-infective specific
to organism

Recurrence of infection (chronic)
Reflux into ureters

Infection ascends into the
upper urinary tract

Pyelonephritis
Pyelitis

Vesicoureteral Reflux

Vesicoureteral reflux is defined as a retrograde (or backflow) of urine into the ureters. The age at diagnosis for VUR rarely occurs after five years of age. The etiology of VUR is categorized into two types, primary and secondary reflux. Primary reflux is due to an inadequate valvular mechanism at the ureterovesical junction and is not associated with any obstruction or neurogenic bladder. The inadequate valve in primary reflux is due to the shortened submucosal tunnel which shortens bladder filling. Secondary reflux occurs secondary to obstruction (50% of cases in infants are due to posterior urethral valves) or neurogenic bladder. Important risk factors associated with VUR include: age, urinary tract infection (UTI), and reflux. The International Classification System has defined five grade variations of VUR. These five grade variations describe the degree of reflux from the bladder into the upper urinary tract structures. The following effects of unrepaired reflux have been identified: defect in urine concentration ability; urine concentration ability is inversely proportional to the grade of reflux; glomerular function is usually not affected unless there is parenchymal damage; renal scarring; developmental arrest is associated with reflux; lower-weight percentiles (in physical growth); hypertension, proteinuria and those with bilateral scarring have an increased risk of developing end stage renal failure (as high as 30%). In the majority of children with a reflux grade of I or II, will disappear spontaneously without surgical intervention if infection is controlled. The primary reflux is unlikely to spontaneously resolve in children with a reflux grade of V or in the adolescent age group. Management of reflux for grades I to III includes antibacterial therapy for infection control. Management of reflux for grade IV and V usually includes surgery (ureteral reimplantation). The expected success rate for surgical intervention is 95% to 99%.

MEDICAL CARE

Diagnostic Evaluation
Ultrasound and Contrast VCUG: is the current recommended initial diagnostic tests for VUR.

Ultrasound: is a useful screening tool for the older child with UTI and as a means to measure renal growth and parenchymal volume.
Voiding Cystourethrography (VCUG): visualizes bladder outline and urethra, reveals reflux of urine into ureters, and shows complications of bladder emptying.
IVP: provides information about the integrity of the kidneys, ureters and bladder. It is recommended after an abnormal ultrasound, especially if anatomy is poorly defined.
Renal scan: is more accurate than the IVU in assessing patients with reflux.

Medical Management
Ureteral reimplantation surgery: antireflux surgery, consists of reimplantation of ureters into the bladder.
Antibacterial therapy: commonly used antibacterials include: nitrofurantoin, sulfas, and sulfa-trimethoprim suspensions (they may be administered for short-term or long-term usage).
Follow-up evaluation: children with reflux should be evaluated at a clinic at 3-month intervals. VCUG: is recommended again, at 2 to 6 months postoperatively.
Analgesics: acetaminophen (Tylenol tablets or syrup, Liquiprin solution), codeine (Methelmorphine) PO or IM postoperatively to control pain postoperatively.
Antispasmodics: flavoxate hydrochloride (Urispas) propantheline (Banlin), PO, belladonna and opium (BSO) SUPP. to relax smooth muscle of bladder and reduce discomfort caused by bladder irritation and spasms.
Urine culture: reveals infectious agent and basis for antibacterial therapy or need for modification of therapy.

NURSING CARE PLANS

Essential nursing diagnoses and plans associated with this condition:

Risk for fluid volume deficit (222)

Related to: Loss of fluid through abnormal routes, deviations affecting intake of fluid
Defining characteristics: NPO status pre and postoperatively, urinary catheter (Foley or suprapubic), dry skin and mucous membranes, poor skin turgor, decreased urinary output via catheter or stents, temperature elevation

Risk for impaired skin integrity (397)

Related to: External factor of surgical incision
Defining characteristics: Disruption of skin surface, catheter site irritation and discomfort

Hyperthermia (112)

Related to: Illness (presence of infection)
Defining characteristics: Increase in body temperature above normal range, evidence of infection at surgical or catheter site, or renal/urinary infection

SPECIFIC DIAGNOSES AND CARE PLANS

Knowledge deficit

Related to: Lack of exposure to information about disorder
Defining characteristics: Expressed need for information about continuous medical regimen to control renal/bladder infection and measures to prevent infection

Outcome Criteria

Absence or control of recurrent urinary infections

Interventions	Rationales
Instruct parent(s) and child in antibacterial administration including information on action, dose, form, time, frequency, how to take, side effects to report	Promotes compliance with the medication regimen for long-term therapy to prevent recurrent or relapse of urinary infection
Instruct parent(s) and child to develop strategies for administration of medications including the development of an organized plan using pill dispensers, alarms on a clock or watch, check-off list, reminder notes to prevent omissions	Assists to ensure compliance to prescribed regimen
Instruct parent(s) and child to write a contract with a mutual agreement on expectations and consequences related to prescribed medical care	Promotes compliance and independence and prevents constant reminding by parent to take medication
Inform and instruct parent(s) and child of need to obtain urine cultures by mid-stream and taking to a laboratory or use of dip slide or strip to use at home	Reveals presence of urinary infection and assists to regulate antibacterial therapy

Discharge or Maintenance Evaluation

- Complies with medication regimen
- Complies with urine testing for infectious process
- Absence of recurrent urinary infection

Anxiety

Related to: Change in health status, change in environment (hospitalization for surgery)
Defining characteristics: Expressed apprehension and concern about surgery (ureteral reimplantation) and pre and postoperative procedures and care

Outcome Criteria

Reduced anxiety verbalized by parent(s) and child

Interventions	Rationales
Assess source and level of anxiety and need for information and interventions that will relieve it	Provides information about anxiety level and need to relieve it; source for parent includes the procedure and care of child pre and postoperatively; source for child includes separation from parent(s), unfamiliar environment, and painful procedures
Allow expression of concerns and time to ask questions about need of surgery, procedure to be done, procedures to prepare for surgery, procedures, care and recovery after surgery	Provides opportunity to vent feelings and fears and to feel secure in the environment

Interventions	Rationales
Answer questions calmly and honestly, use pictures, drawings, models and therapeutic play	Promotes trust and a calm and supportive environment
Encourage and allow parent(s) to stay with child and assist in care	Allows parent(s) to care for and support child and continue parental role and increases child's comfort by having a familiar caretaker
Allow as much input into decisions about care and usual routines as possible by parent(s)	Allows for more control over situations and maintains a familiar routine for care
Orient and introduce child to the surgical unit preoperatively	Reduces anxiety caused by fear of the unknown

Information, Instruction, Demonstration

Interventions	Rationales
Inform parent(s) and child about abnormal functioning ureter and reason for surgical repair, that the ureter will be reimplanted to prevent urine from backing up in the ureter and continuing problems with infections	Provides information that will enhance understanding about surgery to reduce anxiety
Inform parent(s) and child and prepare for preoperative procedures and tests necessary for visualization and diagnosis	Allays anxiety and provides accurate information of what to expect
Inform parent(s) and child that catheter and/or stent will be in place and where they will be placed, that they will be irrigated and receive special care, that urine output will be noted and measured for any abnormalities or complications, that a surgical dressing will be in place to protect the incision and in case of young child, restraints may be in place on	Provides information of what to expect following surgery

Interventions	Rationales
arms and legs, and that medications will be given to control pain	
Inform parent(s) and child that surgery and catheters will not affect sterility or sexual orientation	Provides information that may cause anxiety
Inform parent(s) that if child is discharged with catheter, care will be demonstrated and taught to maintain patency	Provides anticipatory information to reduce concern and anxiety

Discharge or Maintenance Evaluation

- Verbalizes reduction in anxiety about pre and postoperative procedures and care
- Verbalizes positive effects of surgical procedure
- Participates in care and support of child before and after surgery
- Verbalizes what to expect when child returns from surgery

Pain

Related to: Physical injuring agent (surgery)
Defining characteristics: Communication of pain descriptors, crying, irritability, restlessness, withdrawal, flank pain, ureteral edema from surgery, bladder spasms

Outcome Criteria

Absence or control of pain following surgery

Interventions	Rationales
Assess verbal and nonverbal behavior, type and location and severity of pain depending on age	Provides information about pain as a basis for analgesic therapy
Administer analgesic and possibly sedative based on pain assessment and before pain becomes severe	Reduces pain and promotes rest to reduce stimuli and restlessness
Place in a comfortable position; avoid unnecessary movement or manipulation of suprapubic catheter	Promotes comfort and decreases bladder spasms that cause pain

Interventions	Rationales
Administer antispasmodic PO or SUPP as ordered	Reduces bladder spasms caused by irritation of suprapubic catheter
Maintain catheter patency by ensuring placement, checking flow and presence of kinks or obstruction	Reduces pain caused by distention as a result of catheter clogging or displacement
Provide distractions and reassurance when spasms occur and stay with child when they occur to inform the child that the pain is temporary	Reduces anxiety which tends to increase pain

Information, Instruction, Demonstration

Interventions	Rationales
Inform parent(s) and child that pain will subside 24-48 hours following surgery and teach measures taken to control pain	Provides knowledge about duration of pain and causes of pain

Discharge or Maintenance Evaluation

- Absence or control of pain
- Administers medications to control pain or factors that predispose to pain
- Controls pain provoking actions when giving care

Risk for infection

Related to: Urinary tract infection (acute, chronic or postoperatively); invasive postoperative drainage tubes (i.e., Silastic stents, urethral Foley or suprapubic tube)
Defining characteristics: Redness, abnormal drainage, and/or swelling at incision site; UTI symptoms (burning on voiding, cloudy and foul smelling urine); positive urine or wound culture; temperature elevation (38.5°C or higher)

Outcome Criteria

Absence of infection at any site
Wound intact and healing

Interventions	Rationales
Assess wound for redness, swelling, purulent drainage on dressing, healing	Indicates presence of infectious process or poor healing
Assess catheter site for redness, edema, irritation; urine collected in drainage system for cloudiness and foul odor	Indicates infectious process at catheter site or in urinary bladder
Collect urine for culture and sensitivities	Reveals presence of urinary infection and sensitivity to specific antibacterial agent
Administer antibacterial as ordered	Treats specific microorganism or prevents infection when catheter is in place
Encourage increased fluid intake daily depending on age requirements when PO fluids are allowed	Promotes dilution of urine to prevent infection and encourage voiding after catheter is removed
Use sterile technique when changing dressings, giving catheter care or emptying drainage bag	Prevents contamination of wound or urinary tract by the introduction of pathogens
Maintain catheter and collection bag below level of bladder and maintain a closed, patent system free of kinks or obstructions	Prevents backflow or urine into bladder or retention of urine which predisposes to infection
Provide suprapubic catheter care by cleansing with peroxide solution after removing any meatal crusting, catheter care by washing perineum with mild soap and water, rinsing and applying antiseptic ointment	Promotes comfort and prevents infection at suprapubic or meatal site
Change dressings when soiled or wet 24 hours after surgery	Promotes comfort and allows for wound assessment

Information, Instruction, Demonstration

Interventions	Rationales
Instruct and demonstrate catheter care, irrigation, emptying of drainage system using sterile technique and allow for return demonstration	Provides information and skill in caring for and maintaining catheter patency to prevent infection if child is to be discharged with catheter in place
Inform parent(s) of signs and symptoms of infection to report	Allows for early intervention if infection is present

Discharge or Maintenance Evaluation

- Absence of urinary tract infection
- Absence of wound infection with healing in progress
- Complies with preventative measures and anti-infective therapy
- Maintains sterile technique in procedures and catheter patency

Risk for injury

Related to: External physical factor of catheter displacement; internal factor of complications of surgical trauma
Defining characteristics: Catheter obstruction, postoperative bleeding catheter dislodgement, bladder distention, reduced urine output, dysuria, frequency, retention following removal of catheter

Outcome Criteria

Absence of catheter complications or complications of surgical trauma
Urinary output of 1 ml/kg/hr within 24 hours after surgery

Interventions	Rationales
Assess output via catheter and note characteristics of urine, passage of blood clots, color of urine and return to clear color; and if clots or return to red color occurs after a period of normal characteristics	Provides information about possible complication of bleeding or obstruction

Interventions	Rationales
Notify physician immediately if red color returns	Allows for immediate interventions to treat hemorrhage
Immobilize arms and legs with restraints, remove periodically; use bed cradle following surgery	Prevents accidental dislodgement or removal of catheter
Secure catheter to abdomen or leg with tape stents to catheter and avoid placing tension on the catheter when in place by gently holding it when performing care	Prevents movement or manipulation of catheter that may cause displacement
If catheter becomes displaced, notify physician for replacement (have a suprapubic catheter on hand at all times)	Ensures continued drainage of urine
Measure I&O qh for an output of 1 ml/kg/hr and notify physician if less	Provides information to ensure adequate output via catheters
Note first voiding after catheter removed, time of voiding and amount, difficulty, presence of abdominal distention	Provides information about return of urinary pattern, presence of retention
Support during first voiding (warm water over perineum, sitting or standing position) and privacy	Prevents embarrassment and promotes voiding
Encourage increase in fluid intake according to age requirements	Promotes voiding

Information, Instruction, Demonstration

Interventions	Rationales
Inform parent(s) and child that physician should be notified if urinary pattern or characteristics change or if unable to void after catheter is removed	Allows for early interventions if needed

Interventions	Rationales
Inform parent(s) of measures taken to ensure that catheters remain in place and patent (use of restraints, anchoring catheters, irrigations) and that this is a temporary situation	Informs parent(s) of need for measures to prevent displacement of catheter
Inform parent(s) of potential complications and preventative measures to take to avoid or treat them	Relieves anxiety and promotes understanding
Instruct child to void frequently after catheter removal	Prevents stasis of urine leading to urinary infection

Discharge or Maintenance Evaluation

- Maintains placement and patency of catheters
- Urinary output of 1 ml/kg/hr
- Return of urinary elimination pattern and adequate amount after removal of catheters
- Prevents and reports risk of complications
- Absence of signs and symptoms of urinary retention or dysfunction

Vesicoureteral Reflux

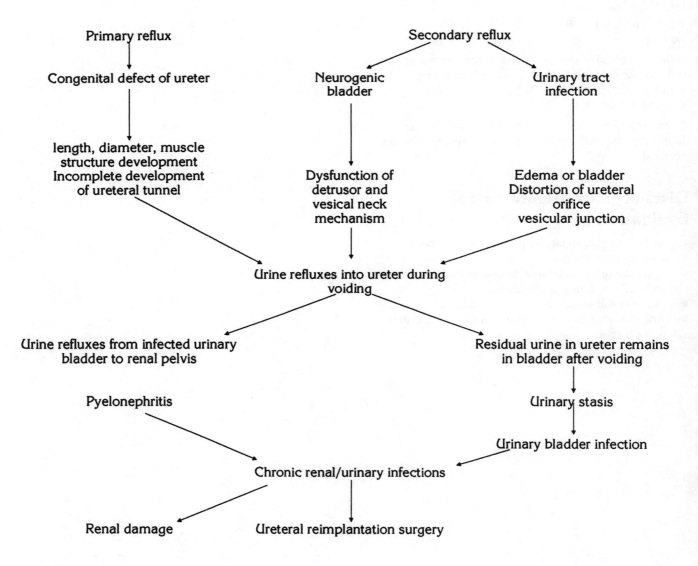

Primary reflux

Congenital defect of ureter

length, diameter, muscle
structure development
Incomplete development
of ureteral tunnel

Secondary reflux

Neurogenic
bladder

Urinary tract
infection

Dysfunction of
detrusor and
vesical neck
mechanism

Edema or bladder
Distortion of ureteral
orifice
vesicular junction

Urine refluxes into ureter during
voiding

Urine refluxes from infected urinary
bladder to renal pelvis

Residual urine in ureter remains
in bladder after voiding

Urinary stasis

Pyelonephritis

Urinary bladder infection

Chronic renal/urinary infections

Renal damage

Ureteral reimplantation surgery

Wilms Tumor

Wilms tumor (or nephroblastoma) is identified as the most common pediatric malignant renal tumor in children. Incidence of Wilms tumor is slightly less frequent in boys than in girls. The mean (or average) age at diagnosis with unilateral tumors is 41.5 months and with bilateral tumors is 29.5 months. Children with Wilms tumor may have associated anomalies and chromosomal abnormalities, such as: aniridia (congenital absence of the iris); hypospadias; cryptorchidism; Beckwith-Wiedemann syndrome; Denys-Drash syndrome; Perlman and the Soto syndrome. The appearance of the Wilms tumor is usually referred to as the "pushing type" (or adjacent renal parenchyma, enclosed by a distinct intra-renal pseudocapsule). The most frequent initial clinical presentation of most children with Wilms tumor is abdominal swelling or the presence of an abdominal mass. This initial presentation is usually first noticed by a parent while bathing or dressing the child. Other frequent findings at diagnosis include: abdominal pain, gross hematuria, fever, and hypertension. The most common sites of metastases of Wilms tumor are the lungs, the regional lymph nodes, and the liver. Histology classifies the tumor into: (1) favorable- or unfavorable-histology; (2) 3 cell types: triphasic or biphasic; with blastemal, stromal and epithelial elements; and (3) 10% have anaplastic or unfavorable histologic findings, including anaplastic Wilms tumor, clear cell sarcoma of the kidney, rhabdoid tumor of the kidney. Other histologic patterns include: nephrogenic rests, congenital mesoblastic nephroma, and renal cell carcinoma. An unfavorable histology is associated with a poor prognosis and more extensive chemotherapy. Prognosis of Wilms tumor is determined by the pathologic staging of Wilms tumor, defined by the National Wilms Tumor Study Group. Both the histology classification and the pathologic staging of Wilms tumor determine the type and length of time for administration of chemotherapy agents and radiation treatments.

MEDICAL CARE

Diagnostic Evaluation: complete peripheral blood count (including a differential white blood cell count platelet count); liver function test (SOOT, SGPT, bilirubin); urinalysis, renal functions tests (BUN, creatinine) and serum calcium determination. Elevated serum calcium is associated with a rhabdoid tumor of the kidney or congenital mesoblastic nephroma.

Abdominal ultrasound examination: can distinquish whether the abdominal mass is intrarenal or estrarenal; unilateral or bilateral; unifocal or multifocal; or solid or cystic.

Contrast-enhanced computed tomography of the abdomen: to evaluate the nature and extent of the mass; and whether the tumor has extended into adjacent structures such as the liver, spleen or colon.

Supine x-ray film of the abdomen: is necessary for planning and review of radiation therapy.

Real-time ultrasonography: determines the patency of the inferior vena cava vessel (when the tumor is identified within this vessel, the proximal extent of the thrombus must be established before the operation).

Chest x-ray and chest CT scan: to determine whether pulmonary metastases are present (are only performed if an unfavorable histology of the tumor is identified).

Radio nuclide bone scan and x-ray skeletal survey: should be performed on all postoperative children with clear cell sarcoma of the kidney, presence of pulmonary or hepatic metastases.

Brain imaging: should be obtained on all children with clear cell sarcoma of the kidney or with rhabdoid tumor of the kidney, both of these tumors are associated with intracranial metastases.

Bone marrow aspiration & biopsy: are usually not performed since bone marrow involvement is rare.

No change for the following tests: renal angiogram; scans of kidney, liver and bone; ESR; albumin; enzymes; CBC and urinalysis.

Therapeutic Management
Chemotherapy and radiation therapy protocol:
Favorable Histology (FH): Stage 1. Vincristine actinomycin-D (no radiation); Stage 2. Vincristine actinomycin-D (with or without Doxorubicin and no radiation); Stage 3. Vincristine, actinomycin-D, Doxorubicin (with radiation).

Unfavorable Histology (UH) any stage (all Stage 4 for both FH and UH; Anaplastic Wilms tumor Stage 2-4): Vincristine, actinomycin-D, Doxorubicin, (with or without Cyclophosphamide, with radiation).

UH (rhabdoid tumor of the kidney and recurrent disease): poor prognosis (no satisfactory treatment has been identified). Usually administer a combination of Cisplatin, etoposide (VP-16) and ifosfamide.

Renal angiogram: reveals renal function and extent of involvement.

Scans of kidney, liver, bone: reveals involvement of these organs if metastasis is present.

Inferior venacavagram: reveals involvement adjacent to the vena cava if the tumor has grown to a large size.

Erythrocyte sedimentation rate (ESR): reveals increases as serum protein levels change.

Albumin: reveals decreases with renal involvement.

Enzymes: reveals increases in alanine aminotranferase (ALT), aspartate aminotransferase (AST), lactic dehydrogenase (LDH) with liver involvement; alkaline phosphatase (ALP) with bone involvement.

Complete blood count: reveals increases in RBC as tumor excretes more erythropoietin.

Urinalysis: reveals characteristics that indicate change in renal function caused by tumor, uric acid, erythropoietin increases.

NURSING CARE PLANS

Essential nursing diagnoses and plans associated with this condition:

Altered nutrition: Less than body requirements (168)

Related to: Inability to ingest and digest food, side effects from cyclophosphamide therapy and radiation therapy

Defining characteristics: Anorexia, nausea and vomiting from chemotherapy, obstruction postoperatively from chemotherapy causing adynamic ileus stomatitis (rare), abdominal cramping

Risk for fluid volume deficits (222)

Related to: Altered intake, excessive losses through normal routes, nausea and vomiting caused by chemotherapy and radiation therapy

Defining characteristics: Diarrhea, vomiting from radiation

Diarrhea (171)

Related to: Side effects of actinomycin-D, or Etoposide (VP-16; infrequent side effect), and radiation therapy

Defining characteristics: Increased frequency of bowel sounds and loose, liquid stools

Constipation (173)

Related to: Gastrointestinal obstructive lesions postoperatively, side effects of Vincristine

Defining characteristics: Adynamicileus, decreased bowel sounds, abdominal distention, frequency less than usual pattern

Risk for impaired skin integrity (397)

Related to: Side effects of actinomycin-D, Cyclophosamide, or Etoposide (VP-16); (rare side effect) and radiation therapy; secondary effects of chronic diarrhea

Defining characteristics: Erythema or hyperpigmentation of previously irradiated skin; local phlebitis; transverse ridging of nails; redness and excoriation of perianal area from chronic diarrhea

SPECIFIC DIAGNOSES AND CARE PLANS

Anxiety

Related to: Change in health status, threat of death, threat to self- concept

Defining characteristics: Increased apprehension and fear of diagnosis, expressed concern and worry about preoperative procedures and preparation, postoperative care and effects of therapy, possible metastasis of disease

Outcome Criteria

Reduced anxiety verbalized as information is given regarding disease and treatment

Interventions	Rationales
Assess source and level of anxiety and need for information and support that will relieve it	Provides information about degree of anxiety and need for interventions and support; sources for parent(s) may be guilt and uncertainty about surgery, treatments and recovery, possible loss of child; sources for the child may be the multiple procedures of diagnosis and surgery and the effects of postoperative treatments
Allow expression of concerns and inquiries about disease and possible consequences of surgery and prognosis	Provides opportunity to vent feelings, secure information needed to reduce anxiety

Interventions	Rationales
Allow parent(s) to stay with the child or open visitation, provide a telephone number to call for information about condition of child	Promotes care and support of child by parent(s)
Provide continuing nurse assignment with the same personnel; encourage parent(s) to participate in care	Promotes trust and comfort and familiarity with staff giving care
Orient child to the surgical and ICU unit, equipment, noises and staff	Reduces anxiety caused by fear of unknown

Information, Instruction, Demonstration

Interventions	Rationales
Inform parent(s) and child of the disease process, surgical procedure, what to expect with procedures done preoperatively and what will be experienced postoperatively including radiation and chemotherapy and its benefits and effects (alopecia, stomatitis, nausea, vomiting, diarrhea are a possibility but are temporary)	Promotes knowledge and understanding of pre and postoperative treatments and effect on disease and self-image
Explain all procedures and care in simple, direct, honest terms and repeat as often as necessary; reinforce physician information if needed and provide specific information as needed	Prevents overwhelming child and parent(s) with information in small amount of time as diagnosis and procedures usually carried out within a short period of time and anxiety will prevent ability to comprehend
Inform parent(s) and child of the extent of surgery with the removal of a kidney and the staging process; discuss their understanding of the pathology report postoperatively and clarify information as needed	Reduces anxiety when knowledge and support is given and child and parent(s) will not feel betrayed by inadequate preparation of procedures and treatments

Interventions	Rationales
Utilize therapeutic play, drawings, models for instruction of child	Provides aids to assist child to understand what will be experienced and to express their feelings
Provide parent(s) and child with information about community agencies and support groups	Provides emotional support by those who have experiences with the effects of the disease

Discharge or Maintenance Evaluation

- Expresses reduction in anxiety as information and explanation are given
- Participates in care and support of child
- Asks questions, clarifies information about procedures and care before and after surgery
- Reveals concern and vents feelings about seriousness of the disease and postoperative medical regimen and effects
- Expresses positive effects of surgery and major benefits of therapy
- Verbalizes effects of therapy on self-concept and physical well-being

Risk for injury

Related to: Internal biochemical factors of regulatory function, abnormal blood profile; internal physical factor of broken skin
Defining characteristics: Intestinal obstruction from Vincristine-induced adynamic ileus; radiation-induced edema; postsurgical adhesion formation; stomatitis (infrequent side effect of VP-16 and cyclophosphamide)

Outcome Criteria

Absence of complications caused by removal of kidney, metastasis or radiation and chemotherapy regimen

Interventions	Rationales
Assess blood pressure for increases pre and postoperatively q2h, changes in pulse and respirations	Provides information about vital signs caused by renal function abnormality preoperatively or by nephrectomy postoperatively, postoperative atelectasis

Interventions	Rationales
Avoid any palpation of abdominal mass; post sign on bed stating not to palpate preoperatively	Prevents trauma to tumor site and possible metastasis by dissemination of cancer cells
Assess bowel activity postoperatively for elimination pattern, bowel sounds, bowel distention	Provides information about possible adynamic ileus from chemotherapy causing bowel obstruction
Assess incision site for redness, swelling, drainage, intactness and healing and change dressing when soiled or wet; assess oral and perineal area	Indicates infectious process resulting from invasive procedure or inflammation resulting from immunosuppressive therapy for stomatitis or skin breakdown or inflammation and provide oral care and anal care after elimination; provide postoperative pulmonary care
Assess urinary output for presence of cloudy, foul smelling urine; collect specimen for culture analysis and report any change in renal function (hypertension, headache irritability, weight gain, behavior changes)	Indicates possible renal impairment and/or urinary bladder infection; renal involvement alters renin excretion which increases BP and immunosuppressive therapy leads to infection
Maintain reverse isolation if leukopenia present or according to agency dictate	Prevents transmission of infective agents to the immunosuppressed child
Assess and document frequency of bowel movements; document a description of all bowel movements; measure abdominal girth	To assess potential intestinal obstruction from Vincristine-induced adynamic ileus
Give stool softeners (as prescribed)	To prevent straining with bowel movements

Information, Instruction, Demonstration

Interventions	Rationales
Inform parent(s) and child of all assessments and procedures and reason for isolation precautions	Promotes understanding and cooperation

Interventions	Rationales
Inform parent(s) of potential for complication of surgery and therapy protocols	Promotes compliance and participation in preventative measures
Inform parent(s) to avoid exposing child to infectious agents; limit visitors	Prevents exposure to possible pathogens in the immunosuppressed child
Advise parent(s) to dress child appropriate to weather conditions and to avoid rough activities or sports	Prevents respiratory infections associated with exposure or trauma to the abdominal site preoperatively and surgical site postoperatively
Instruct parent(s) and child in mouth care (rinsing and swabbing with solutions, cleansing and drying after bowel elimination)	Prevents or treats skin and mucous membrane damage as a result of therapy
Inform parent(s) and child of importance of radiation and chemotherapy protocol and desired and untoward effects and compliance with therapy and follow-up visits to physician	Promotes compliance with postoperative regimen
Inform parent(s) and child to report any changes in urinary pattern or characteristics or renal function promptly	Allows for immediate attention to any genitourinary problems in remaining kidney

Discharge or Maintenance Evaluation

- Absence or resolution of signs and symptoms of pre or postoperative complications; monitors for potential complications
- Maintains safe environment with absence of infection or injury
- Verbalization of type of complications and risks associated with care and treatments preoperatively and radiation/chemotherapy postoperatively
- Meets protective needs of child pre and postoperatively

Altered oral mucous membrane

Related to: Medication (chemotherapy)
Defining characteristics: Stomatitis, oral ulcers, hyperemia, oral pain or discomfort, oral plaque

Outcome Criteria

Absence or control or oral mucosal changes and discomfort

Interventions	Rationales
Assess oral cavity for pain ulcers, lesions, gingivitis, mucositis or stomatitis and effect on ability to ingest food and fluids	Provides information about effect of chemotherapy
Administer medication before meals and offer bland, smooth foods that are not hot or spicy	Permits eating with more comfort
Administer an antiseptic mouth rinse (nystatin) 30 minutes before any food or fluid intake	Promotes comfort of oral mucosa and maintains integrity
Provide oral hygiene (30 minutes before or after meals): mouthwashes (i.e., Peridex, or normal saline solution); nystatin (swish and swallow); instruct patient not to eat or drink for 30 minutes after oral hygiene is completed	To prevent oral mucositis
Use soft-sponge toothbrush or sponge toothette or gauze to provide Peridex mouth rinse	To avoid oral trauma
Administer local anesthetics to oral area (i.e., Chloraseptic lozenges Ulcerase, or apply an ice cube to affected area); administer these before meals	May be effective in temporary pain relief from oral lesions; permits eating with decreased oral pain
Avoid oral temperatures	To avoid oral trauma
Avoid use of viscous lidocaine	To avoid risk of aspiration (viscous lidocaine may cause depression of the gag reflex or seizures)
Avoid use of lemon glycerin swabs to oral lesions	Lemon may increase irritation to oral lesions
Offer moist, soft, bland foods	To minimize irritation to oral ulcers; it may also be better tolerated by the child

Interventions	Rationales
Avoid foods which are hot, spicy, or which include ascorbic acid	To minimize irritation to oral ulcers; these foods may increase pain and irritation to oral areas

Information, Instruction, Demonstration

Interventions	Rationales
Instruct parent(s) in effect of chemotherapy on oral mucosa and in treatments to decrease discomfort in oral cavity	Promotes understanding of side effects that occur and temporary nature of the side effects
Instruct parent(s) in mouth rinses and topical application of medications	Promotes effective care of oral cavity to relieve discomfort and prevent mucosa breakdown and increased inflammation
Instruct to use soft brush or swabs to clean mouth	Prevents trauma to mucosa

Discharge or Maintenance Evaluation

- Oral mucous membranes intact and reduced inflammation
- Complies with measures to prevent trauma or breakdown of mucosa
- Controls discomfort associated with impaired oral mucosa
- Progressive return to oral mucous membrane baseline following chemotherapy protocol

Altered protection

Related to: Drug therapy (antineoplastics): abnormal blood profile (leukopenia, thrombocytopenia, anemia, coagulation); treatments (radiation)
Defining characteristics: Altered clotting, bone marrow suppression, deficient immunity against infection, petechiae, bleeding from nose, gums, hematuria (25% of cases will display preoperatively), hemorrhagic cystitis (a common side effect of cyclophosphamide)

Outcome Criteria

Absence of bleeding from any source
Protection from exposure to pathogenic microorganisms

Interventions	Rationales
Assess for bleeding from any site, WBC, platelet count, Hct, absolute neutrophil, count and febrile episodes	Provides information about frank bleeding or blood profile abnormalities that predispose to bleeding caused by bone marrow suppression and immuno-suppression resulting from chemotherapy
Administer blood transfusion as ordered for severe blood loss and monitor patency, vital signs, chills, fever, urticaria, rash, dyspnea, diaphoresis, headache throughout transfusion and terminate if any of these changes occur	Replaces blood loss when symptoms of anemia appear (dizziness, pallor, fatigue, increased pulse and respirations) or when Hct is less than 20% or platelet count less than 20,000/cu mm
Pad sides of bed, avoid trauma with use of hard toothbrush or dental floss, apply pressure for 5 minutes after IV administration, discontinue taking rectal temperatures or performing unnecessary invasive procedures	Prevents bleeding caused by trauma during chemotherapy administration which alters platelets and clotting factor
Carry out handwashing technique before giving care, use mask and gown when appropriate, provide a private room, monitor for any signs and symptoms of infection	Prevents transmission of pathogens to a compromised immune system during chemotherapy if the absolute neutrophil count is less than 1000/cu mm

Information, Instruction, Demonstration

Interventions	Rationales
Inform parent(s) and child to avoid rough play or sports, straining at defecation, blowing nose hard	Prevents trauma that causes bleeding
Inform parent(s) and child to avoid persons with upper respiratory infection or any illness	Prevents risk for infection in the highly susceptible child
Instruct parent(s) to report any fever, behavior changes, headache, dizzi-	Indicates a complication associated with abnormal blood profile

Interventions	Rationales
ness, fatigue, pallor, slow oozing of blood from any area, exposure to communicable diseases	
Impress on parent(s) the need for compliance in laboratory tests and physician appointments	Monitors effect of chemotherapy on child and need for modification of therapy
Instruct and allow for return demonstration of urine and stool testing for blood using dipstick and hematest	Identifies presence of bleeding in gastrointestinal or urinary tract

Discharge or Maintenance Evaluation

- Absence of excessive bleeding or infection during chemotherapy or radiation
- Complies with measures to prevent bleeding and infection based on blood profile
- Reports signs and symptoms of complications to physician
- Complies with laboratory blood testing and follow-up visits to physician

Wilms Tumor

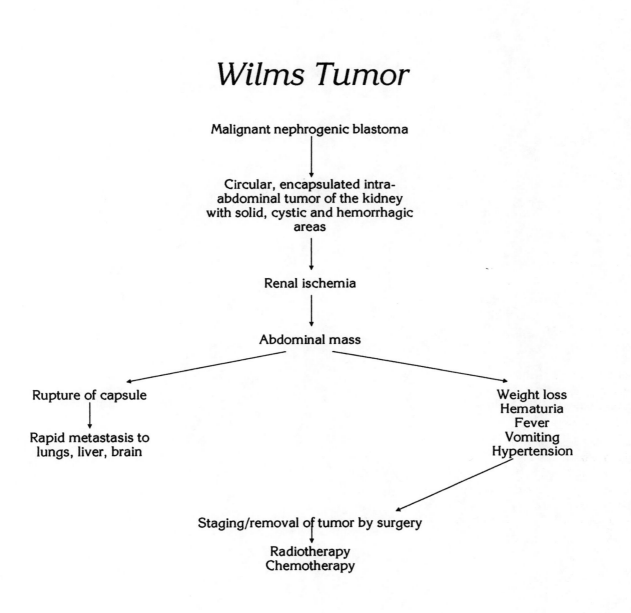

Malignant nephrogenic blastoma

↓

Circular, encapsulated intra-
abdominal tumor of the kidney
with solid, cystic and hemorrhagic
areas

↓

Renal ischemia

↓

Abdominal mass

Rupture of capsule

↓

Rapid metastasis to
lungs, liver, brain

Weight loss
Hematuria
Fever
Vomiting
Hypertension

Staging/removal of tumor by surgery

Radiotherapy
Chemotherapy

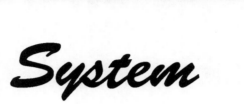

Musculoskeletal System

The musculoskeletal system includes components that are needed for supportive and protective framework for the body. The system functions to provide the movement that is essential for interacting and adapting to the child's environment and is especially vulnerable to forces in the environment. The system includes bones which compose the skeletal system, muscles which compose the muscular system, joints which compose the articular system, tendons and ligaments. Tendons and ligaments with muscle attach to the surfaces of bones and the combination of all of the components allows for ambulation, personal care, and play. The problems encountered in these systems are classified as traumatic (most common) and long-term disability (degenerative disease), and any problem and abnormality that affects this system commonly affects the function of one or more other organ systems. The functional disruption that occurs as a result of a musculoskeletal problem that requires immobilization leads to physical and emotional alterations in a child who is usually active and curious. With growth and development of the system structures and gross and fine motor development, the child progressively functions within adult parameters for movements and activities of daily living.

GENERAL MUSCULOSKELETAL CHANGES ASSOCIATED WITH PHYSICAL GROWTH AND DEVELOPMENT

Bone, muscle, joint, tendon, ligament structure

- Spine in the newborn is rounded or has a convex curvature with the lumbar curve developed by 12-18 months of age; cervical spine is concave; thoracic spine is convex; and lumbar spine is concave after 18 months of age with the double S curve developed in the older child

- Muscles are completely formed at birth with size increasing by hypertrophy and strength increasing with muscular functions of walking, climbing, running, and jumping which is well established by 3 years of age
- Muscle development and bone growth continue to mature with skeletal lengthening and muscle strengthening increases throughout childhood
- Bone ossification is continuous with 25 new ossification centers appearing during the second year and bones continue to ossify until maturity is reached
- Bone growth occurs in the epiphysis at the end of long bones until it closes, at which time growth ceases
- Height and rate of skeletal growth increases at a slower rate with age with the toddler increasing 3-5 inches/year
- Feet of the infant and toddler appear flat and an arch develops with walking
- Height averages vary with age and sex

	Boys	Girls
6 mo	26 3/4 in	26 in
1 yr	30 in	29 1/4 in
2 yr	34 1/4 in	34 1/4 in
3 yr	37 1/4 in	37 in
4 yr	40 1/2 in	40 in
6 yr	45 3/4 in	45 in
8 yr	50 in	49 3/4 in
10 yr	54 1/4 in	54 1/2 in
12 yr	59 in	59 3/4 in

Musculoskeletal function

- Gross and fine motor function and muscle strength and refinement continue in preschool and schoolage child
- From the beginning of walking through toddler stage, legs are usually bowlegged until back and leg muscles develop and wide stance and waddle or toddling gait is apparent until 2-2 1/2 years of age; by schoolage the legs become closer together and walking and posture is sturdy and balanced
- Bones in the child resist pressure and muscle pull less than the adult, so injury by trauma is common
- Bones heal faster in children since the bones are still in the process of ossification and growth

ESSENTIAL NURSING DIAGNOSES AND CARE PLANS

Impaired physical mobility

Related to: Intolerance to activity; decreased strength and endurance
Defining characteristics: Inability to purposefully move within physical environment, including bed mobility, transfer and ambulation, limited range of motion, decreased muscle strength, control and/or mass, fatigue, bedrest

Related to: Pain and discomfort
Defining characteristics: Reluctance to attempt movement, limited range of movement, painful and/or swollen joints, fracture, surgical procedure, infectious process

Related to: Neuromuscular impairment
Defining characteristics: Inability to purposefully move within physical environment, including bed mobility, transfer and ambulation, decreased muscle strength, control and/or mass, impaired coordination, paralysis (paraplegia or quadraplegia), progressive deterioration, inadequate gross and fine motor skills, diminished musculoskeletal responses

Related to: Musculoskeletal impairment
Defining characteristics: Inability to purposefully move within physical environment, including bed mobility, transfer and ambulation, reluctance to attempt movement, limited range of motion, decreased muscle strength, control and/or mass, imposed restrictions of movement including mechanical (cast, traction, splint, brace, or bedrest), contractures, fracture, joint disease and destruction inflammation, congenital disorders

Outcome Criteria

Optimal mobility within disease and developmental limitations
Independence in ambulation and activities of daily living
Absence of complications associated with musculo-skeletal disorder or in mobility

Interventions	Rationales
Assess muscle tone, strength, mass; joint mobility, pain, stiffness, swelling; ability to move and activity level in performing ADL	Provides information about musculoskeletal condition and function
Assess bedrest status, activity restrictions, imposed immobility by braces, casts, traction, splints	Maintains rest during acute stages to promote healing and restoration of health
Assess sensory (diminished sensation and numbness) and motor (gait and balance) function of extremities; presence of paralysis, fracture, surgical correction of musculoskeletal abnormalities	Provides information about conditions or treatments that affect mobility
Assess physical effects of immobilization on body systems; constipation, skin breakdown, urinary retention, hypercalcemia, loss of muscle strength, contractures, circulatory stasis, stasis of pulmonary secretions, anorexia, renal calculi, decreased metabolism and energy, loss of nerve innervation	Prevents complications of immobility by monitoring and intervening when needed; mobility provides important contributions to development and physical health
Assess psychologic effect of immobilization; reduce body image, inability to reduce stress, loss of stimuli, loss of independence and mastery, anxiety, regressive behavior, anger and aggression, passive and submissive behavior, crying, irritability, temper tantrums	Provides information about behavior and deprivation resulting from immobilization which prevents children from dealing with feelings and expression of anxiety and tensions
Avoid restriction in activities unless ordered; encourage and allow for as much movement as possible in performing daily activities; administer analgesic before activity	Promotes mobility and activity synonymous with health and life; allows for autonomy and control for normal development

Interventions	Rationales
Encourage all age-appropriate activities that facilitate mobility, allow infant to crawl	Promotes mobility according to limitations of illness and provides outlet for frustration of imposed immobility
Provide quiet play and progress in ambulation by scheduling dangling at bedside, standing with support, ambulation with support with increases daily and praise for all attempts regardless of progress	Maintains large and small muscle strength as condition permits
Transport/transfer infant/child by Hoyer lift, stroller, wheelchair, bed outside of room/hospital	Provides stimulation by interacting in a different environment in absence of mobility
Provide and apply brace, splint; use of aids including wheelchair, crutches, supportive reading, eating, and other aids for ADL as needed	Promotes independence and support in mobility and activities
Maintain body alignment on bedrest, reposition q2h or as needed; use a drawing for child to follow for position and where to lie in bed	Prevents contractures and physical deformity and preserves joint function
Coordinate rest with periods of mobility	Prevents fatigue and conserves energy
Perform muscle strengthening exercises, passive stretching exercises, joint mobilizing exercises if ordered or as appropriate	Preserves muscle strength or prepares for use of crutches or other mobility aids
Apply special shoes, split or appliance for day or night use	Maintains position at night and prevents deformity and allows for locomotion by increasing gait efficiency during day use
Prepare for physical and/or occupational therapy during recuperative period as ordered	Promotes and maintains optimal function and mobility of child

Information, Instruction, Demonstration

Interventions	Rationales
Inform parent(s) and child of hazards of immobility and importance of compliance with medical and exercise regimen	Promotes compliance with program to maintain mobility and understanding of effects of immobility
Instruct parent(s) and child in use of devices or aids for mobility and ADL	Promotes safe use of aids and apparatus and increased security
Inform parent(s) and child to provide clear pathways, removal of rugs, environmental modifications as needed	Provides safe environment for mobility
Inform parent(s) and child of activities for large muscle strengthening (tricycle, swimming, running, skipping rope), and small muscle strengthening (games, puzzles, crayons, coloring books)	Promotes strengthening of muscles as condition improvement
Inform child of expected progress in ambulation and ADL	Provides child with a goal to strive for and achieve
Instruct parent(s) and child in ROM, strengthening exercises as appropriate	Maintains muscle and joint function
Inform parent(s) and child of importance of therapy and follow-up care, short- or long-term depending on need	Promotes compliance with prescribed therapy especially if needed to ensure mobility or health maintenance in chronic disorders

Discharge or Maintenance Evaluation

- Maximum mobility and participation in ADL according to developmental level
- Correct application and use of appliances, aids, devices to promote mobility and activities
- Absence of complications of immobility

- Compliance with exercise regimen, rest, and energy preservation
- Perform play activities for diversion, development, and mobility
- Comply with physical and/or occupational therapy schedule
- Maintain bedrest of activity restrictions if appropriate with gradual return of mobility and self-care activities

Fractures

A fracture is a break in a bone which is usually caused by a fall or injury. They are common in children because of their activity and continual changes and growth in their gross motor function. Injury of this type in an infant or very small child is usually the result of physical abuse. The most common type of fracture in children under 3 years of age is the greenstick which is an incomplete fracture and results in a compression of one side causing it to bend and the other side to fail. A bend fracture is the result of the bone bending and straightening on its own because of the flexibility of the bone at a young age. A buckle fracture is raised bulging of the bone resulting from compression of the bone near its most porous part. A complete fracture is a division in the bone with or without attachment of a periosteal hinge remaining. The most common sites of fractures in children are the femur, humerus, clavicle, ulna, radius, tibia, and fibula. Treatment includes reduction (open or closed), and immobilization by casting and/or traction depending on the type and severity of the fracture. Healing is faster in the child and takes place within 3-4 weeks. Remodeling is usually completed within 9 months depending on the type and site on the fracture, amount of fragmentation, and the age of the child.

MEDICAL CARE

Analgesics: codeine (Methylmorphine), acetaminophen (Tylenol tablets, Liquiprin, solutions, or drops) given PO for pain control depending on severity.

Bone x-ray: reveals trauma site, separation of the epiphysis in older child.

Enzymes: reveals increases in alkaline phosphatase (ALP), lactic dehydrogenase (LDH), creatine phosphokinase (CPK), aspartate aminotransferase (AST) with bone, and muscle damage.

Complete blood count (CBC): reveals increased WBC and neutrophils if infection present, decreased RBC, Hct, Hgb with destruction of RBC caused by muscle, bone and soft tissue injury.

NURSING CARE PLANS

Essential nursing diagnoses and plans associated with this condition:

Impaired physical mobility (278)

Related to: Pain and discomfort, musculoskeletal impairment (fracture)

Defining characteristics: Intolerance to activity, decreased strength and endurance, inability to purposefully move within physical environment including bed mobility, transfer and ambulation, reluctance to attempt movement, imposed restrictions of movement including mechanical medical protocol (cast, traction), inability to participate in activities and socializing

Altered tissue perfusion, peripheral (6)

Related to: Interruption in arterial and venous flow

Defining characteristics: Cold, pallor or blue color of extremity, decreased peripheral pulse, cast tightness

Risk for impaired skin integrity (397)

Related to: External factor of physical immobilization, pressure of cast, traction apparatus, presence of surgical incision from open reduction; internal factors of altered circulation and sensation

Defining characteristics: Disruption of skin surface, invasion of bony structures, redness, irritation of skin at cast edges or pressure areas, numbness or tingling of casted extremities

Constipation (173)

Related to: Inadequate physical activity or immobility

Defining characteristics: Frequency less than usual, hard formed stool, decreased bowel sounds, straining at defecation

SPECIFIC DIAGNOSES AND CARE PLANS

Pain

Related to: Physical injuring agents (bone fracture); surgery to realign fracture

Defining characteristics: Communication of pain descriptors, guarding and protective behavior to injured part, crying, irritability, restlessness, swelling of part, muscle spasms

Outcome Criteria

Absence or control of pain

Interventions	Rationales
Assess site for pain including type, severity, and duration using a pain scale if appropriate; pain as a result of surgical open reduction	Provides information about pain as a basis for analgesic and muscle relaxant therapy
Administer analgesic, muscle relaxant, or both; IV initially and wean to PO administration when appropriate and note response	Reduces pain and promotes rest following injury or surgery
Apply ice to fracture if ordered	Treats pain and edema by vasoconstriction
Apply splint or Jones dressing (cotton wrapping over area covered by an Ace bandage)	Relieves pain and prevents further damage by protecting and immobilizing limb
Elevate limb above heart level, maintain alignment of limb when positioning	Promotes venous return to relieve edema which causes pain and prevents contractures
Support limb above and below injured area when moving and positioning; use smooth movements and avoid abrupt movement of limb	Prevents pain caused by movement

Information, Instruction, Demonstration

Interventions	Rationales
Inform parent(s) and child of pain medications and expected results and importance of reporting pain before it becomes too severe	Provides information about expected effects of analgesic therapy during acute stages of pain and as pain subsides with healing
Inform parent(s) and child of ways to move and position limb, importance of maintaining immobilization of extremity, and to avoid weight-bearing until advised	Prevents undue pain caused by movement of limb

Discharge or Maintenance Evaluation

- Absence of pain and associated responses
- Controls pain provoking actions when giving care or changing positions
- Administers analgesics/muscle relaxants correctly, then monitors responses

Risk for injury

Related to: Internal factors of sensory dysfunction, tissue hypoxia, altered mobility resulting from cast application
Defining characteristics: Change in color, temperature, edema, movement of fingers/toes; tingling or numbness of fingers/toes; drainage or musty odor from under cast; skin irritation at cast edges; moist, wet, or broken cast, foreign objects inserted between cast and skin

Outcome Criteria

Absence of complications resulting from cast application
Neurovascular competency maintained during immobilization by cast

Interventions	Rationales
Assess pulses in casted upper or lower extremity, swelling, coolness, inability to move digits, pallor or cyanosis, numbness of areas distal to the cast q2h	Provides information about the neurovascular status of an extremity following cast application as swelling continues causing the cast to become tight and compromise circulation; a bivalved cast treats excessive edema to prevent tissue damage
Allow cast to dry thoroughly using a fan, turning q2h, support on pillows and use palm of hands to lift or handle cast exposing as much of the cast to the air as possible	Prevents indentations in the cast which may cause pressure areas, allows cast to dry from inside out for 1/2 hour or more depending on substance used for cast and type of cast
Do not use a heated fan or dryer	Heat causes the cast to dry on the outside but stay wet underneath, or may cause burns from heat conduction through the cast
Elevate casted part on pillow until completely dry and when at rest for a few days	Promotes venous return to reduce swelling

Interventions	Rationales
Provide quiet play for a few days and exercise muscle and joints above and below	Maintains muscle and joint function
Remove small articles or food that may be put into the cast	Prevents pressure to injury and infection if skin is broken under the cast
Clean plaster cast with vinegar and water; fiberglass casts are cleaned with mild soap and water	Maintains cleanliness of the cast
Petal cast if rough edges are present; massage skin near cast edges and note any reddened or abrasive areas	Protects skin from irritation and breakdown
Outline area of drainage on cast with pen; and include date and time.	Monitors increases in drainage under the cast
Provide muscle strengthening exercises, ROM of unaffected parts, isometric exercises appropriate	Prepares for crutch walking if appropriate and maintains joint and muscle mobility

Information, Instruction, Demonstration

Interventions	Rationales
Inform parent(s) and child of type of cast, type of fracture and how it heals	Provides information about injury and type of immobilization to allow for healing process
Instruct parent(s) and child to restrict activities according to physician advice, to avoid placing articles, such as a coat hanger for scratching, into the cast	Prevents damage to the cast and skin that may lead to infection or impair the desired effect of the cast
Instruct parent(s) and child to avoid allowing limb to hang down and maintain elevation of the limb when sitting and support limb with a sling when standing; avoid standing for prolonged periods of time	Maintains return venous flow and prevents fatigue from heavy cast

Interventions	Rationales
Instruct parent(s) to note and report any pain, swelling, musty odor from cast; changes in neurovascular status in casted extremity, tightness or looseness of cast	Indicates presence of infection or neurovascular compromise that may require a cast change
Instruct parent(s) to massage skin at cast edges, avoid use of lotions and powder in these areas, and pad cast edges if needed	Toughens skin to prevent breakdown and prevents infection by providing media for bacterial growth
Instruct child in use of crutches or application of sling	Allows for mobility and participation in activities
Inform parent(s) and child of length of cast presence, need for physical therapy if appropriate, and method of maintaining clean cast (plaster or plastic)	Permits planning for continuing care if appropriate

Discharge or Maintenance Evaluation

- Maintains immobilization by casting
- Maintains neurovascular competency during immobilization by cast
- Verbalizes and provides appropriate cast care
- Avoids activities that damages cast and affects immobilization of casted part
- Protects skin, tissue, and joints from impairment caused by cast and immobilization
- Participates in activities with proper protection to cast and extremity

Risk for injury

Related to: Internal factors of sensory dysfunction, altered mobility resulting from skin or skeletal traction
Defining characteristics: Redness, swelling, pain at pin site, change in neurovascular status of extremity, malfunction of traction apparatus, ineffective traction, contractures or weakness of joint and muscles

Outcome Criteria

Maximum effectiveness of traction without complications
Neurovascular, skin and musculoskeletal integrity maintained during traction
Appropriate function for each component of the traction apparatus

Interventions	Rationales
Assess type and purpose of traction, extremity or body part involved	Provides information about use of traction to realign bone ends, provide immobilization of a part, reduce muscle spasms, correct a deformity, provide rest for an extremity; traction may be manual as in cast application, skin in which the pull is attached to the skin with bandages or straps, or skeletal in which the pull is attached to a pin, wire, or tongs inserted into the bone at a distal position to the fracture
Assess functioning part of the traction apparatus including correct weight amount and hanging, ropes in tract with secure knots, pulleys in original site with movable wheels, position of frames, splints	Provides information needed to ensure correct traction applied to body part
Assess skin color, pulses, numbness, or changes in movement of body part; weakness or contractures of uninvolved muscles and joints: neurochecks q2-4h	Indicates neurovascular changes resulting from traction; muscular changes resulting from immobilization
Assess pressure points noting any redness or breakdown and reposition if possible; massage uninjured skin areas	Prevents prolonged pressure on skin that results in breakdown and decreased blood flow to area
Maintain bed position as ordered with head or foot elevated	Provides desired amount of pull and counter-traction
Maintain correct body alignment especially in hips, legs, arms, and shoulders; realign after the child has moved or changed position	Promotes comfort and prevents deformity

Interventions	Rationales
Perform ROM to unaffected joints, apply foot plate if appropriate	Prevents contractures and foot drop
Maintain nonadhesive straps or bandages used; do not remove or change unless permitted while someone maintains traction; note tightness or looseness that may cause ineffective traction	Supplies attachment for pull in skin traction
Cleanse and dress pin site daily; apply antiseptic ointment if ordered; check skin for infection at site; examine screws within metal clamp for proper attachment of clamp to traction; do not remove traction	Supplies attachment for pull in skeletal traction and treats pin site to prevent infection
Assist child to perform ADL activities independently as much as possible; facilitate self-care with assistive aids	Promotes independence in self-care within limitations of age and immobilization
Provide diversionary activities and encourage visits from family and friends, move bed to area of activity with peers	Provides and promotes social interactions

Information, Instruction, Demonstration

Interventions	Rationales
Inform parent(s) and child as appropriate for age about reason for traction and length of time traction must be in place	Provides information to assist with coping with immobility
Inform child of amount and type of movement allowed while in traction	Ensures that amount of activity is not exceeded and will not affect traction
Inform parent(s) that traction will assist in the healing of fracture	Promotes positive response to treatment
Suggest activities such as hobbies, TV, reading, games while in tradition	Allows for movement without disturbing traction

Discharge or Maintenance Evaluation

- Verbalizes type of traction and purpose
- Maintains maximum effect of traction
- Prevents malfunction or complications of traction apparatus
- Provides pin site care, ROM, and exercises to muscles and joints
- Promotes independence in self-care activities and social interaction

Fractures

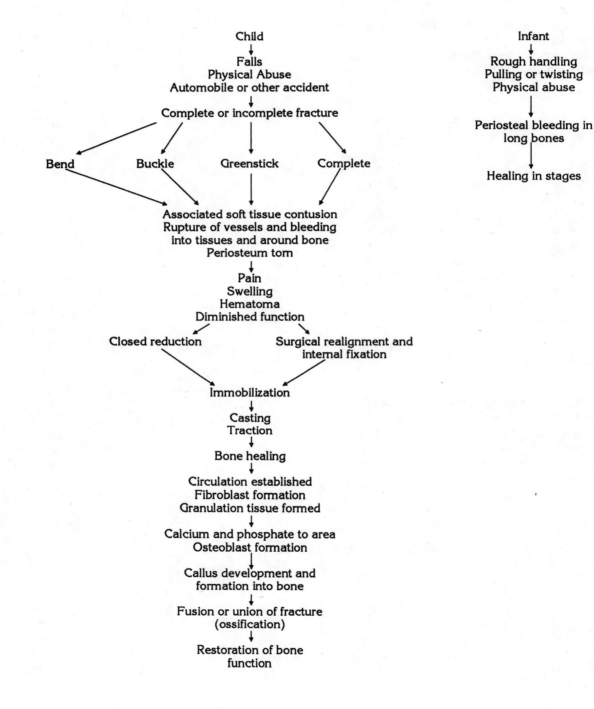

Child
↓
Falls
Physical Abuse
Automobile or other accident
↓
Complete or incomplete fracture

Bend   Buckle   Greenstick   Complete

Associated soft tissue contusion
Rupture of vessels and bleeding
into tissues and around bone
Periosteum torn
↓
Pain
Swelling
Hematoma
Diminished function

Closed reduction   Surgical realignment and
internal fixation

Immobilization
↓
Casting
Traction
↓
Bone healing
↓
Circulation established
Fibroblast formation
Granulation tissue formed
↓
Calcium and phosphate to area
Osteoblast formation
↓
Callus development and
formation into bone
↓
Fusion or union of fracture
(ossification)
↓
Restoration of bone
function

Infant
↓
Rough handling
Pulling or twisting
Physical abuse
↓
Periosteal bleeding in
long bones
↓
Healing in stages

Developmental Dysplasia of the Hip (DDH)

Developmental dysplasia of the hip (DDH) describes a group of disorders related to abnormal hip development. The abnormalities include hip instability, preluxation (shallow acetabulum), subluxation (incomplete dislocation of the hip), and dislocation (femoral head not in contact with the acetabulum). It usually involves one hip, but may involve both. It occurs 6 times more often in females than males. It is usually identified in the newborn period and responds to treatment best if initiated before 2 months of age. Therefore, it is important to examine every infant for DDH from birth to 12-months of age. Treatment is dependent on the age of the child and the degree of abnormality, and ranges from application of a reduction device, to traction and casting, to surgical open reduction. Casting and splinting with correction is usually impossible after 6 years of age.

MEDICAL CARE

Pelvic x-ray: reveals outward femoral displacement with upward slope of the roof of the acetabulum in infant/child over 4 months of age.
Ultrasound: reveals cartilaginous head displacement in infant under 1-4 months of age.
Ortolani test: a maneuver abducting the infant's leg (1-4 months) that, in the event of DDH, causes the femoral head to enter the acetabulum and is identified by a "clunk" as this occurs.
Barlow's test: a maneuver adducting the infant's leg (14 months) that, in the event of DDH, causes the femoral head to exit the acetabulum and is palpable by the examiner as a clunk.

NURSING CARE PLANS

Essential nursing diagnoses and plans associated with this condition:

Impaired physical mobility (278)

Related to: Musculoskeletal impairment (hip defect)
Defining characteristics: Imposed restriction of movement by harness, cast, traction, or splint; inability to purposefully move within physical environment including bed mobility; ambulation

Risk for impaired skin integrity (397)

Related to: External factor of physical immobilization; internal factor of altered circulation; sensation by pressure of device, cast, traction
Defining characteristics: Edema, tight appliance or cast, change in skin color and temperature proximal to spica cast or device or pin site, skin irritation at pin site or cast edges, numbness proximal to cast

Constipation (173)

Related to: Musculoskeletal impairment, inadequate physical activity or immobility
Defining characteristics: Frequency less than usual, hard formed stool, decreased bowel sounds, straining at defecation

Altered growth and development (419)

Related to: Effects of physical disability (immobilization)
Defining characteristics: Environmental and stimulation deficiencies, inability to perform self-care activities appropriate for age, isolation with long-term immobilization

SPECIFIC DIAGNOSES AND CARE PLANS

Risk for injury

Related to: Internal physiological factor of untreated or improper treatment for dislocation
Defining characteristics: Late onset dislocation, absence of early recognition and intervention for correction, muscle contracture, muscle shortening, femoral and acetabulum deformity, tight spica cast, inappropriate traction or malfunctioning traction

Outcome Criteria

Early detection and effective treatment for hip displacement

Absence of cast syndrome or incorrect traction function

Interventions	Rationales
Assess infant up to 2 months of age for frank breech birth, caesarean birth, hip joint laxity or dislocation (Ortolani or Barlow test), degree of dysplasia or dislocation, shortened limb on the affected side (telescoping), broadened perineum, asymmetry of thigh and gluteal folds with increased number of folds and flattened buttocks	Provides information about the presence and degree of dysplasia; may be preluxation, subluxation, or dislocation (luxation) and involve a laxity of the capsule or an abnormal acetabulum; identification of the presence of the deformity at this age results in the highest success rate in complete correction
Assess child's shortened leg affected with telescoping; palpation of femur when thigh is extended and pushed toward the head and pulled in distal direction; delayed walking and a limp that causes lurching toward affected side; downward tilt of pelvis toward unaffected side if weight-bearing on affected side when standing (Trendelenberg Sign); lordosis and waddling gait if both hips affected	Provides information about the presence of deformity in one or both hips in the older infant or toddler and preschool age group; usually identified when the child begins to walk or stand, and limb is shortened and adductor and flexor muscle contracture has occurred; requires closed reduction (traction and cast) or open reduction (surgery, cast, splint) to correct
Apply Pavlik harness splinting device to infant up to 6 months of age to be worn continuously for 3-6 months to ensure hip stability; apply double or triple diapers or Frejka pillow if this is treatment ordered	Maintains abducted, reduced position for maintaining the femur in the acetabulum; other methods to correct unstable hip may be used to stretch legs and maintain abducted position depending on decree of deformity
Maintain skin traction in presence of abduction contracture in the infant up to 6 months of age and spica cast if applied fol-	Promotes hip abduction until stable; applies with a spica cast if unable to maintain stable reduction of the hip for 3-6 months;

Interventions	Rationales
lowing the traction; maintain skin traction for gradual reduction of the hip adductor and flexor muscles with a spica cast application for immobilization in child 6-10 months of age	removal of the spica cast is followed by an abduction brace for protection
Provide traction care including correct alignment of extremity, correct amount of weights, free hang of weights, correctly functioning pulleys with secure knots, neurologic and circulatory checks q4h for color, warmth, sensation	Maintains safe, effective traction to affected hip(s) with child's response to traction monitored
Provide spica cast care including support of cast when moving, removing crumbs and small articles that may get into cast, petal cast edges, avoiding insertion of anything into cast to scratch, clean cast when needed, allow to dry completely, protect cast from soiling and dampness from elimination or bathing; neurologic and circulatory checks q4h for color, peripheral pulse, warmth, capillary refill, sensation; nausea and vomiting resulting from cast syndrome	Maintains safe, effective immobilization to ensure permanent stability of hip with child's response to cast monitored for cast syndrome caused by tight spica cast compressing the superior mesenteric artery of the duodenum
Provide diaper change frequently and as needed; use disposable diapers or plastic protection over diaper	Maintains clean harness brace, or cast

Information, Instruction, Demonstration

Interventions	Rationales
Inform parent(s) of type and degree of deformity and cause and treatment plan for correction and	Provides information about abnormality, its classification, medical and/or surgical regimen which is deter-

Interventions	Rationales
prognosis by reinforcing physician information; inform of proposed operative reduction in older child or if obstruction of joint development by soft tissue is present in the young child	mined by age and severity of the deformity
Instruct parent(s) to apply splint or harness correctly over the diaper and shirt, use disposable diapers or water proof undergarment to protect appliance; on removal of harness for bathing if allowed or sponge bathing child with harness in place, padding shoulder straps, changing position q2h; to avoid adjusting the harness	Promotes and maintains reduction of hip to correct deformity
Instruct parent(s) in traction care including reason and purpose for traction, amount of movement that the child is allowed, performing neurovascular assessment and what to report, correct weight for amount and hanging with pulleys and knots if present, maintaining body alignment	Ensures correct traction for gradual reduction of the hip and/or preoperative if surgery anticipated
Instruct parent(s) in spica cast care including reason and purpose; support of the cast during movement; maintaining clean, dry cast and protecting it from stool and urine with waterproof tape or plastic cover; padding cast edges; avoid lifting by crossbar; disallowing small objects or crumbs to enter cast; cast signatures without leaving white space between writing; instruct in diapering or bedpan/toilet use; use of a diaper tucked into the perineal opening on cast; feeding infant in supine	Ensures correct cast care for immobilization of hip following reduction of the hip; traction or surgical correction may be used for reduction or reconstruction of the acetabulum

Interventions	Rationales
position (head elevated propped with pillows or while being held in upright position on lap or in a car seat); inform parent(s) that specially made car seats for infants with casts/harness are available and must be used if the child rides in a car; refer to social worker if cost prevents access to the seats	
Inform parent(s) of crippled children or other community agencies available	Provides information and support services to the child and family
Inform parent(s) of method to monitor for cast syndrome	Provides for early treatment of this complication

Discharge or Maintenance Evaluation

- Early detection of defect noted, and treatments begun
- Applies diapers, pillow splint, and harness correctly and maintains correct reduction of hip over prescribed periods of time
- Provides effective traction and/or cast care as appropriate over prescribed periods of time
- Verbalizes causes of deformity, reason and purpose of treatment, prognosis of condition
- Verbalizes knowledge of deformity and promotes corrective therapy
- Controls possible complications of traction or cast application
- Complies with follow-up supervision of medical regimen to correct deformity
- Absence of cast syndrome and traction functioning correctly

Impaired social interaction

Related to: Limited physical mobility
Defining characteristics: Change in pattern of interaction, lengthy treatment and immobilization, boredom, inability to engage in usual activities for age group, environment that lacks diversion

Outcome Criteria

Participation in activities despite immobilizing treatments

Interventions	Rationales
Provide age appropriate toys to be used in bed while in a prone or sitting position depending on type of treatment and degree of immobilization	Promotes social and developmental activities and reduces boredom during long-term treatment
Provide exposure to other children by moving bed near areas of activity or near a window; wheel on a stretcher, wheelchair, or stroller; allow to walk with cast or brace if permitted	Provides environmental stimulation and social interaction; promotes social interaction with others during long-term treatment and reduces boredom
Encourage family and friends to visit or stay with child	Promotes social interaction with others during long-term treatment and reduces boredom
Place toys and other articles within reach	Provides access to diversion activities when needed

Information, Instruction, Demonstration

Interventions	Rationales
Inform parent(s) to include infant/child in family activities	Promotes feeling of acceptance and well-being as part of the family
Inform of devices available or methods of converting aids used for mobility to fill needs of child with a cast or appliance	Promotes exposure to a variety of activities and changes of environmental stimuli
Inform parent(s) to allow as much independence if self-care by child as possible	Promotes independence and allows some control over the situation

Discharge or Maintenance Evaluation

- Participates in positive interaction with peers and family members
- Maintains age appropriate stimulation and play activities
- Participates in family activities
- Promotes a variety of activities contributing to growth and development needs

Hip Dysplasia

Genetic factor/
In utero development
↓
Defective acetabulum
Femoral head is out of joint and
positioned posterior and superior
to acetabulum
↓
Abnormal development of hip
↓
Affected leg shorter in older infant
and child
Inability to abduct leg
↓
Unstable hip and weight bearing
↓
Delayed walking with a limp
Contracture of hip adductor and
flexor muscles
↙ ↘
Surgical reduction   Reduction by traction
and spica cast   and casting

Environmental factor
↓
Intrauterine malposition
Breech birth/Cesarean birth
Ligament-relaxing hormone by
mother prior to birth
↓
Joint laxity in young infant
↓
Femoral head in contact with
acetabulum
↓
Splinting of hip with
femur in acetabulum
↓
Pavlik harness
Double/triple diapering

Lupus Erythematosus

Lupus erythematosus is a chronic systemic inflammatory disease of the collagen or supporting tissues and affects any organ in the body. It is classified into a transient type affecting neonates and a type with an onset after infancy that is the same as systemic lupus erythematosus affecting adults. The disease is characterized by remissions and exacerbations and may appear in children as young as 6 years of age but is most commonly seen in those 10 years of age and older. Disease manifestations include lesions or rash on face, neck, trunk and extremities; pleurisy; pericarditis; kidney failure; arthritis; anemia; gastrointestinal abnormalities; and enlarged lymph nodes. Prognosis is dependent on the response to the medical regimen and prevention of exacerbations and severe complications of the renal system.

MEDICAL CARE

Anti-inflammatories (Nonsteroidal): aspirin (acetylsalicylic acid) given PO to relieve joint pain by decreasing inflammation.

Anti-inflammatories (Steroidal): prednisone (Deltasone) given PO and prednisolone sodium phosphate (Hydeltrasol) given IV in large doses to relieve severe manifestations of the disease; oral dose is tapered to lowest effective amount to control symptoms.

Immunosuppressants: azathioprine (Imuran) given PO in combination with an anti-inflammatory to reduce amount of steroids.

Antimalarials: hydroxychloroquine sulfate (Plaquenil sulfate), chloroquine (Aralen) given PO as second line therapy to relieve symptoms caused by skin, joint, and renal complications and to reduce amounts of steroids needed.

Antibiotics: given PO specific to identified microorganisms and sensitivity to tested antibiotics.

Anticonvulsants: phenytoin (Dilantin-30 Pediatric) given PO to control or prevent seizure activity if central nervous system affected.

Antihypertensives: propranolol (Inderal), methyldopa (Aldomet) given PO with a diuretic to lower blood pressure if needed.

Diuretics: chlorathiazide (Diuril) given PO to promote diuresis and elimination of sodium by preventing reabsorption if renal function affected or if blood pressure elevated.

Electrocardiogram: reveals changes and arrhythmias if cardiac output decreased.

Blood urea nitrogen (BUN): reveals increases in impaired renal function.

Creatinine: reveals increases in impaired renal function.

Complete blood count: reveals increased WBC in presence of infection, decreased Hgb, and platelet and RBC decreases.

Urinalysis: reveals protein, RBC with renal impairment.

Guaiac test: reveals occult blood in stool.

NURSING CARE PLANS

Essential nursing diagnoses and plans associated with this condition:

Risk for impaired skin integrity (397)

Related to: Internal factors of altered pigmentation, circulation, immunological
Defining characteristics: Disruption in skin surface; scaly erythematmous blush or patchy area over nose and cheeks in the shape of a butterfly; sensitivity to cold in hands and feet with or without cyanosis; dry, cracked skin; alopecia

Impaired physical mobility (278)

Related to: Intolerance to activity, decreased strength and endurance, pain and discomfort
Defining characteristics: Generalized weakness; joint swelling, stiffness, and pain; limited range of motion; generalized aching; arthralgia; fatigue

Hyperthermia (112)

Related to: Illness (inflammation)
Defining characteristics: Increase in body temperature above normal range, low grade elevation

Altered thought processes (116)

Related to: Physiological changes
Defining characteristics: Forgetfulness, changes in consciousness, excitability, seizures, psychosis, irritability, nystagmus, diplopia, disorientation

Risk for fluid volume deficit (222)

Related to: Failure of regulatory mechanisms (renal failure)
Defining characteristics: Increased urine output, altered intake, weight loss or gain, edema, dry skin and mucous membranes, thirst, hypotension, increased pulse rate, proteinuria

Decreased cardiac output (3)

Related to: Mechanical factor of alteration in preload, electrical factor of altered conduction
Defining characteristics: Variations in hemodynamic readings, arrhythmias, ECG changes, cyanosis, skin and mucous membrane pallor, decreased peripheral pulses, rales, dyspnea, orthopnea, restlessness

Altered nutrition: Less than body requirements (168)

Related to: Inability to ingest, digest, and absorb nutrients
Defining characteristics: Anorexia, nausea, vomiting, diarrhea, abdominal discomfort

SPECIFIC DIAGNOSES AND CARE PLANS

Body image disturbance

Related to: Biophysical and psychosocial factors
Defining characteristics: Verbal and nonverbal responses to change in body appearance (alopecia, skin rashes, steroid side effects), negative feelings about body, multiple stressors and change in daily living limitations and social relationships

Outcome Criteria

Body image improved, preserved, and maintained
Accommodations made for and adaptation to long-term needs and limitations of chronic illness

Interventions	Rationales
Assess child for feelings about multiple restrictions in lifestyle, chronic illness, difficulty in school and social situations, inability	Provides information about status of self-concept and body image that require special attention

Interventions	Rationales
to keep up with peers and participate in activities	
Encourage expression of feelings and concerns and support communications with parent(s), teachers, and peers	Provides opportunity to vent feelings and reduce negative feelings about changes in appearance
Avoid negative comments and stress positive activities and accomplishments	Enhances body image and confidence
Note withdrawal behavior and signs of depression	Reveals responses to body image changes and possible poor adjustment to changes
Note hair loss, skin rashes or changes, weight gain and shift in body fat distribution, hirsutism, edema and effect on child	Reveals side effects of steroid therapy and disease manifestations that affect body image
Show support and acceptance of changes in appearance of child; provide privacy as needed	Promotes trust and demonstrates respect for child

Information, Instruction, Demonstration

Interventions	Rationales
Inform parent(s) of importance of maintaining support for child regardless of their needs	Encourages acceptance of the child with special needs (long-term steroid therapy and side effects, risk for infection and bleeding tendency, lifelong activity restrictions)
Inform parent(s) of use of wig, scarf, makeup, clothing selection	Supports child during body image changes involving skin, hair, edema, weight gain, hirsutism
Instruct parent(s) of need for flexibility in care of child and need to integrate care and routines into child to participate in peer activity even though after-effects may be felt as long as the risk of damage is not great	Promotes well-being of child and sense of belonging and control of life events

Interventions	Rationales
Inform parent(s) and child about how to deal with peer and school perceptions of appearance and how to tell others about change in appearance	Prevents stigmatization of child by those who are not apprised of the child's disease; attitudes of others will affect child's body image

Discharge or Maintenance Evaluation

- Verbalizes improved body image and sense of well-being
- Participates in family, school, and social activities as appropriate
- Verbalizes feelings about special needs in positive terms
- Supports positive body image and promotes adjustment to chronic illness
- Modifies appearance with special clothing, wig, cosmetics to cover and/or protect skin; alopecia; weight gain

Pain

Related to: Biological injuring agents (inflammatory process)
Defining characteristics: Communication of pain descriptors, joint pain, achiness, joint swelling and stiffness

Outcome Criteria

Absence or control of joint pain with return of mobility

Interventions	Rationales
Assess severity of joint pain, location, duration, remissions, and exacerbations and what precipitates pain such as weight gain, activity; affect on mobility and participation in ADL; presence of joint deformity	Provides information symptomatic of the effect of the disease on the musculoskeletal system; allows for analgesic selection and better management of activity involvement
Administer analgesic and anti-inflammatories and assess effect of medications in relieving pain	Relieves pain and the inflammatory process associated with the pain
Apply warm compresses or packs to painful areas	Promotes circulation to the area by vasodilation to relieve pain

Interventions	Rationales
Provide 1-2 rest periods during day and quiet environment for sleep	Decreases stimulation that increases pain, and it promotes rest
Allow to assume position of comfort	Promotes comfort and rest for joints to reduce pain
Provide toys, TV, books, games, for quiet play during painful episodes	Promotes diversionary activity to detract from pain

Information, Instruction, Demonstration

Interventions	Rationales
Explain cause of pain to child and measures that should be taken to relieve pain	Provides reasons for treatments and medications
Inform child of factors that exacerbate pain episodes and to express or report presence of pain at the onset	Promotes opportunity to avoid those situations or activities that contribute to pain and to provide for immediate relief

Discharge or Maintenance Evaluation

- Pain relieved or controlled
- Limits or avoids factors that initiate or increase pain
- Analgesic therapy based on severity of pain and age with desired results
- Decreasing need for analgesic administration
- Complies with long-term anti-inflammatory therapy

Knowledge deficit of parent(s), child

Related to: Lack of information about chronic illness
Defining characteristics: Request for information about disease and the special needs associated with the disease; prevention of exacerbation and complications of the disease; risk of noncompliance with multiple preventative precautions

Outcome Criteria

Adequate knowledge of parent(s) and child for long-term compliance of medical regimen
Adjustment of family and child to treatment regimen

Interventions	Rationales
Assess knowledge of disease, type of treatments, effect on all systems, importance of compliance with medical regimen	Provides information needed to understand this complex disease and adjust long-term treatment and restrictions
Inform parent(s) and child of the disease process, effect on connective tissue and all systems, and treatment regimen needed to maintain remission	Provides information about known facts related to the disease to enhance knowledge of potential for exacerbations which may lead to early death
Instruct parent(s) and child in the administration and side effects of anti-inflammatories and immunosuppressant drugs, the importance of strict compliance to the medication protocol without decreasing or skipping the dose if side effects appear, and the need to adjust dosage during stressful situations	Promotes compliance to long-term medication regimen even when affected by undesirable side effects; an abrupt withdrawal of the medication may cause a serious physiological complication
Instruct parent(s) and child in activity restrictions or moderate activities allowed and how to weigh one activity against another as appropriate for the child	Prevents exacerbation of the symptoms while considering the long-term difficulty the child faces when activities are restricted
Instruct parent(s) and child to avoid sun exposure directly, through clouds, or reflected from water or snow; to use special sun screen or brimmed or visored hat to protect face	Prevents skin eruptions/reactions common to this disease when exposed to the sun
Inform parent(s) and child of child's need to take naps and have 8 hours of sleep/night; avoid fatigue or stressful situations; avoid medications such as sulfonamides, tetracyclines, anticonvulsants, and others that cause an exacerbation	Prevents exacerbations of the disease symptoms
Inform parent(s) and child to report bruising, petechiae, elevated temper-	Provides for early interventions if complications occur

Interventions	Rationales
ature, blood in urine or stool, increased irritability, vomiting, inability or remission in taking medications, respiratory or urinary changes	
Inform of community agencies or American Lupus Society for contact and support	Provides information and support for families and children to assist in adjusting to the disease and its lifelong limitation

Discharge or Maintenance Evaluation

- Complies with lifelong medical regimen to prevent exacerbations and complications
- Verbalizes disease process, affects to each system, treatments and limitations imposed by the disease
- Complies strictly to medication and activity protocols
- Prevents risk of exacerbations by avoiding factors that precipitate signs and symptoms
- Utilizes community agencies for assistance, information, and support
- Reports untoward signs and symptoms to physician
- Monitors VS, weight, urine and fecal testing as instructed

Ineffective individual coping

Related to: Multiple life changes, personal vulnerability
Defining characteristics: Alteration in social participation, inappropriate use of defense mechanisms (denial, regression, projection), withdrawal, intolerance of new experiences, lifelong hardships of medical regimen and limitations

Outcome Criteria

Increased ability to deal with stressful and restrictive requirements of medical regimen

Interventions	Rationales
Assess coping behaviors of child and factors that induce use of defense mechanisms, response to stressful situations (avoidance behavior, cooperation or resistance, aggression, regression, delaying tactics, inappropriate humor)	Provides information about child's coping mechanisms and pattern and use of coping strategies

Interventions	Rationales
Allow child to express feeling and provide outlet for release of feeling in an accepting environment	Promotes independence and control over a situation
Provide therapeutic play including throwing ball or balloons, pounding board, hand painting, water play	Provides expression of feelings and outlet to release aggression
Involve child in care decisions and encourage independence in as much of the care as possible	Promotes active participation in care with assistance as needed
Identify and support coping mechanisms during play, social interactions, painful procedures, restrictions, and bedrest	Allows for experiences which gives the child an opportunity to practice successful coping behaviors which enhance development of one's self-esteem
Encourage parent(s) to participate in child's care and support	Increases feelings of security when the child must deal with new situations

Information, Instruction, Demonstration

Interventions	Rationales
Inform child of behaviors that are positive and negative and about the factors that influence coping pattern (age, development, past experiences, ability to adapt, support, perception of what is happening, inner resources)	Promotes understanding of coping pattern and reasons for behavior
Inform child of any procedures well before scheduling and that support will be given to assist through the event	Promotes coping with new and painful experiences
Suggest psychological consultation if appropriate	Assists child to deal constructively with frustration and compliance with medical regimen for lifelong illness

Discharge or Maintenance Evaluation

- Identifies and uses positive coping mechanisms
- Engages in decision making and expression of feelings about illness
- Participates in therapeutic play and other activities that allow expression of frustration
- Verbalizes meaning of behaviors and factors that contribute to them
- Develops new coping mechanisms that are acceptable for age and level of development
- Initiates counseling services when needed

Lupus Erythematosus

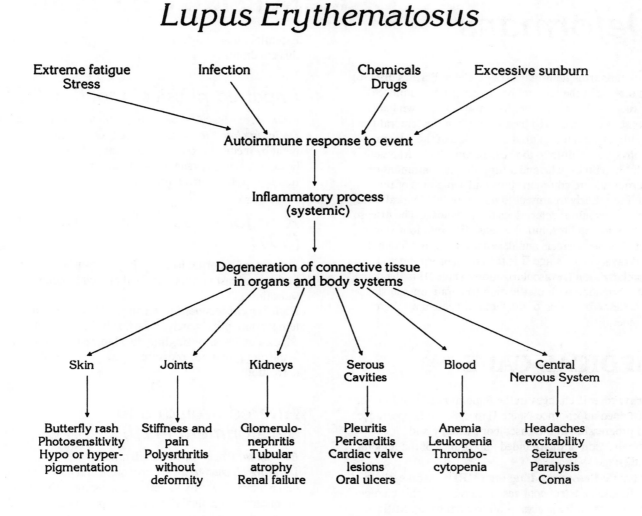

Extreme fatigue
Stress

Infection

Chemicals
Drugs

Excessive sunburn

Autoimmune response to event

Inflammatory process
(systemic)

Degeneration of connective tissue
in organs and body systems

Skin	Joints	Kidneys	Serous Cavities	Blood	Central Nervous System
Butterfly rash Photosensitivity Hypo or hyper- pigmentation	Stiffness and pain Polysrthritis without deformity	Glomerulo- nephritis Tubular atrophy Renal failure	Pleuritis Pericarditis Cardiac valve lesions Oral ulcers	Anemia Leukopenia Thrombo- cytopenia	Headaches excitability Seizures Paralysis Coma

Osteochondritis Deformans

Osteochondritis deformans (Legg-Calve-Perthes disease) is a disease of the femoral head occurring in children between 3-12 years of age. Its cause is unknown but the disease is characterized by a necrosis of the femoral head resulting from an impaired circulation of the femoral epiphysis extending to the acetabulum. Joint dysfunction with hip pain or ache and a limp that is continuous or intermittent are common signs and symptoms of the condition. Early treatment to maintain the femoral head in the acetabulum determines the prognosis. The disease progression and resolution is classified into four stages: stage I is the necrosis and degeneration of the femoral head (avascular); stage II is the bone absorption and vascularization (revascularization); stage III is the new bone formation with ossification (reparative); and stage IV is the reformation of the femoral head to a sphere (regenerative).

MEDICAL CARE

X-ray: reveals changes in the femoral head and hip from a flattened appearance (stage I) to a mottled appearance and progressing to increased bone density and normalization of the rounded appearance of the femoral head (stage IV).

Magnetic Resonance Imaging (MRI): useful early in the disease to detect changes since radiographic changes are not present for several months after onset. MRIs are useful later in assessing containment of the femoral head in the acetabulum.

Abduction traction: used to increase the range of motion in a child who has developed limited hip motion due to pain and spasm. Abduction traction is gradually increased on a daily basis to a point comfortably tolerated by the child. Traction may be used prior to surgical intervention and may be used in a home-based program.

Serial casting: casting of the hips in an abducted position with weekly cast changes using a progressively longer bar until full range of abduction is achieved. Casting also contains the femoral head in the acetabulum. The cast may be bi-valved later and used as a splint.

Osteotomy: surgical re-alignment of the femur so that the head of the femur is securely contained within the acetabulum. Requires 6-8 weeks of a hip spica cast after surgery and may be preceded by traction.

NURSING CARE PLANS

Essential nursing diagnoses and plans associated with this condition:

Impaired physical mobility (278)

Related to: Musculoskeletal impairment (femoral head)
Defining characteristics: Imposed restrictions of movement by medical protocol of corrective device (cast, brace, traction), reluctance to attempt movement, restriction in weight-bearing, limited ROM, bedrest

Risk for impaired skin integrity (397)

Related to: External factor of physical immobilization, pressure of cast or appliance and altered circulation, sensation
Defining characteristics: Change in skin color and temperature proximately to cast, skin irritation at cast edges, numbness or tingling distal to cast, redness on skin from prolonged pressure, break in skin from surgical correction

Altered growth and development (419)

Related to: Effects of immobilization
Defining characteristics: Environmental and stimulation deficiencies, inability to perform self-care activities appropriate for age, inability to participate in school and social activities

SPECIFIC DIAGNOSES AND CARE PLANS

Knowledge deficit of parent(s), child

Related to: Lack of information about the disease
Defining characteristics: Request for information about initial and long-term treatment, management of the therapy, and modification of activities

Outcome Criteria

Adequate information for compliance of medical protocol for corrective measures needed to ensure positive ultimate outcome

Interventions	Rationales
Assess knowledge of pathology of the disease and its four stages, treatment and prognosis, signs and symptoms	Provides information needed to develop a plan of instruction to ensure compliance of the medical regimen for correction; usually lasts 1-4 years and affects children 3-12 years of age with each stage lasting approximately 9-12 months; the younger the child at the time of diagnosis, the more positive the results and prognosis
Inform parent(s) and child that hip pain or stiffness that is constant or intermittent with involvement of the knee or thigh, limited ROM of the hip joint, a limp on the affected side may indicate aseptic necrosis of the femoral capital epiphysis with degenerative changes in the femoral head	Reveals signs and symptoms of the disease usually noted in the second stage
Inform parent(s) and child of use and purpose of traction if used	Applied to stretch adductor muscles before abduction cast is used, or before surgery
If home traction is used, refer parent(s) to a home health agency; child should be visited day of or day after discharge from hospital and 1-2 times per week while in traction	Home traction allows child to be in comfortable, familiar surroundings while maintaining therapeutic regimen; visits from home nurse allow evaluation of treatment and provision of family support and education
For surgical correction, inform parent(s) that child will need prophylactic antibiotics, will receive IV narcotics for pain for 2-3 days after surgery, will	Decreases anxiety about the surgical procedure through knowledge of post-operative care

Interventions	Rationales
have a hip spica cast applied, and will be discharged to home 4-5 days after surgery	
Inform and instruct parent(s) in purpose and application of an abduction splint; after ROM achieved, demonstrate and allow for return demonstration of application	Provides containment of the position of the femur while allowing for supported weight-bearing during healing, and is removable for bathing
Inform parent(s) and child of importance of avoiding weight-bearing on the affected limb (except as prescribed by physician) and need to be relatively inactive; advise activities suitable to stage of condition such as hobbies, crafts, games, museums, events of interest	Prevents degeneration of the hip joint caused by femoral damage resulting from weight-bearing activities; prolonged bedrest is no longer required
Inform parent(s) to advise school of activities that are allowed for learning and peer interactions	Provides special needs of child in order to continue school attendance and activities that may be adapted to appliance to promote feeling of acceptance
Instruct parent(s) in care of cast or splint including cleaning, tightness, and alignment with joints	Promotes proper function of appliance used and prevents complications associated with its use
Instruct parent(s) and child in use and care of crutches if used including swing through gait; monitor for repair needs as presence of loose screws and worn tips	Promotes safe use of crutches for mobility
Inform parent(s) to maintain pathways clear of clutter or toys	Prevents falls and injury
Inform parent(s) to prepare for attendance at special activities by calling in advance for special transportation, use of wheelchairs or other aids	Provides for participation in outside activities to enhance growth and development needs in long-term therapy

Discharge or Maintenance
Evaluation

- Complies with long-term medical regimen to correct disorder
- Maintains correct position of hip joint; applies splint correctly
- Prevents complications resulting from cast or appliance
- Verbalizes signs and symptoms of disease, cause of disease, length of treatment, type of treatment, prognosis, and projected outcome
- Complies with follow-up care requirements to monitor healing
- Prevents risk of degeneration by weight-bearing or noncompliance of medical regimen
- Allows for continuing school and activities adapted to appliance within disease limitations
- Included in family activities with necessary preparations made to accommodate restrictions of disease/appliance
- Devises new activities and interests within restrictions of mobility

Osteochondritis Deformans

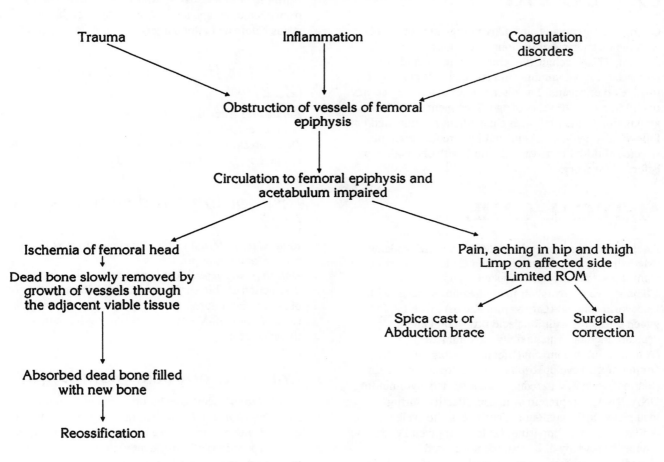

Trauma   Inflammation   Coagulation disorders

Obstruction of vessels of femoral epiphysis

Circulation to femoral epiphysis and acetabulum impaired

Ischemia of femoral head

Dead bone slowly removed by growth of vessels through the adjacent viable tissue

Absorbed dead bone filled with new bone

Reossification

Pain, aching in hip and thigh
Limp on affected side
Limited ROM

Spica cast or Abduction brace

Surgical correction

Osteogenic Sarcoma

Osteogenic sarcoma is a primary malignancy of the bone with the metaphysis of the long bones most commonly affected. These include the femur, humerus, and tibia. Metastasis most commonly affects the lungs but may involve other organs. The disease most commonly occurs in children over 10 years of age. Treatment consists of amputation of the limb with chemotherapy before and/or following surgery, or a bone and joint replacement in selected children to salvage the limb with chemotherapy before the surgery.

MEDICAL CARE

Analgesics: morphine sulfate (MS) given SC, codeine (Methylmorphine), acetaminophen (Tylenol) given PO to control postoperative pain depending on severity.
Chemotherapy protocol: methotrexate (Mexate) with leucovorin calcium (Citrovorum Factor) given IV, PO which interferes with folic acid production and to decrease methotrexate toxicity, doxorubicin (Adriamycin), bleomycin (Bienoxane), dactinomycin (Actinomycin) cyclophosphamide (Cytoxan), cisplatin (Platinol) given IV to reduce tumor activity by inhibiting DNA, RNA, and protein synthesis effective during metaphase or throughout the entire cell life cycle.
Antigout agent: allopurinol (Zyloprim) given IV, PO to reduce the severity of hyperuricemia caused by chemotherapy which promotes nucleic acid degradation causing increased plasma uric acid levels.
Bone x-ray: reveals bone lesion, fracture caused by tumor invasion.
Bone scan: reveals presence of bone lesions and size.
Bone biopsy: reveals presence of malignant tumor.
Computerized tomography (CT): reveals metastasis of bone and other organs.
Enzymes: alkaline phosphatase (ALP): reveals increased caused by abnormal osteoblastic activity or bone cell production; also reveals presence of isoenzymes (ALP2) of bone origin.

NURSING CARE PLANS

Essential nursing diagnoses and plans associated with this condition:

Altered nutrition: Less than body requirements (168)

Related to: Inability to ingest and digest food, chemotherapy
Defining characteristics: Anorexia, nausea, vomiting from chemotherapy, anxiety, grieving, weight loss, NPO status before and after surgery

Risk for fluid volume deficit (222)

Related to: Altered intake; excessive losses through normal routes
Defining characteristics: Diarrhea, vomiting from chemotherapy, NPO status before and after surgery

Risk for impaired skin integrity (397)

Related to: External factors for chemotherapy IV, surgical site, and use of prosthesis
Defining characteristics: Disruption of skin surfaces, destruction of skin surfaces, redness, edema, excoriation of stump site, improper fit or application of prosthesis, extravasation of IV site with swelling skin, redness, and tissue necrosis

Impaired physical mobility (278)

Related to: Musculoskeletal impairment (amputation)
Defining characteristics: Inability to move within physical environment, reluctance to attempt movement, imposed restrictions of movement with loss of limb, inability to adapt to prosthesis or brace, use of crutches or wheelchair

Diarrhea (171)

Related to: Chemotherapy
Defining characteristics: Increased frequency of bowel sounds and loose, liquid stools

SPECIFIC DIAGNOSES AND CARE PLANS

Anxiety of parent(s) and child

Related to: Change in health status, threat of death, threat to self-concept

Defining characteristics: Increased apprehension and fear of diagnosis; expressed concern and worry about preoperative procedures and preparation, postoperative effects of therapy on physical and emotional status, possible metastasis of disease, loss of limb and use of prosthesis

Outcome Criteria

Reduced anxiety verbalized as information regarding disease, treatment, and prognosis

Interventions	Rationales
Assess level of anxiety of parent(s) and child and how it is manifested; the need for information that will relieve anxiety	Provides information about source and level of anxiety and need for interventions to relieve it; sources for the child may be procedures, fear of mutilation or death, unfamiliar environment of hospital and may be manifested by restlessness, inability to play or sleep or eat
Assess possible need for special counseling services for child	Reduces anxiety and supports child dealing with illness and promotes adjustment to lifestyle changes
Allow open expression of concerns about illness, procedures, treatments, and possible consequences of surgery	Provides opportunity to vent feelings and fears to reduce anxiety
Communicate with child at appropriate age level and answer questions calmly and honestly; use pictures, models, and drawings for explanations	Promotes understanding and trust
Allow child as much input in decisions about care and routines as possible	Allows for more control and independence in situations
Allow parent(s) to stay with child or open visitation; provide a telephone number to call for information	Promotes care and support by parent(s)
Provide continuing nurse assignment with the same personnel	Promotes trust and comfort and familiarity with staff giving care

Interventions	Rationales
Orient child to surgical and ICU unit, equipment, noises, and staff	Reduces anxiety caused by fear of unknown

Information, Instruction, Demonstration

Interventions	Rationales
Inform parent(s) and child of the disease process, surgical procedure, what to expect preoperatively and postoperatively including chemotherapy and its benefits and side effects (nausea, vomiting, diarrhea, stomatitis, alopecia, and others are possibilities but are temporary; phantom pain)	Provides information to promote understanding that will relieve fear and anxiety; understanding of preoperative and postoperative treatments and effect on body image
Explain all procedures and care in simple, direct, honest terms and repeat as often as necessary; reinforce physician information if needed and provide specific information as requested	Supplies information about all diagnostic procedures and tests such as CBC, platelets with chemotherapy and scans and x-rays for diagnosis
Inform parent(s) and child of the extent of surgery with the removal of a limb that a temporary prosthesis will be fitted immediately following surgery, and a permanent one will be fitted in 6-8 weeks; that recreational and physical therapy will be undertaken following amputation	Reduces anxiety when knowledge and support is given, and child and parent(s) will not feel betrayed by inadequate preparation of procedures and treatments
Introduce child to another who has same disease and amputation	Provides information and support from a peer with the same condition and who would have empathy
Provide information about contacting American Cancer Society	Provide resource for information and support groups

Discharge or Maintenance Evaluation

- Expresses reduction in anxiety as information and explanations are given
- States concerns and reason for anxiety and behavior
- Verbalizes and participates in preoperative and postoperative procedures
- Explores and notes anger about diagnosis and proposed changes in body structure and function
- Utilizes existing and new support systems
- Participates in decision making regarding care and postoperative rehabilitation

Altered oral mucous membrane

Related to: Medication (chemotherapy)
Defining characteristics: Stomatitis, oral ulcers, hyperemia, oral pain or discomfort, oral plaque

Outcome Criteria

Absence or control of oral mucosal changes and discomfort

Interventions	Rationales
Assess oral cavity for pain ulcers, lesions, gingivitis, mucositis or stomatitis and effect on ability to ingest food and fluids	Provides information about effect of chemotherapy
Provide mouth rinses, cleansing with swabs or soft toothbrush	Provides mouth care without irritating oral mucosa
Administer medication topically (xylocaine) before meals and offer bland, smooth foods that are not hot or spicy	Permits eating with more comfort
Administer an antiseptic mouth rinse (nystatin) 30 minutes before any food or fluid intake	Promotes comfort of oral mucosa and maintains integrity
Encourage child to select foods that are allowable and that they prefer	Allows for independence and control over situation to reduce helplessness and increase nutrition

Information, Instruction, Demonstration

Interventions	Rationales
Instruct parent(s) in effect of chemotherapy on oral mucosa and in treatment to decrease discomfort in oral cavity	Promotes understanding of side effects that occur and temporary nature of the side effects
Instruct parent(s) in mouth rinses and topical application of medications	Promotes effective care of oral cavity to relieve discomfort and prevent mucosa breakdown and increased inflammation
Instruct to use soft brush or swabs to clean mouth	Prevents trauma to mucosa

Discharge or Maintenance Evaluation

- Oral mucous membranes intact and reduced inflammation present
- Complies with measures to prevent trauma or breakdown of mucosa
- Controls discomfort associated with impaired oral mucosa
- Progressive return of oral mucous membrane baseline following chemotherapy protocol

Altered protection

Related to: Drug therapy (antineoplastics): abnormal blood profile (leukopenia, thrombocytopenia, anemia, coagulation)
Defining characteristics: Altered clotting, bone marrow suppression, deficient immunity against infection, hematoma, petechiae, bleeding from nose or gums, hematemesis, blood in stool

Outcome Criteria

Absence of bleeding from any source
Protection from exposure to pathogenic microorganisms

Interventions	Rationales
Assess for bleeding from any site, WBC, platelet count, Hct, absolute neutrophil count, and febrile episodes	Provides information about frank bleeding or blood profile abnormalities that predispose to bleeding caused by bone marrow suppression and

Interventions	Rationales
	immunosuppression resulting from chemotherapy
Avoid trauma by use of hard toothbrush or dental floss, taking rectal temperatures, performing unnecessary invasive procedures	Prevents bleeding caused by trauma during chemotherapy which alters platelet and clotting factors
Carry out handwashing technique before giving care, use mask and gown when appropriate, provide a private room, monitor for any signs and symptoms of infections, especially pulmonary	Prevents transmission of pathogens to a compromised immune system during chemotherapy if neutrophil count is less than 1000/cu mm

Information, Instruction, Demonstration

Interventions	Rationales
Inform parent(s) and child to avoid rough play or sports, straining at defecation, forcefully blowing nose	Prevents trauma that causes bleeding
Instruct parent(s) and child to avoid those with upper respiratory infection or an illness	Prevents risk for infection in the highly susceptible child
Instruct parent(s) to report any fever, behavior changes, headache, dizziness, fatigue, pallor, slow oozing of blood from any area, exposure to a communicable disease	Indicates a complication associated with an abnormal blood profile
Impress on parent(s) the need for compliance in laboratory testing and physician appointments	Monitors effect of chemotherapy on child and need for modification of therapy or care
Instruct and allow for return demonstration of urine and stool testing for blood using dipstick and hematest	Identifies presence of bleeding in gastrointestinal or urinary tract

Discharge or Maintenance Evaluation

- Absence of excessive bleeding or infection during chemotherapy
- Complies with measures to prevent excessive bleeding or infection based on blood profile
- Reports signs and symptoms of complication to physician
- Complies with laboratory blood testing and follow-up visits to physician

Risk for injury

Related to: Internal physical factor of broken skin and altered mobility; external physical factor of prosthesis use
Defining characteristics: Amputation of a limb, changes in stump incision (redness, irritation, swelling, drainage), improper fit of prosthesis and failure to adapt to it, improper positioning and alignment of the stump, psychosocial maladaption to prosthesis

Outcome Criteria

Absence of complications at surgical site
Progressive adaptation to a limb prosthesis
Compliance with physiotherapy regimen
Preservation and maintenance of body image

Interventions	Rationales
Assess child for type of surgery and condition and healing of the stump, type of bandaging or cast, presence of drains, type of prosthetic device and fit	Provides information about amputation needed to provide specific care of stump and rehabilitation
Assess dressing for bleeding, redness, pain, drainage at stump area q2-4h; maintain dressing (pressure) or wrapping of stump as ordered; change dressing only if ordered	Indicates infection or risk of hemorrhage at amputation
Maintain Trendelenburg and prone position; avoid elevation (with pillow), external rotation, or abduction of stump	Prevents deformities and contractures caused by hip flexion
Perform ROM daily and exercises recommended by physical therapist	Promotes mobility and healing of the stump and prevents contractures

Interventions	Rationales
Cleanse stump and socket daily with mild soap and warm water, rinse and pat dry	Promotes adaptation to device and prevents infection caused by pathogens transmitted via the prosthetic device
Support expressions about loss of lifestyle and permanent disability adjustment difficulties (age appropriate)	Promotes venting of feelings and assists to cope with change in body image

Information, Instruction, Demonstration

Interventions	Rationales
Instruct parent(s) and child in stump care, toughening exercises, application of stocking and prosthesis, care of device	Promotes adaptation to loss and correct care of stump and prosthesis
Instruct child in stump positioning and exercising, ROM of muscles and joints	Prevents muscle or joint complications and enhances mobility
Inform child of importance of daily activities to perform and those to avoid and explain reasons for restrictions	Promotes mobility and return to former activities within limitation imposed by amputation and use of prosthetic device
Impress on parent(s) and child the importance of continued chemotherapy and rehabilitation therapy	Promotes compliance of medical regimen
Discuss modification of clothing and instruct in crutch walking and how to get around in room, at home, and at school	Enhances body image and return to limited activities
Inform child that feelings of anger, denial, and hostility are normal following such a loss	Promotes acceptance of child while grieving for loss

Discharge or Maintenance Evaluation

- Maintains appropriate and effective care of stump and prosthetic device
- Complies with exercises and physical therapy regimen
- Surgical site is healing and free of infection
- Proper fit and use of prosthesis with progressive mobility
- Adapts daily to loss of a limb and dependence on prosthesis
- Provides changes in lifestyle and appearance necessary to preserve body image
- Resumes preoperative activities gradually
- Utilizes aids (crutches, wheelchair) until healing and prosthesis use and competency realized

Osteogenic Sarcoma

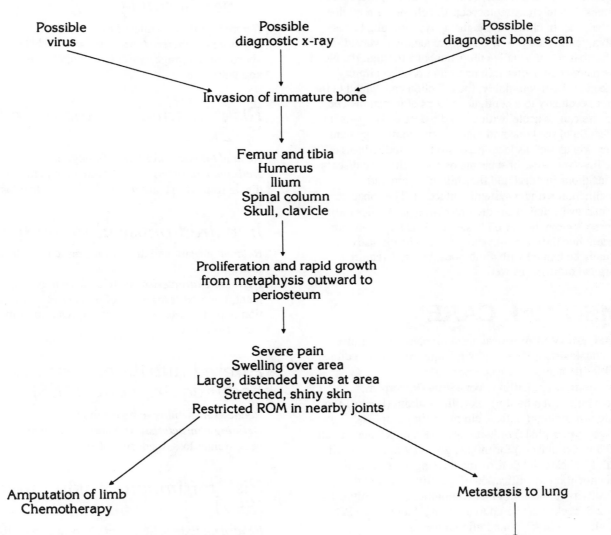

Possible
virus

Possible
diagnostic x-ray

Possible
diagnostic bone scan

Invasion of immature bone

Femur and tibia
Humerus
Ilium
Spinal column
Skull, clavicle

Proliferation and rapid growth
from metaphysis outward to
periosteum

Severe pain
Swelling over area
Large, distended veins at area
Stretched, shiny skin
Restricted ROM in nearby joints

Amputation of limb
Chemotherapy

Metastasis to lung

Chemotherapy
Radiation therapy

Osteomyelitis

Osteomyelitis is an infection of the bone caused by any infectious agent, but most commonly by Staphylococcus aureus, Hemolytic streptococci, E. coli, or Hemophilus influenzae. In children, the metaphyses of long bones (tibia, femur) are the sites most frequently involved. The infectious agent usually enters the bone through the blood (hematogenous) after trauma or an upper respiratory infection. Less commonly, the infection can spread to the bone secondary to a contiguous focus of infection. The disease can be acute, with a rapidly destructive pyogenic infection of the bone and marrow and signs of systemic infection as well as local pain, swelling and redness of the involved area. In subacute osteomyelitis, the disease is insidious in onset and the child has pain and dysfunction without systemic infection. The subacute form may be due to children receiving antibiotics during a presymptomatic period. Osteomyelitis most commonly occurs in children 5-14 years of age. The disease can usually be treated with antibiotics, but may require surgical drainage as well.

MEDICAL CARE

Analgesics/Antipyretics: acetaminophen (Tylenol tablets, Pedric wafers or elixir, Liquiprin solution drops) PO for pain and to reduce fever.
Antibiotics: Penicillin G potassium (Pfizerpen), methicillin (Staphcillin), oxacillin sodium (Bactocill) or nafcillin sodium (Nafcil), clindamycin phosphate (Cleocir Phosphate) or kanamycin (Kantrex), gentamicin sulfate (Garamycin) for infants given IV to inhibit cell wall synthesis and destroy infective agent; selection dependent on identification of infective agent and sensitivity to the antibiotic. Antibiotics usually given IV for 2-3 weeks (can be up to 6 weeks), followed by PO administration for 3-4 additional weeks.
Bone x-ray: shows lytic changes in the involved area after the first 2 weeks.
Computerized tomography (CT): reveals bone changes early in the disease.
Bone scan: reveals infectious process in bone by increased uptake of radionucleotides.
Erythrocyte sedimentation rate (ESR): reveals increases in acute stage.
Complete blood count (CBC): reveals increased WBC during infectious process.
Blood/wound cultures: reveals organisms responsible for infection by culture of site.

NURSING CARE PLANS

Essential nursing diagnoses and plans associated with this condition:

Hyperthermia (112)

Related to: Illness (infection)
Defining characteristics: Increase in body temperature above normal range, warm to touch, increased respiratory and pulse rate

Risk for fluid volume deficit (222)

Related to: Excessive losses through normal routes
Defining characteristics: Elevated temperature, diaphoresis, thirst, altered intake, insensitive losses

Impaired physical mobility (278)

Related to: Pain and discomfort, musculoskeletal impairment
Defining characteristics: Reluctance to attempt movement, imposed restrictions of movement by immobilization of part by cast and/or bedrest, restriction in weight-bearing

Altered nutrition: Less than body requirements (168)

Related to: Inability to ingest food
Defining characteristics: Anorexia, irritability, restlessness, weight loss, inadequate food intake

Risk for impaired skin integrity (397)

Related to: External factor of physical immobilization, pressure of cast and altered circulation, sensation
Defining characteristics: Change in color and temperature of skin proximal to cast or device, skin irritation at cast edges, numbness distal cast, prolonged pressure on an area with redness present, break in skin from surgical wound

SPECIFIC DIAGNOSES AND CARE PLANS

Anxiety of parent(s) and child

Related to: Change in health status, change in environment (hospitalization)

Defining characteristics: Expressed apprehension and concern about prolonged hospitalization resulting from spread of infection, possible surgical drainage of infected area

Outcome Criteria

Reduced anxiety verbalized by parent(s) and child
Verbalizes positive effects of treatments and/or surgical drainage
Acceptance of long-term antibiotic therapy

Interventions	Rationales
Assess source and level of anxiety and need for information that will relieve anxiety	Provides information about anxiety, its effect and need to relieve it; sources may include prolonged immobilization and hospitalization, long-term IV antibiotic therapy, possible surgical drainage and antibiotic instillation into wound, risk of complications from disease and high-dose medication therapy
Allow expression of concerns and time to ask questions about condition, procedures, prognosis, recovery time by parent(s) or child	Provides opportunity to vent feelings and fears to reduce anxiety
Answer questions calmly and honestly; use pictures, drawings, and models for information and demonstrations	Promotes trust and a secure, supportive environment
Encourage parent(s) to stay with child during hospitalization, and encourage to assist in care; encourage visits from friends and relatives	Allows parent(s) to care for and support child, continue parental role and promote security for the child

Interventions	Rationales
Give parent(s) and child as much input into decisions about care and usual routines as possible	Allows for more control over situations and maintains familiar routines for care

Information, Instruction, Demonstration

Interventions	Rationales
Inform parent(s) and child of cause and course of the disease, extent of the infectious process, and treatment modalities	Provides information that will enhance understanding of the disease to relieve anxiety
Inform parent(s) and child of tests and procedures to be done and the reasons for them; include surgical procedure if planned	Provides rationale for diagnostic procedures and surgery to prepare for these experiences and reduce fear of unknown which increases anxiety
Inform parent(s) and child of reason for antibiotic therapy IV to be followed by PO administration when acute stage subsides	Provides rationale for long-term therapy to control infectious process and prevent its spread to reduce anxiety
Inform parent(s) and child of treatment to expect following surgery including presence of cast on the affected extremity, antibiotic therapy instillation into the wound, and continuous removal of drainage from the wound by low suction	Provides information about postoperative care to reduce anxiety
Inform parent(s) and child that although weight-bearing will be disallowed until healing is well established, appetite, quiet activity, and improved sense of well-being will be increased as acuity of the disease is reduced	Promotes comfort and positive attitude and reduces anxiety level when expectations are known
Inform parents that physical therapy may be prescribed after infection subsides, acute healing assured	Permits optimal function of affected extremity and allows for feeling of positive outcome

Discharge or Maintenance Evaluation

- Verbalizes reduction in anxiety about disease, diagnostic procedures, and treatments
- Verbalizes positive effects of surgical intervention and postoperative treatments
- Participates in care and support of child and decision making during hospitalization

Pain

Related to: Physical injuring agent (inflammation/infection)

Defining characteristics: Communication of pain descriptors, crying, irritability, restlessness, withdrawal, reluctance to use or move affected limb, tenderness

Outcome Criteria

Absence or control of pain

Interventions	Rationales
Assess site for pain on movement of extremity; resistance of muscles to passive movement, holding extremity in semi-flexion; severity, type, and duration of pain using a pain scale if appropriate	Provides information about pain as a basis for analgesic therapy
Administer analgesic and sedative as ordered and note response	Reduces pain and promotes rest to reduce stimuli that causes pain
Place extremity in position of comfort and support with pillows at 30 degrees elevation	Promotes comfort and reduces or prevents pain by reducing edema when venous return is enhanced
Move extremity with smoothness and care	Prevents pain caused by careless handling or abrupt movement of affected part
Provide diversionary activities and quiet play during acute stage	Diverts attention from the pain

Information, Instruction, Demonstration

Interventions	Rationales
Inform parent(s) and child of analgesic medications and expected results when administered properly either for acute infection or post-operative pain	Provides information about effects expected from analgesic therapy to relieve pain until acute stage subsides or healing is underway
Inform parent(s) and child of ways to move, position extremity; importance of maintaining immobilization of the extremity and avoiding any weight-bearing until advised	Prevents undue pain caused by movement of affected area

Discharge or Maintenance Evaluation

- Absence of pain and associated responses
- Controls pain provoking actions when giving care or changing position
- Administer analgesics and sedatives correctly and monitor responses

Risk for injury

Related to: Internal factors of infection spread, immobilization, effects of cast application

Defining characteristics: Changes in color and temperature, tactile perception of casted extremity, increased body temperature, purulent drainage, edema, erythematic infection site, musty odor under cast, increased WBC, positive wound culture

Outcome Criteria

Progressive resolution of infection with absence of infection spread with or without surgical wound
Positive response from antibiotic therapy and local treatments

Interventions	Rationales
Assess presence of localized pain, swelling, and warmth over the affected bone; purulent drainage with a musty odor from open wound, under cast, or over the infected area that is left open for observation	Provides information about site of infection(s) which may be open wound, bone, or surgical drainage wound; inadequate treatment may result in chronic osteomyelitis or persistence and spread of infection
Administer antibiotics IV based on culture and sensitivity results and physician orders; administer antibiotics PO following acute phase of the disease; administer via IV heparin lock if therapy is long-term	Treats infectious process and prevents spread of infection by preventing cell wall synthesis of the invading bacteria; IV therapy may last for 2-3 weeks or longer depending on the response to treatment
Administer antibiotic solution into the wound, if present, via an IV administration set at a regulated rate; provide wound drainage by connecting tubes from wound to low suction	Treats open wound infections and ensures continuous wound drainage
Place in isolation or maintain body fluid precautions (wound and skin) if wound is open and draining	Prevents wound contamination or spread of infection; agency policy dictates measures for precautions
Maintain sterile technique for all procedures and dressing changes; cleanse, pack wound as ordered	Prevents introduction of infectious organisms
Measure limb circumference when assessing infectious process	Reveals changes caused by edema
Monitor WBC, ESR, and antibiotic levels as appropriate	Increases in WBC and ESR found in infections and antibiotic levels reveal if therapeutic levels are maintained for effective treatment
Provide immobilization of limb by maintaining cast, splint, and bedrest status monitor color, temperature, sensation, and motion of digits	Maintains limb alignment, limits spread of infection, and prevents possible fraction or complications resulting from neurovascular problems

Information, Instruction, Demonstration

Interventions	Rationales
Instruct parent(s) and child in proper technique for handwashing, wound care and handling contaminated articles/supplies	Prevents transmission of microorganisms to or from child
Instruct parent(s) of PO antibiotic administration including action, dose, time, frequency, side effects, and expected results; length of time that antibiotic therapy may last	Ensures compliance of long-term therapy to ensure effective results
Inform parent(s) of importance of laboratory testing if ordered	Monitors infectious process and need for change in therapy
Instruct parent(s) and child of need for measures to maintain immobility and reason for isolation precautions	Prevents further spread of infection and possible damage to affected area and surrounding tissue
Instruct parent(s) in care of cast or splint including petaling edges, maintaining dry and clean cast or splint, preventing small particles or objects from entering cast or splint	Ensures effective immobilization and prevents complications caused by whole or bivalve cast or splint
Inform parent(s) and child that physical therapy may follow healing and resolution of infection	Ensures optimal functioning of affected limb

Discharge or Maintenance Evaluation

- Absence of infection spread
- Administers antibiotic therapy correctly; IV, PO, or wound instillation as appropriate
- Maintains isolation or wound and skin precautions
- Performs handwash and proper technique during care and procedures
- Maintains safe, effective cast or splint care for immobilization
- Reports and prevents complications of immobilization or medication administration

Impaired social interaction

Related to: Limited physical mobility, therapeutic isolation

Defining characteristics: Change in pattern of interaction, lengthy treatment and immobilization, boredom, inability to engage in usual activities for age group, environment that lacks diversion

Outcome Criteria

Participation in activities despite immobilizing treatments

Interventions	Rationales
Provide age-appropriate toys that can be used in bed while in a prone or sitting position depending on type of treatment and degree of immobilization	Promotes social and developmental activities and reduces boredom during long-term treatment
Provide exposure to other children by moving bed near areas of activity or near a window; wheel on a stretcher or in a wheelchair or stroller, allow to walk with cast or splint when permitted	Provides environmental stimulation and social interaction
Encourage family and friends to visit or stay with child; if in isolation provide frequent interactions or someone to stay with child	Promotes social interaction with others during long-term treatment and reduces boredom
Place toys and other articles within reach	Provides access to diversion activities when needed

Information, Instruction, Demonstration

Interventions	Rationales
Inform parent(s) to include infant/child in family activities	Promotes feeling of acceptance and well-being as part of the family
Inform of devices available or methods used for mobility to fit needs of child with a cast or splint	Promotes exposure to various activities and changes of environmental stimuli

Interventions	Rationales
Inform parent(s) to allow as much independence in self-care by child as possible	Promotes independence and allows some control over the situation

Discharge or Maintenance Evaluation

- Participates in positive interaction with peers and family members
- Maintains age appropriate stimulation and play activities
- Participates in family activities
- Promotes a variety of activities contributing to growth and development needs

Osteomyelitis

Older child → Haemophilus influenzae

Younger child → Staphylococcus aureus

Exogenous sources
Direct invasion of bone by penetrating wound,
fracture, surgical contamination
Secondary invasion from abscess or burn

Hematogenous sources
Furuncles, tonsillitis, otis media, pyelonephritis,
impetigo, upper respiratory infection
↓
Infective emboli circulated
↓
Increased vascularity
Edema with accumulation of leukocytes in area
↓
Thrombosis and Ischemia
↓
Bone destruction and death
Abscess formation
↓
Pus ruptures into subperiosteal space
↓
Periosteum stripped
↓
Spread of infection beneath periosteum with necrosis
↓
Thrombosis of vessels

Antibiotic therapy
Immobilization

Surgery

New bone formed in young
children with the cortex
of bone deprived of blood supply

Resolution
↓
Physical therapy to
restore function

↓
Necrotic bone formed
↓
Infected dead bone separated
from living bone (sequestrum)
↓
New Bone formation around
dead bone
↓
Chronic osteomyelitis
with exacerbations

Rheumatoid Arthritis (Juvenile)

Rheumatoid arthritis of the juvenile type is a chronic inflammatory disease that involves the synovium of the joints resulting in effusion and eventual erosion and destruction of the joint cartilage. It is classified into different types and characterized by remissions and exacerbations with the onset most common between 2-5 and 9-12 years of age. Pauciarticular arthritis involves only a few joints, usually under five; polyarticular arthritis involves many joints, usually more than four; and systemic arthritis involves the presence of arthritis and associated high temperature, rash, and affects other organs such as the heart, lungs, eyes, and those located in the abdominal cavity. Prognosis is based on the severity of the disease, type of arthritis, and response to treatment with the most severe complications of the permanent deformity, hip disease, and iridocyclitis with visual loss.

MEDICAL CARE

Anti-inflammatories (Nonsteroidal): aspirin (acetylsalicylic acid), indomethacin (Indocin), naproxen (Naprosyn), tolmetin sodium (Tolectin) given PO for analgesia, antipyretic action as well as anti-inflammatory and antirheumatic effects; may be used in combination with steriods and gold salts; action thought to be the inhibition of prostaglandin synthesis.

Anti-inflammatories (Steroidal): prednisone (Deltasone) given PO to suppress inflammatory responses and reactions, also reduces antibody titers and inhibits phagocytosis and release of allergic substances.

Antirheumatics (Slow acting): penicillamine (Depen) given PO, gold sodium thiomalate (Myochrysine) given IM to inhibit collagen formation or alter immune responses and inhibit prostraglandin synthesis in the treatment of rheumatic diseases.

Immunosuppressants: cyclophosphamide (Cytoxan), methotrexate (MTX) given PO to treat rheumatoid arthritis when response to other anti-inflammatory drugs are not effective if the disease is severe and debilitating; usually used in combination with other drugs.

Joint x-ray: reveals widened joint spaces with later joint destruction and fusion, evidence of osteoporosis and inflammation at affected joint sites.

Erythrocyte sedimentation rate (ESR): reveals increases in systemic type but may be increased or decreased depending on the degree of inflammation.

Antinuclear antibodies: reveals presence in 75 percent of rheumatoid factor with a positive result in 25 percent; positive or negative result depending on type of arthritis.

Rheumatoid factor: reveals presence in those with later onset type with a positive result in pauciarticular type.

Complete blood count: reveals increased WBC in early stages.

Synovial fluid culture: reveals absence of infectious process and confirms absence of other conditions by joint aspiration of fluid for examination.

NURSING CARE PLANS

Essential nursing diagnoses and plans associated with this condition:

Impaired physical mobility (278)

Related to: Musculoskeletal impairment, pain, and discomfort
Defining characteristics: Reluctance to attempt movement, limited range of motion, imposed restrictions of movement by medical protocol, resting or immobilization of joint(s) by splinting and positioning, fatigue, malaise

Risk for impaired skin integrity (397)

Related to: External factor or physical immobilization
Defining characteristics: Skin irritation under splint(s), redness from prolonged pressure, break in skin from surgery if done, macular rash on extremities and trunk areas

Altered growth and development (419)

Related to: Effects of physical disability
Defining characteristics: Environmental and stimulation deficiencies, inability to perform self-care activities appropriate for age, growth retardation during active disease, reduced peer relationships

Hyperthermia (112)

Related to: Illness of inflammation
Defining characteristics: Increase in body temperature above normal range, chills, low grade temperatures or high elevations late in day or twice a day

Altered nutrition: Less than body requirements (168)

Related to: Inability to ingest food
Defining characteristics: Anorexia, weight loss or poor gain, weakness, fatigue, irritability

SPECIFIC DIAGNOSES AND CARE PLANS

Chronic pain

Related to: Chronic physical disability
Defining characteristics: Verbalization or observed evidence of pain experienced for more than 6 months, guarded movement, fear of reinjury, altered ability to continue activities, physical and social withdrawal. Single or multiple joint involvement, joint stiffness, loss of motion, edema, and warmth in joint(s) and painful to touch

Outcome Criteria

Control or relief of joint pain by reduction of inflammation
Movement with minimal pain

Interventions	Rationales
Assess severity of joint(s) pain, location, duration, remissions and exacerbations, stiffness and what precipitates pain such as weight gain, activity, fatigue; effect on mobility and participation in ADL; presence of joint deformity	Provides information symptomatic of the effect of the disease on the musculoskeletal system: allows for analgesic/anti-inflammatories selection and better management of activity involvement; inflammatory process cause pain with the edema resulting from joint effusion and synovial thickening and limited motion resulting from muscle spasms; joint deformity results from joint destruction
Administer NSAIDS, SHARDS, steroid anti-inflammatories as ordered and assess effect of medications in relieving pain	Relieves pain and the inflammatory process associated with the pain; drugs may be administered alone or in combination including the nonsteroidal anti-inflammatory drugs which

Interventions	Rationales
	act as analgesic, antipyretic and anti-inflammatory; slower acting antirheumatic drugs which may be added for optimal effect if NSAIDs are ineffective; corticosteroid drugs in lowest effective dose for short period of time especially in the presence of a life threatening situation
Apply warm compresses, packs, or soaks to painful areas; paraffin baths and whirlpool as ordered	Promotes circulation to the area by vasodilation to relieve pain; moist heat relieves painful, stiff areas
Provide 1-2 rest periods during day and quiet environment for sleep	Decreases stimulation that increases pain, and it promotes rest, especially during acute episodes
Allow to assume position of comfort; elevate and support painful joints when changing position	Promotes diversionary activity to detract from pain
Apply splints if ordered for night use	Provides immobilization of joints to ease pain during movement

Information, Instruction, Demonstration

Interventions	Rationales
Explain cause of pain to child and measures that should be taken to relieve pain	Provides reasons for treatments and medications
Inform child and parent(s) of factors (stress, climate movement) that exacerbate pain episodes, and to express or report presence of pain at the onset	Promotes opportunity to avoid those situations or activities that contribute to exacerbations of pain and to provide for immediate relief
Instruct parent(s) and child in accurate administration of medications including side effects and importance of compliance with regimen whether taken QID, HS, or BID and side effects to report	Promotes compliance with medical regimen to control pain and inflammation

Interventions	Rationales
Instruct parent(s) to give warm bath daily for 10 minutes or warm wet packs with a towel bath to painful areas	Supplies heat to affected joints to relieve pain and stiffness
Instruct parent(s) and child to avoid over-activity or movement of affected joints	Prevents injury to affected joints during the acute episode when immobilization is important
Instruct child in relaxation techniques, music therapy and diversionary activities such as TV, reading, games	Provides non-pharmacologic interventions to relieve pain

Discharge or Maintenance Evaluation

- Pain and inflammation relieved or controlled
- Limits or avoids factors that initiate or increase pain
- Complies with long-term medication protocol
- Minimal discomfort during movement or activity
- Administers medications properly with meals, reports side effects, complies with laboratory testing as ordered

Body image disturbance

Related to: Biophysical and psychosocial factors
Defining characteristics: Verbal and nonverbal responses to change in body appearance (joint deformity, steroid side effects), negative feelings about body, multiple stressors and change in daily living limitations and social relationships

Outcome Criteria

Body image improved, preserved and maintained
Accommodations made for and adaptation to long-term need and limitations of chronic illness

Interventions	Rationales
Assess child for feelings about multiple restrictions in lifestyle, chronic illness, difficulty in school and social situations, inability to keep up with peers and participate in activities	Provides information about status of self-concept and body image that require special attention

Interventions	Rationales
Encourage expression of feelings and concerns, and support communications with parent(s), teachers, and peers	Provides opportunity to vent feelings and reduce negative feelings about changes in appearance
Avoid negative comments and stress positive activities and accomplishments	Enhances body image and confidence
Note withdrawal behavior and signs of depression	Reveals responses to body image changes and possible poor adjustment to changes
Note presence of joint deformities, need to use splints, weight gain, shift in fat distribution, edema and effect on child	Reveals side effects of steroid therapy and disease manifestations that affect body image
Show support and acceptance of changes in appearance of child; provide privacy as needed	Promotes trust and demonstrates respect for child

Information, Instruction, Demonstration

Interventions	Rationales
Inform parent(s) of importance of maintaining support for child regardless of their needs	Encourages acceptance of the child with special needs (long-term steroid therapy and side effects, lifelong activity restrictions)
Inform parent(s) and child of impact of the disease on body systems and risk for deformity and disabilities; correct misinformation and inform of ways to cope with body changes	Provides correct information to assist in dealing with negative feelings about body
Instruct parent(s) of need for flexibility in care of child and need to integrate care and routines into family activities; to allow child to participate in peer activity even though after effects may be felt as long as the risk of damage is not great	Promotes well-being of child and sense of belonging and control of life events by participating in normal activities for age and enhancing developmental task achievement

Interventions	Rationales
Inform parent(s) and child about how to deal with peer perceptions of appearance and how to tell others about change in appearance	Prevents stigmatization of child by those who are not apprised of the child's disease; attitude of others will affect child's body image
Suggest psychological counseling or child life worker and inform of functions performed by these professionals	Assists to improve self-esteem and to learn coping and problem solving skills
Provide information concerning Juvenile Arthritis Foundation	Promotes support from others and how they handle the changes

Discharge or Maintenance Evaluation

- Verbalizes improved body image and sense of well-being
- Participates in family, school, and social activities as appropriate
- Verbalizes feelings about special long-term needs in positive terms
- Supports positive body image and promotes adjustment to chronic illness
- Identifies need and seeks out social services, psychological counseling as appropriate

Self-care deficit: bathing/ hygiene, dressing/grooming, feeding, toileting

Related to: Pain, discomfort, and musculoskeletal impairment
Defining characteristics: Impaired ability in performance of ADL and maintenance of complete physical care; pain and weakness of joints and intolerance to activity; immobility status; joint deformity and/or contractures

Outcome Criteria

Participation in ADL within limitations imposed by disease
Progressive ability to perform and maintain daily self-care

Interventions	Rationales
Assess abilities and level of care and assistance	Provides information about child's ability to perform self-care and to monitor progress
Allow as much independence in ADL as possible but assist when needed	Promotes independence and control over daily personal care needs without damage to joints
Encourage to perform own care and praise all accomplishments	Promotes sense of accomplishment and independence; motivates to continue progress in ADL
Position articles needed for care within reach; provide physical aids/ devices to assist in performance of ADL (crutches, wheelchair, utensils that are easy to handle, hand bars, handles that are easy to open, clothing that is easy to put on and take off with zippers, velcro, etc.)	Promotes independence and allows child access to aids to enhance independence
Assist parent(s) and child to develop plan and goals for daily ADL and suggest inclusions of actions taught by physical and occupational therapist	Promotes independence and compliance in self-care

Information, Instruction, Demonstration

Interventions	Rationales
Inform parent(s) and child of the activities to avoid in self-care	Prevents the type of strain on joints that may cause damage
Inform parent(s) and child of importance of progressing in self-care and independence	Promotes independence and control over changes that must be made to comply with medical regimen
Instruct parent(s) and child in application and use of aids and devices to accommodate self-care activities	Promotes independence in ADL and self-confidence

Interventions	Rationales
Inform of possible change or adjustments in home and school environment to accommodate child's independence in meeting physical needs (pathways, furniture, doors)	Allows for safe participation in activities that are usually carried out by child on a daily basis

Discharge or Maintenance Evaluation

- Performs ADL within physical abilities without fatigue or injury to joints
- Maximizes capabilities for self-care with use of aids/devices as appropriate
- Plans and schedules ADL with daily progression in independence
- Avoids activities that cause pain or injury to joints
- Contacts Juvenile Arthritis Foundation or local community agencies for information, support, and assistive aids and personnel referral

Ineffective family coping: Compromised

Related to: Inadequate or incorrect information or understanding, prolonged disease or disability progression that exhausts the physical and emotional supportive capacity of caretakers

Defining characteristics: Expression and/or confirmation of concern and inadequate knowledge about long-term care needs, problems and complications, anxiety and guilt, overprotection of child

Outcome Criteria

Development of family coping skills and support for long-term care
Adaptation of family to child's condition and disabilities
Adequate knowledge regarding long-term therapy and interdisciplinary approach to treatment

Interventions	Rationales
Assess family coping methods used and effectiveness, family interactions and expectations related to long-term care, developmental level of	Provides information identifying coping methods that work and the need to develop new coping skills and behaviors, family attitudes; child with special

Interventions	Rationales
family, response of siblings, knowledge and use of support systems and resources, presence of guilt and anxiety, overprotection and/or overindulgence behaviors	long-term needs may strengthen or strain family relationships and an undue degree of overprotection may be detrimental to child's growth and development (disallow school attendance and peer activities, avoiding discipline of child, and allowing child to assume responsibilities for ADL)
Encourage family members to express problem areas and explore solutions responsibly	Reduces anxiety and enhances understanding; provides family an opportunity to identify problems and develop problem solving strategies
Assist family to establish short- and long-term goals for child and to integrate child into family activities, include participation of all family members in care routines	Promotes involvement and control over situations and maintains role of family members and parent(s)
Provide assistance of social worker, counselor, clergy, or other as needed	Provides support to the family faced with long-term care of child with a chronic illness
Suggest community agencies and contact with the Arthritis Foundation or other families with a child with arthritis	Provides information and support to child and family
Allow family members to express feelings, how they deal with the chronic needs of family member and coping patterns that help or hinder adjustment to the problems	Allows for venting of feelings to determine need for information and support, and to relieve guilt and anxiety

Information, Instruction, Demonstration

Interventions	Rationales
Inform family of requested and needed information regarding long-term care and treatments	Enhances family understanding of medical regimen and responsibilities of family members

Interventions	Rationales
Inform family that over-protective behavior may hinder growth and development, and to treat child as normally as possible	Promotes understanding of importance of making child one of the family and the adverse affects of overprotection of the child
Discuss importance of follow-up appointments for physical and occupational therapy, eye examinations, laboratory tests to prevent drug toxicity	Promotes positive outcome when family collaborates with the physician and health team to monitor disease
Inform family of remissions and exacerbations of the disease and that an exacerbation may last for long periods of time (over a period of months); that exacerbations may be precipitated by overactivity, stress, presence of other illnesses, climate changes	Provides a realistic view of the chronic nature of the disease
Inform parent(s) and child of suggestions of unorthodox cures for the disease by friends, and the harmful effects caused by some of them	Prevents injury as well as disappointment when cures don't measure up to expectations

Discharge of Maintenance Evaluation

- Verbalizes and clarifies child's and family's knowledge about long-term needs and care
- Develops and uses coping skills and problem solving techniques effectively
- Supports and cares for child by family members while meeting own needs
- Preserves family relationships and minimizes family stressors with differences resolved
- Progressive adaptation and acceptance of long-term condition and therapy by family
- Implements preventative measures of follow-up care to ensure optimal function and health of child

Rheumatoid Arthritis (Juvenile)

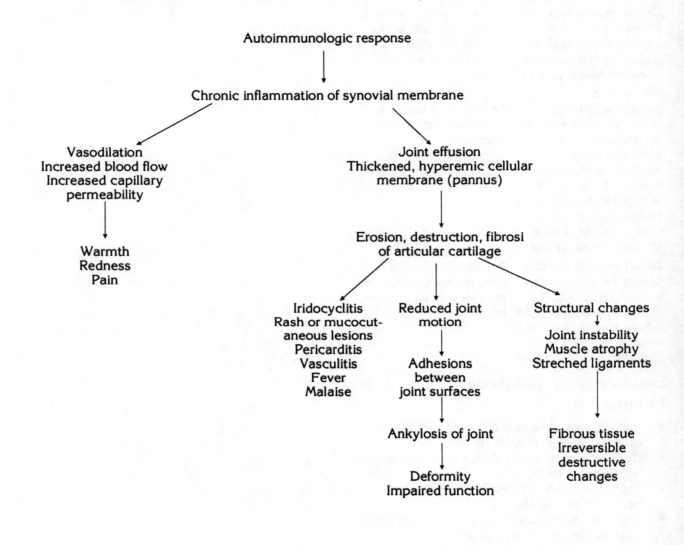

Autoimmunologic response

Chronic inflammation of synovial membrane

Vasodilation
Increased blood flow
Increased capillary
permeability

Warmth
Redness
Pain

Joint effusion
Thickened, hyperemic cellular
membrane (pannus)

Erosion, destruction, fibrosi
of articular cartilage

Iridocyclitis
Rash or mucocut-
aneous lesions
Pericarditis
Vasculitis
Fever
Malaise

Reduced joint
motion

Adhesions
between
joint surfaces

Ankylosis of joint

Deformity
Impaired function

Structural changes

Joint instability
Muscle atrophy
Streched ligaments

Fibrous tissue
Irreversible
destructive
changes

Scoliosis

Scoliosis is a lateral curvature of the spine with the thoracic area being the most commonly affected. It can be classified as functional or structural. Functional scoliosis is the result of another deformity and is corrected by treating the underlying problem. Structural scoliosis is most often idiopathic although it may be congenital or secondary to another disorder. There is a growing body of evidence that idiopathic scoliosis is probably genetic but the etiology is not completely understood. Structural scoliosis is more progressive and causes changes in supporting structures, such as the ribs. Management includes observation, bracing, and surgical fusion. Patients with idiopathic curves of less than 25 degrees are observed for progress until they have reached skeletal maturity. Bracing is recommended for adolescents with curves between 30 and 45 degrees, while curves greater than 45 degrees usually require surgery. The deformity may occur at any age, from infancy through adolescence, with the best prognosis belonging to those who are almost fully grown and whose the curvature is of a mild degree. Idiopathic scoliosis most commonly occurs in adolescent girls.

MEDICAL CARE

Analgesics: morphine sulfate (MS) given SC codeine; (Methylmorphine) given PO; acetaminophen (Tylenol) given PO to control postoperative pain depending on severity.

Spinal x-ray: reveals curvature of the spine via different. views (A, P, and lateral) with head and hips unaligned.

Myelogram: reveals presence of neurologic abnormalities of muscle function.

Scoliometer: reveals deformity of back when in a forward bending position.

Milwaukee brace: a molded pelvic brace with one anterior and two posterior uprights connected to a padded neck ring, generally used to treat higher thoracic curves (above T4). The brace is worn 23 hours per day until skeletal maturity is reached.

Thoracolumbosacral brace (TLSO): an underarm brace of molded plastic fitting from below the rib cage to the lower pelvis to correct thoracolumbar and lumbar curves. This brace is also worn 23 hours per day until skeletal maturity.

Surgical fusion: includes the use of instrumentation and bone grafts to maintain internal fixation to correct severe deformities (greater than 45 degrees). The newer instruments no longer require post-operative casting, but im-

mobility after surgery is maintained through bracing. The instruments include:

Harrington rods: metal rods connected by wires to the vertebrae.

Luque rods: flexible L-shaped metal rod fixed by wires to the bases of the spinous processes.

Dwyer instrumentation: a titanium cable fixed by screws to the vertebrae.

Cotrel-Dubousset (CD) procedure: bilateral segmental fixation using 2 rods and multiple hooks.

Electrical stimulation: an electrical pulse transmitted to muscles on the convex side of the curve causing muscles to contract to straighten the spine. May be used for mild to moderate curves, but the effectiveness of this treatment is not well documented.

NURSING CARE PLANS

Essential nursing diagnoses and plans associated with this condition:

Impaired physical mobility (278)

Related to: Musculoskeletal impairment (curvature of spine)

Defining characteristics: Imposed restrictions of movement by medical protocol of corrective device (brace, traction), bed rest and inability to purposefully move within the physical environment following surgery or with halo traction

Risk for impaired skin integrity (397)

Related to: External factor of physical immobilization, traction, or brace and altered sensation and circulation, surface electrical stimulation

Defining characteristics: Change in skin color and temperature, skin irritation at stimulation, brace, redness on areas from prolonged pressure, break in skin from surgical correction or implantation of stimulators

Altered growth and development (419)

Related to: Effects of immobilization and restricted movement from spinal curvature

Defining characteristics: Environmental and stimulation deficiencies, difficulty participating in self-care and social activities with long-term continuous brace use

SPECIFIC DIAGNOSES AND CARE PLANS

Knowledge deficit of parent(s), child

Related to: Lack of information about correction of functional or structural scoliosis

Defining characteristics: Request for information about treatments for scoliosis, application of brace and surgical procedure to correct scoliosis

Outcome Criteria

Adequate knowledge of parent(s) and child for long-term compliance of corrective therapy
Adjustment of parent(s) and child to treatment regimen

Interventions	Rationales
Assess knowledge of deformity, cause and treatments	Provides information about teaching needs
Inform parent(s) and child of presence of functional or structural defect and methods of treatment modalities specific to age of child and severity of the deformity	Promotes understanding of type of defect and treatment protocol to relieve anxiety; functional scoliosis is corrected by treating the underlying problem, and structural scoliosis is treated with long-term bracing and exercising or surgical fixation to straighten and re-align spine
Instruct parent(s) and child in application care, and removal of brace or orthoplast jacket, and inform that appliance must be worn for 23 hours/day and may be removed for bathing and exercise	Provides nonoperative bracing to prevent progressive curvatures; higher curves are treated with the Milwaukee brace and lower curves with the TLSO brace and both are worn until growth is complete
Instruct child in exercises performed in and out of the brace or other appliance and to perform them daily	Prevents atrophy of muscle of spine and abdomen
Instruct child in maintaining proper posture, use of shoe lifts, exercises, and	Corrects functional scoliosis which is usually caused by poor posture or

Interventions	Rationales
other prescribed treatments for functional scoliosis	unequal length of legs
Instruct parent(s) and child in use of electrical stimulation, application of electrodes, skin protection, connection of leads, operation of machine to be used at night	Provides stimulation to the muscles to prevent progression of curvature
Inform parent(s) and child of operative procedure planned and preoperative preparation required; reinforce physician information and use pictures, models and drawings to aid in teaching	Provides information about option for internal surgical instrumentation of curves over 45 degrees or those which are rapidly progressing to 45 degrees
Inform parent(s) and child of postoperative care, especially activity restrictions, log rolling, progression to ambulation, use of pillows for proper support, maintaining flat position, and possible use of special bed such as Stryker frame	Provides information about what to expect following surgery depending on the type of procedure
Inform parent(s) and child of use of safety belt and walker when ambulating; instruct in safety precautions to take for child wearing brace (clear pathways, handrails, performing ADL using aids)	Prevents trauma caused by fall from postoperative weakness, unassisted ambulation, or wearing of brace causing awkwardness in ambulation and ADL performance
Inform parent(s) and child that physical and occupational therapy will be prescribed after surgery	Provides information and support services
Inform parent(s) and child of agencies to contact for assistance such as National Scoliosis Foundation, community support groups	Promotes optimal physical activity

Discharge or Maintenance Evaluation

- Verbalizes knowledge of spinal defect, cause and treatment
- Compliance and adjustment to long-term therapy regimen
- Appropriate application, removal, and care of brace
- Performs daily exercises appropriate to specific child
- Performs electrical stimulation without complications
- Verbalizes understanding of need for surgical interventions and potential for positive outcome for child
- Absence of accidents or injury with use of brace or during ambulation following surgery
- Complies with physiotherapy until independent in activities
- Absence of complications from cast application, use of brace, or surgical alignment of spine

Body image disturbance

Related to: Biophysical and psychosocial factors of spinal deformity

Defining characteristics: Verbal response to actual change in structure of spine, negative feelings about body, dependence on long-term use of brace, feeling of rejection by peers, inability to participate in some activities

Outcome Criteria

Body image improved, preserved and maintained with adjustment to use of appliance
Accommodations made for and adaptation to long-term needs and limitations of appliance use or other treatments

Interventions	Rationales
Assess child for feelings about wearing brace, long-term treatments, restrictions in lifestyle, inability to keep up with peers and participate in activities	Provides information about status of self-concept and changes in appearance
Encourage expression of feelings and concerns and support child's communications with parent(s), peers and teachers	Provides opportunity to vent and reduce negative feelings about changes in appearance and continuing wearing of an appliance

Interventions	Rationales
Maintain positive environment and promote activities that are allowed (sports, play, games)	Enhances body image and confidence, and promotes trust and respect of child
Assist with plan for independence in ADL, application and removal of appliance, selection of shoes and clothing to wear such as T-shirt	Promotes independence and adjustment to appliance
Assist child to adjust to self-perception of short leg, use of appliance and effect on appearance	Promotes positive self-image and realistic view of appearance
Suggest open communication with school nurse and teacher	Promotes adaptation to school within activity limitations

Information, Instruction, Demonstration

Interventions	Rationales
Inform parent(s) and child that most activities are allowed with use of appliance	Promotes positive feelings about treatment and restrictions imposed by the deformity
Inform child of type of clothing to cover appliance that is stylish and has peer acceptance	Enhances appearance and body image
Inform child of ways to inform others about wearing appliance	Assist child in dealing with questions and curiosity of others about differences caused by deformity
Inform child of activity restrictions that include progression from quiet activities to involvement in those to avoid: contact sports, bike riding, driving, skating, or those that may result in a fall if surgery has been done	Prevents injury following surgical correction of the deformity

Discharge or Maintenance Evaluation

- Verbalizes improved body image and sense of well-being

- Participates in family, school, and social activities as appropriate
- Verbalizes feelings about special long-term needs in positive terms
- Supports positive body image and prompt adjustment to restrictions caused by use of appliance or surgery
- Purchases or adapts clothing to use of appliance
- Avoids activities potentially injurious for spinal correction
- Promotes independence and decision making in ADL

Scoliosis

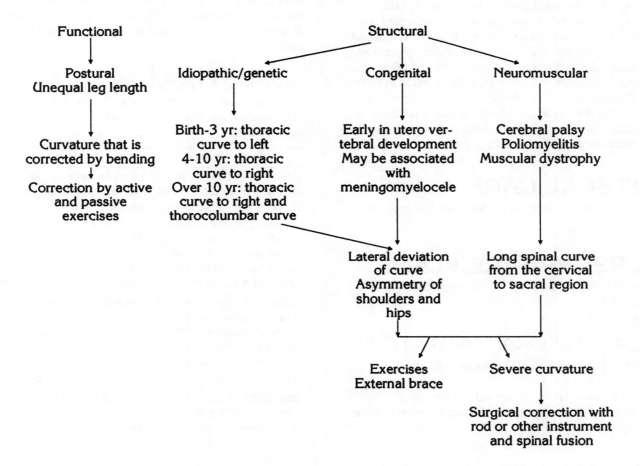

Functional

↓

Postural
Unequal leg length

↓

Curvature that is
corrected by bending

↓

Correction by active
and passive
exercises

Structural

Idiopathic/genetic

↓

Birth-3 yr: thoracic
curve to left
4-10 yr: thoracic
curve to right
Over 10 yr: thoracic
curve to right and
thorocolumbar curve

Congenital

↓

Early in utero ver-
tebral development
May be associated
with
meningomyelocele

↓

Lateral deviation
of curve
Asymmetry of
shoulders and
hips

↓

Exercises
External brace

Neuromuscular

↓

Cerebral palsy
Poliomyelitis
Muscular dystrophy

↓

Long spinal curve
from the cervical
to sacral region

↓

Severe curvature

↓

Surgical correction with
rod or other instrument
and spinal fusion

Talipes

Talipes (club foot) is a congenital disorder of the foot usually with ankle involvement characterized by a twisting out of a normal position that is unable to be manipulated into a different position. The deformity is typed and named according to the position of the foot and include talipes varus (foot inversion), talipes valqus (foot aversion), talipes equines (plantarflexion), and talipes calcaneus (dorsiflexion). Most are a combination of these with the most common deformity known as talipes equinovarus (inversion and plantarflexion of the foot). The defect may occur along or in association with other congenital syndromes or defects.

MEDICAL CARE

Foot/ankle x-ray: reveals abnormal bone deformity or distortion.

NURSING CARE PLANS

Essential nursing diagnoses and plans associated with this condition:

Impaired physical mobility (278)

Related to: Musculoskeletal impairment (talipes deformity)
Defining characteristics: Imposed restrictions of movement by medical protocol of corrective device, serial cast application

Risk for impaired skin integrity (397)

Related to: External factor of physical immobilization by cast(s), internal factors of altered circulation, sensation by cast pressure
Defining characteristics: Edema, rapid growth rate, tight cast or appliance, color change and cool skin proximal to cast

Altered growth and development (419)

Related to: Effects of physical disability (immobilization)
Defining characteristics: Delay in performing motor skills typical of age group during cast applications, lack of stimulation while cast is present

SPECIFIC DIAGNOSES AND CARE PLANS

Knowledge deficit of parent(s)

Related to: Lack of information about condition
Defining characteristics: Request for information about disorder, its cause and treatment for correction, follow-up care

Outcome Criteria

Adequate information for compliance to medical protocol of corrective measures needed to ensure normal foot development

Interventions	Rationales
Assess knowledge of disorder, type of deformity, and if one or both feet are involved; type of immobilization and application and/or care; presence of associated congenital disorders or syndromes	Provides information needed to develop plan of instruction to ensure compliance to medical regimen for correction; usually begins in infancy and lasts for 3-5 months, and most commonly occurs in males
Inform parent(s) of type of talipes deformity and describe the position of the foot and ankle and the stages of corrective treatment	Provides information about how the correction is accomplished, maintained, and re-evaluated to ensure the correction and prevent recurrence of the deformity
Instruct parent(s) in manipulation of feet in one smooth motion, demonstrate and allow for return demonstration	Ensures correct positioning of the feet in preparation for immobilization
Instruct parent(s) in application of Denis-Browne Splints (if used) including applying socks and then shoes attached to the bar, tightening shoes against bar with a key, and maintaining shoe placement on the bar; protect feet with socks; change position q2h and note edema, color change of feet	Ensures correct splinting of deformity for one method that immobilizes feet in high shoes placed on bar to maintain rotation of the ankle
Instruct parent(s) in strapping of feet with adhesive following manipulation, allow for return demon-	Provides another method that ensures immobilization for correction of deformity

Interventions	Rationales
stration; instruct to manipulate feet and restrap q3 days	
Inform parent(s) of casting procedure and type of cast applied (midthigh long led) and that new successive casts will be applied q2-3 days for 1-2 weeks and then ql-2 weeks with the final cast remaining in place for 4-8 weeks	Ensures correction by the most reliable method of manipulation and serial casting to stretch tight structures and contract lax structures; frequent castings allow for rapid growth in infant
Instruct parent(s) in monitoring extremities for color, peripheral pulses, coolness and report changes in these circulatory parameters	Prevents circulation and neurologic impairment from tight casts
Inform parent(s) to use plastic pants or diapers for infant	Prevents soiling or dampness of cast which affects immobilization efficiency of casts by softening them
Inform parent(s) that the splint may be applied for night use and special shoes worn during the day after final cast is removed, and that this over-correction in position may be maintained for 6 months after correction evident	Prevents recurrence of the deformity
Inform parent(s) that if conservative treatment fails or child is older, surgery may be needed to correct deformity by releasing ligaments, lengthening tendons, or correcting bone deformity with casting following immobilization of the feet	Prepares parent(s) for possibility of surgical correction if manipulation is ineffective after 5 months of treatment
Inform parent(s) of importance of follow-up physician evaluations and cast changes	Ensures compliance over long-term correction of deformity by casting or appliance

Discharge or Maintenance Evaluation

- Complies with long-term medical regimen to correct deformity
- Maintains correct position of feet, applies strapping or splint correctly and in appropriate frequency
- Prevents circulatory complications of cast application
- Verbalizes type of deformity, cause, length, and projected outcome of treatment
- Protects casts from damage
- Complies with follow-up care requirements of cast changes
- Prevents risk of recurrence of deformity by prolonged over-correction of deformity

Talipes

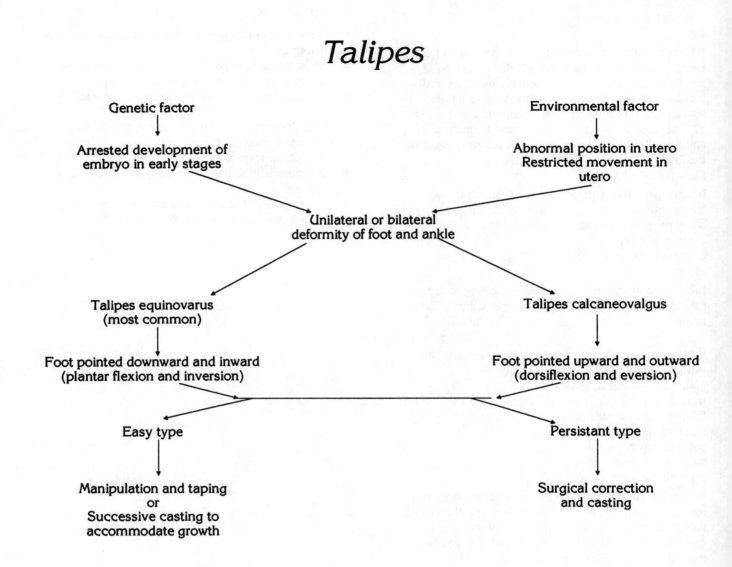

Genetic factor

↓

Arrested development of
embryo in early stages

Environmental factor

↓

Abnormal position in utero
Restricted movement in
utero

Unilateral or bilateral
deformity of foot and ankle

Talipes equinovarus
(most common)

↓

Foot pointed downward and inward
(plantar flexion and inversion)

Talipes calcaneovalgus

↓

Foot pointed upward and outward
(dorsiflexion and eversion)

Easy type

↓

Manipulation and taping
or
Successive casting to
accommodate growth

Persistant type

↓

Surgical correction
and casting

Hematologic System

Hematologic System

The hematologic system includes the blood (plasma and cells) and the blood-forming tissues/organs (red bone marrow, lymph, lymph nodes, spleen, thymus, and tonsils). The cellular portion of the blood contains the erythrocytes (RBC), leukocytes (WBC), and thrombocytes (platelets). The plasma portion contains water and solutes, which include albumin, electrolytes, and proteins (clotting factors, fibrinogen, globulins, and antibodies). The system provides the body with cells that have certain functions in the transport of oxygen, nutrients, and substances to all the tissues; assists in clotting to prevent blood loss; regulates heat to maintain body temperature; and provides protection to the body from infectious agents (immunologic function). Changes in the hematologic system occur throughout the infant/child's development until adult parameters are reached. These changes make the child more vulnerable to disorders common to the system such as anemia, immunologic disorders, hemostatic problems, and malignancies involving the lymphatic system and blood cell production. Further disturbances in the function of any cellular or transport activities in children cause a multiple number of disorders and pathologies that affect all organ systems of the body.

GENERAL HEMATOLOGIC/IMMUNOLOGIC CHANGES ASSOCIATED WITH PHYSICAL GROWTH AND DEVELOPMENT

Hematologic and immunologic component structure and content

- Blood volume of full-term newborn is 80-85 m/m/kg; averages 300 ml, with as much as 100 ml added to the volume depending on amount of placental transfer
- Fetal hemoglobin is present for 5 months, with adult hemoglobin forming at 13 weeks of age
- Infant hemoglobin is at its lowest between 4 and 6 months of age because maternal iron stores in the infant are present for 5-6 months and then decrease, which accounts for the lower hemoglobin at 6 months of age
- Erythrocyte production increases rapidly after birth, resulting in an increase in reticulocytes (immature RBC)
- The life span of a RBC is 120 days, of a granulocyte 4-5 days, of an agranulocyte a half-life of 60-90 days, and of a platelet 8-10 days
- Cell-mediated immune responses are deficient in the infant; immunoglobulin A (IgA) appears in the blood serum at 1 month of age, with adult levels being reached at 10 years of age
- Phagocytic action of neutrophils and monocytes is not at full strength in the newborn, so inflammatory response is less effective than in an older infant or child
- By 5 months of age, immunoglobulin level is based on antibodies made by the infant's own system, but the child/adult level is not attained until 1 year of age
- Lymphoid tissue (thymus, tonsils, adenoids, spleen, lymph nodes) grows rapidly during infancy and reaches peak growth at 12 years of age; it filters and traps pathogens before they enter blood stream

Acquired Immunodeficiency Syndrome

Acquired Immunodeficiency Syndrome (AIDS) is caused by HIV. The term human immunodeficiency virus (HIV) type I is the official name of the HIV virus. HIV has been found in blood and bodily fluids (semen, saliva, vaginal secretions, urine, breast milk, and tears). Transmission of HIV can occur by 3 primary modes: horizontal exposure by sexual contact, parenteral exposure to blood, or vertical exposure from an HIV-infected mother to infant (during vaginal birth). In children and adolescent age groups 3 populations have been identified: 1) children exposed in utero to an infected mother; 2) children who have received blood products, especially children treated with hemophilia (before testing of blood products began in 1985); and 3) adolescents who are infected after engaging in high-risk behaviors (i.e., sharing of needles for injection of drug use; accidental needle sticks; unprotected sex and multiple sexual partners). The majority of children with AIDS are less than 5 years of age (85% of resulted from perinatal transmission, 11% resulted from blood transfusions). HIV virus cultures and polymerase chain reaction (PCR) tests are very accurate in detecting HIV in infected infants (30% shortly after birth and 100% at 3 to 6 months of age). Diagnosis of AIDS in children under 13 years of age, based on the Center of Disease Control (CDC) criteria, include the presence of one of the following: (1) confirmed HIV in blood or tissues; (2) symptoms meeting the CDC criteria; or (3) HIV antibody and one or more of the following disorders: secondary infectious diseases, recurrent bacterial infections, or secondary cancers. Diagnosis of AIDS in children over 13 years of age and above are based on the CDC adult criteria. Children with HIV infection usually have detectable HIV antibody 6-12 after exposure (except for infants of HIV positive mothers). Difficult diagnosis process for infants of HIV seropositive mothers, in the first 15 months of life, due to presence of maternal antibody. Infants with perinatal acquired AIDS are normal at birth but may develop symptoms within the first 18 months of life. Clinical manifestations in children include: fever; decreased CD4 count; anemia; decreased WBC count (of less than 3000 cells/mm3); neutropenia (absolute neutrophil count of less than 1500 cells/mm 3); thrombocytopenia; myelosuppression; Vitamin K deficiency; hepatitis; pancreatitis; stomatitis and esophagitis;

meningitis; retinitis (common with low CD4 counts); otitis media and sinusitis (chronic or recurrent); lymphadenopathy; hepatosplenomegaly; recurrent bacterial infections (especially, Streptococcus pneumoniae and Haemophilus influenzae); Mycobacterium infections (MAC) or tuberculosis; cytomegalovirus (CMV); failure to thrive (in infants); chronic diarrhea; neurologic involvement (seen in 75% to 90% of children with HIV, displayed as developmental delays and microcephaly in infants, or loss of motor skills in the older child); and pulmonary infections {two-thirds will develop Pneumoncystis carinii (PCP), and lymphocytic interstitial pneumonitis (LIP), and pulmonary lymphoid hyperplasia (PLH)}. Kaposi sarcoma, a hallmark of adults with HIV, is rare in children with HIV (seen in less than 1% of cases). A major success in pediatric HIV is the recognition that a majority of vertical transmissions can be prevented with prophylactic zidovudine given to mother and child.

MEDICAL CARE

Diagnostic tests for HIV in children: enzyme-linked immuno-absorbent assay (ELISA) detects HIV antibodies; Western blot, (detects serum antibody bound to specific HIV antigens); Immunofluorescence assays. Because of the presence of maternal antibodies, the following specific tests are required: polymerase chain reaction (PCR assay); HIV-p24 antigen; CD4 T-lymphocyte counts; and virus cultures.

Medical Management: there is no cure for HIV. Medical care is directed at slowing the virus, preventing and treating the opportunistic infections, nutritional support, and symptomatic treatment. Combination drug therapy with antiviral therapy is recommended, with at least two antiviral drugs.

Antiviral Drugs include:

Zidovudine {AZT or Retrovir (360-720 mg/m²/d, every 6 hrs.)}: is a synthetic dideoxynecleoside (a thymidine analogue), which inhibits replication of some retroviruses, (can be given PO or IV, dosage is based on CD4 cell count). Reported benefits: improvement in encephalopathy, decrease in p24 antigen, transient increase in CD4 counts, and weight gain.

Didanosine {DDI or Videx (270-360mg/m²/d, bid or tid)}: is a synthetic purine dideoxynecleoside, which inhibits replication of retroviruses, used when intolerant or resistant to AZT, (can be given PO). Reported benefits: sustained increase in CD4 counts; decrease in p24 antigen, and weight gain.

3TC {Lamivudine (4-8 mg/kg/d, bid)}: Treatment of MAC infections: should include at least three drugs (clarithromycin or azithromycin, ethambutol, rifampin).

Additional agents to be used include: amikacin, clofazimine, and diprofloxacin. Reported benefit: decrease in p24 antigen, decrease in viral plasma RNA, weight gain, subjective increase in energy and appetite.
Investigational antiviral drugs (dosage not yet established in children, limited available data in children; currently, only approved for use in adults):
Dideoxyinosie (ddC): Reported benefit: decrease in p24 antigen, increase in CD4 counts, alternating schedule with AZT may reduce myelotoxicity.
Stavudine (D4T): Reported benefit: increase in CD4 counts, decrease in p24 antigen.
Nevirapine (RG-BI-587): Reported benefit: rapid decrease in viral serum RNA, decrease in p24 antigen.
Adjunct Prophylactic Therapy:
G-CSF (granulyctye colony stimulating factor): (given subcutaneous) is effective in the treatment and prevention of neutropenia.
IVIG (intravenous gamma globulin): should be given every 4 weeks to patients with hypogammaglobulinemia (to reduce or prevent infections, and it may be helpful to compensate for the deficiency of B-lymphocytes and to treat thrombocytopenia).
Trimethoprim (TMP)-sulfamethoxasole (SMX) {also called Bactrim or Septra}: used for prevention/treatment of opportunistic infections (i.e., Pneumoncystis carinii). {given PO for 2 months}.
Pentamidine {also called NebuPent or Pentam 300}: (can be given per monthly aerosolized route; IM or IV for 14 to 21 days): used for prevention/treatment of opportunistic infections (i.e., Pneumoncystis carinli).
Immunizations: all immunizations should be given as recommended for all children. Exceptions: give inactivated poliovirus (IPV) instead of oral poliovirus (OPV); pneumococcal and influenza vaccine are recommended; Varicella zoster immune globulin should be given within 96 hours of chickenpox exposure; MMR vaccine should be given within 72 hours of exposure to measles.
Acyclovir: as prophylaxis for herpes infections.
Antituberculosis in infants, children and adolescents: Ethambutol (PO), Isoniazid (PO), Pyrazinamide (PO), Rifambin (PO), and Streptomycin (IM).
Complete blood count (CBC): reveals increased WBC in infections, decreased T-helper lymphocytes.
Immunoglobulins (Ig): reveals increased levels.

NURSING CARE PLANS

Essential nursing diagnoses and plans associated with this condition:

Ineffective airway clearance (42)

Related to: Infection, obstruction, secretions, decreased energy, and fatigue
Defining characteristics: Abnormal breath sounds; changes in rate, ease, and depth of respirations; tachypnea; fever; weakness; ineffective cough with or without sputum

Ineffective breathing pattern (45)

Related to: Illness (infection)
Defining characteristics: Increase in body temperature above normal range, increased respiratory rate, tachycardia

Diarrhea (171)

Related to: Inflammation, irritation of bowel
Defining characteristics: Chronic, increased frequency of loose, liquid stools; cramping; abdominal pain

Altered nutrition: Less than body requirements (168)

Related to: Inability to ingest, digest, or absorb nutrients
Defining characteristics: Anorexia, weight loss, lack of interest in feeding, failure to thrive, child's growth begins to slow or weight begins to decrease

Altered growth and development (419)

Related to: Neurologic involvement (75% to 90% of HIV infected children)
Defining characteristics: Developmental delays or, after achieving normal development, loss of motor milestones; microcephaly (in HIV infected infants); and abnormal neurologic examination findings

SPECIFIC DIAGNOSES AND CARE PLANS

Anxiety of parent(s) and child

Related to: Change in health status, threat of death, threat to self-concept, fear of interpersonal transmission and contagion
Defining characteristics: Increased apprehension and fear of diagnosis; expressed concern and worry about

early death, effect of lifestyle changes on physical and emotional status, possible opportunistic infections

Outcome Criteria

Reduced or manageable anxiety level verbalized as information about disease, treatment, and prognosis is given

Interventions	Rationales
Assess level of anxiety of parent(s) and child and how it is manifested; and need for information that will relieve anxiety	Provides information about source and level of anxiety and need for interventions to relieve it; sources for the child may be procedures, fear of mutilation or death, unfamiliar environment of hospital, and may be manifested by restlessness and inability to play, sleep or eat
Assess possible need for special counseling or social services for child	Reduces anxiety, supports child's dealing with illness, and promotes adjustment to lifestyle changes
Allow open expression of concerns about illness, procedures, treatments, and prognosis	Provides opportunity to vent feelings and fears to reduce anxiety
Communicate with child at appropriate age level and answer questions calmly and honestly; use pictures, models, and drawings for explanations	Promotes understanding and trust
Allow child as much input in decisions about care and routines as possible	Allows child more control and independence in situations
Allow parent(s) to stay with child or have open visitation, provide a telephone number to call for information	Promotes parental care and support

Information, Instruction, Demonstration

Interventions	Rationales
Inform parent(s) and child of the disease process, treatments, and therapy; include effect on lifestyle and possible stigma associated with the disease	Promotes understanding that will relieve fear and anxiety
Explain all procedures, treatments, and care in simple, direct, honest terms, and repeat as often as necessary; reinforce physician information if needed; provide specific information as needed	Supplies information about all diagnostic procedures and tests
Inform parent(s) and child that all information about the disease will be kept confidential	Decreases anxiety associated social attitudes about the disease and those infected with it
Inform of local and national AIDS groups and agencies to contact for assistance	Provides information and support from those in similar circumstances

Discharge or Maintenance Evaluation

- Expresses reduction in anxiety as information and explanations are given
- States concerns and reason for anxiety and behavior
- Verbalizes knowledge of and participates in decision making regarding care
- Explores and notes anger and sorrow about diagnosis, prognosis, and proposed changes in lifestyle
- Utilizes existing and new support systems

Anticipatory grieving

Related to: Perceived potential loss of infant/child by parent(s), perceived loss of physiopsychosocial well-being by child
Defining characteristics: Expression of distress at potential loss, fatal prognosis of the disease, premature death of child

Outcome Criteria

Progressive grief resolution over presence of fatal illness
Management of stages of grieving process

Interventions	Rationales
Assess stage of grief process, problems encountered, feelings regarding long-term illness and potential loss	Provides information about stage of grieving time to work through the process varies with individuals as they move toward acceptance
Provide emotional and spiritual comfort in an accepting environment and avoid conversations that will cause guilt or anger	Provides for emotional needs of parent(s) and child as appropriate, and helps them to cope with illness and its implications without adding stressors that are difficult to resolve
Allow for parent(s) and child's responses and expressions of feelings such as concern, fear, anxiety, or guilt	Promotes ventilation of feelings
Assist in identifying and using effective coping mechanisms and in understanding situations over which they have no control	Promotes constructive use of coping skills
Allow for discussion of likelihood of child's death with parent(s) and child, if appropriate, and encourage them to discuss this with family members, friends	Presents realistic view of probable outcome of illness
Refer to social, psychological, clergy services, or counseling as appropriate	Provides support and information to child and family if need assistance

Information, Instruction, Demonstration

Interventions	Rationales
Inform parent(s) of stage of grieving process and of behaviors that are acceptable in resolving grief	Promotes understanding of feelings and behaviors that are manifested by grief
Instruct parent(s) and child in coping skills, problem-solving skills, and approaches that may be used	Promotes coping ability over period of prolonged illness and assists in resolving family stress

Interventions	Rationales
Inform of AIDS groups and agencies for social, economic, legal aid; family and friends for support	Provides support for family and child as needed

Discharge or Maintenance Evaluation

- Verbalizes understanding of grief process and responses
- Shares feelings with professionals, family members, friends
- Secures assistance from support groups and individuals
- Identifies and uses coping skills with a positive effect
- Discusses death and dying with appropriate professionals and friends

Risk for infection

Related to: Inadequate secondary defenses (immunosuppression), insufficient knowledge to avoid exposure to pathogens
Defining characteristics: Presence of infective organism, opportunistic infectious process and malignancy, expressed need for information about transmission prevention

Outcome Criteria

Absence of evidence of infectious process in child
Prevention of spread of disease to others

Interventions	Rationales
Assess CBC lab values; assess CD4 T-lymphocyte counts; assess blood culture for opportunistic infections; assess vital signs, as ordered, to identify changes in respirations or lung sounds	To identify abnormal range of lab values relate to infection or anemia; early recognition of organisms will expedite appropriate treatment of infections; early recognition of signs of pulmonary infections will expedite treatment for pulmonary changes
Assess for fever, malaise, fatigue, night sweats, weight loss, chronic diarrhea, oral infection or lesions, pain in joints and muscles, lymphadeno-	Provides information about signs and symptoms of infection during the (podromal) stage of AIDS with responses that are age-dependent at onset of

Interventions	Rationales
pathy, upper and lower respiratory infections	AIDS in infants/children: long-term opportunistic infections, including Pneumocystis carinii pneumonia, Kaposi's sarcoma, and lymphoma
Provide protective isolation for immunosuppressed child; use gloves, mask, and gown for visitors; and during care, proper handwashing when needed	Protects child from contact with infectious process in others
Wear gloves for all care, especially when in contact with body fluids (changing diapers, handling any secretions or excretions); avoid recapping needles; clean all spills and disinfect article or area; use bleach solution in home; wash, disinfect, or dispose of all contaminated articles used; double bag all linens and specimens with proper precautionary labeling	Prevents transmission of virus to personnel or caretaker; follows guidelines published by the Centers for Disease Control
Use medical or surgical asepsis for all procedures and care as appropriate	Prevents transmission of pathogens to child
Administer medications as ordered to control disease progression or treat any infection as ordered	Prevents or treats infectious process, compensates for immunosuppression by improving functioning of immune system
Restrict contact with persons with infections or illnesses, have child to share room with another child who does not have an infection	Prevents transmission of infection to child

Information, Instruction, Demonstration

Interventions	Rationales
Inform parent(s) and child of possible source for infection and risk of spread or transmission of infection	Promotes understanding and cooperation in treatments and procedure, prevent spread of existing infection or risk of new infection

Interventions	Rationales
Inform parent(s) and child that isolation is needed to prevent contact with sources of potential infections (i.e., infected persons or contaminated articles)	Promotes compliance with isolation techniques
Inform parent(s) and child of diagnostic and reporting methods, signs and symptoms of specific diseases, risk factors in acquiring or transmitting disease and potential complications	Provides information about the disease causes, treatment, and preventative measures
Instruct parent(s) and child in high-calorie protein diet by showing with food selections and sample menus	Assists in maintaining nutritional status necessary to fight infection
Inform parent(s) and child to avoid family members, friends, peers, or others with infections or illnesses	Prevents exposure to others with infection that may be transmitted to child with a compromised immune system
Instruct parent(s) and child in handwashing technique and methods to maintain medical asepsis	Prevents transmission of pathogens via the hands
Using written guidelines offered by Centers for Disease Control, instruct in care of bodily fluids, use of gloves, cleansing and care of articles used, disposal methods, care of linens, clothing, specimens, mode of transmission to others	Prevents transmission of virus to others
Inform parent(s) to contact school nurse and discuss child's needs and guidelines for school attendance	Promotes safety of child and possible contacts; attendance is recommended by physician as long as child has control of body secretions, and does not bite or have open lesions
Inform parent(s) and child of immunization needed to prevent infectious disease	Protects child from infectious diseases (pneumonia and influenza)

Interventions	Rationales
If appropriate, inform child of precautions to take if sexually active (condom use) or if using drugs (not sharing needles)	Prevents transmission of virus to others by taking appropriate precautions

Discharge or Maintenance Evaluation

- Absence or control of opportunistic infections
- Prevents transmission of the virus to others
- Provides precautions to prevent infection in child
- Follows Center for Disease Control guidelines and Universal Precaution in care of child to prevent infection or transmission of disease to others
- Administers medications correctly to prevent progression of disease and treat infections if present
- Verbalizes risk factors in acquiring or transmitting disease
- Attends school within limitations imposed by the disease
- Verbalizes precaution to prevent disease by sexual contact or IV drug use
- Provides immunizations for child

Social isolation

Related to: Altered state of wellness, unaccepted social behavior, low blood count precautions, repeated hospitalizations, social stigma of HIV, physical limitations
Defining characteristics: Protective isolation; absence of support by family, friends, others; seeks to be alone; expresses feelings of rejection, indifference of others; aloneness; withdrawal; displays behavior unaccepted by dominant culture; evidence of altered state of wellness

Outcome Criteria

Maintenance of peer, family group acceptance and support
Reduction in feelings of isolation

Interventions	Rationales
Assist child to identify personal strengths to facilitate enhanced coping	To increase child's self-competence and increase child's self-esteem
Assess child and family for feelings about stigma associated with the disease, rejection by others	Provides information about extent of isolation felt by the family and child

Interventions	Rationales
Provide accepting, warm environment for child and parent(s) to express their feelings	Promotes trust and comfort to enhance adaptation to presence of positive testing or actual symptoms of the disease
Encourage child to interact with peers, attend school and activities	Promotes feeling of belonging, and provides growth and development

Information, Instruction, Demonstration

Interventions	Rationales
Inform peers, school nurse and personnel about AIDS and safe activities for child and other children	Provides information and education about AIDS
Discuss with child and parent(s) misconceptions that the public has and ways to correct the situation by providing information about causes and mode of transmission and by answering questions and concerns	Promotes correct information dissemination and dispels myths about the disease, thereby reducing fear and rejection by others
Inform parent(s) and child that confidentiality will be maintained at school and elsewhere if needed	Protects child from stigma associated with the disease

Discharge or Maintenance Evaluation

- Participates in family and peer activities, including school
- Exhibits a positive, secure feeling in child
- Verbalizes feeling of acceptance

Acquired Immunodeficiency Syndrome

Hemophilia requiring
Factor VIII treatment

High risk behavior
of older child

Perinatal transmission

Transmission of HTLV, type III
(human T-cell lymphotropic virus)

Impaired T-lymphocyte function
with

Decreased helper T-lymphocytes
Increased suppressor T-lymphocytes

Reverse helper:suppressor T-cell ratio

Increased immunoglobulins that are nonfuctional

Altered immune state

opportunistic infections

Pneumocystis carinii
Parotitis
Mucosal candidiasis
Chronic diarrhea
Progressive encephalopathy
Kaposi's sarcoma (low incidence)

Anemias

Anemia is identified as the most common group of hematologic disorders of infancy and childhood. The term anemia refers to a reduction in either the total number of circulating red blood cells (RBC) or a decrease in the concentration of hemoglobin (Hgb). The etiology of anemia is divided into 3 categories: 1) excessive blood loss (acute or chronic hemorrhage), 2) increased destruction of RBCs (or hemolysis), or 3) impaired or decreased rate of production (or bone marrow failure). The following three types of anemia will be discussed: iron deficiency, sickle cell anemia and aplastic anemia. Iron deficiency is primarily due to an inadequate intake of dietary iron. The iron stores of the full-term infant normally meet the infant's nutritional needs until 6 months of age. In comparison, the iron stores for the premature infant normally is depleted by 2 to 3 months of age. Treatment consists of iron supplementation and optimum nutrition. Sickle cell anemia (Hgb SS) is referred to as a genetic disease of autosomal dominant inheritance (and a sickling hemoglobinopathy syndrome). Hgb SS is due to the substitution of a single amino acid (valine replaces glutamic acid) at the sixth position of the B-chain. It occurs primarily in the black race and symptoms appear usually after 4 to 6 months of age due to the presence of fetal hemoglobin. Treatment consists of prevention/treatment of sickle cell pain crisis; and supportive/symptomatic measures. Aplastic anemia is defined as bone marrow failure characterized by the reduction or absence of the solid elements of the blood (red cells, white cells, and platelets). There are two types: primary (congenital or Fanconi anemia, an inherited autosomal recessive trait) or secondary (acquired, caused by exposure to toxins in the environment or a complication of an infection). Symptoms occur in the acquired type (after exposure to a toxin or infection); and in the congenital type (usually after 17 months of age). Treatment is directed at restoration of bone marrow function, by two approaches: 1) immunosuppressive therapy and 2) replacement of the bone marrow through bone marrow transplantation.

MEDICAL CARE

Diagnostic Evaluation for Iron Deficiency Anemia:
Red Cell Smear: examines the red cell shape and content (i.e., MVC and MCH).
Free erythrocyte protoporphyrin (FEP): elevated FEP is associated with an inadequate iron supply.

Serum-iron concentration (SIC): measures circulating iron (normal: 70% ug/dl in infants).
Total iron-binding capacity (TIBC): measures transferrin (iron-binding globulin) for iron transport. Transferrin saturation: divide the SIC by the TIBC and multiplying by 100; (10% — suggests anemia).
Treatment for Iron Deficiency Anemia:
Iron supplements (POI): ferrous sulfate (i.e., tablets, drops, elixir, syrup) for prevention/treatment of iron deficiency (give in 2 divided doses in a straw, absorption is enhanced with foods with ascorbic acid; avoid ingestion of milk, tea, bran, egg yolks or antacids because these foods may interfere with iron supplements).
Vitamin C Supplements (oral): {200 mg per 30 mg iron}; may enhance iron absorption.
Diagnostic Evaluation for Sickle Cell Anemia:
Stained blood smear: will reveal a few sickled RBCs; it is not 100% accurate.
Sickle-turbidity test (Sickledex): a reliable screening method for the sickle cell trait or disease.
Hemoglobin electrophoresis: is an accurate, rapid, and specific test for detecting the homozygous and heterozygous forms of sickle cell anemia.
Treatment for Sickle Cell Anemia:
Hydration (PO or IV): given for hemodilution to treat/prevent sickle cell crisis.
Hydroxyurea (PO): (a myelosuppressive agent), enhances production of fetal hemoglobin (hemoglobin F); it has also been helpful in decreasing pain crisis episodes.
Penicillin V Potassium (PO): recommended as prophylactic treatment, initiate after 2 to 3 months of age.
Analgesics: to prevent/treat pain crisis; (IV morphine is given in the hospital; PO Tylenol is given at home). (Avoid giving Demerol because of increased risk of normeperidine-induced seizures); Ketorolac (a potent analgesic, with no side effects of respiratory depression). Patient-controlled analgesia (PCA), has been very effective and safe in the administration of morphine to the pediatric patient with SCD.
Immunizations: should receive all recommended childhood immunizations; should also receive: pneumococcal (at 2 years of age and a booster at 5 years of age); Haemophilus influenza type B (is given to all infants at 2 months of age); and meningococcal vaccine (at 2 years of age).
Folate replacement: is given for the treatment of aplastic type of sickle cell crisis.
Blood transfusions: packed RBC transfusions are used to replace prematurely destroyed red cells and to diminish the percentage of hemoglobin S (sickled hemoglobin). It is primarily used with severe complications (ie., stroke, progressive hypoxia, pulmonary disease, or in severe hemolysis).

Deferoxamine (Subcutaneous or IV): to prevent iron overload (hemosiderosis), a complication of blood transfusions.

Diagnostic Evaluation for Aplastic Anemia:

Red cell indices: examines an elevated MCV (mean corpuscular volume of the RBC).

Hgb electrophoresis: will reveal an abnormally high fetal hemoglobin.

Chromosomal studies: will reveal multiple chromosomal abnormalities.

CBC: evaluation of lab values characteristic of anemia, leukopenia, and decreased platelet count.

Bone marrow aspiration: examination confirms hypocellularity and fatty replacement of bone marrow (conversion of red bone marrow to yellow, fatty bone marrow).

Treatment for Aplastic Anemia:

Antilymphocyte globulin (ALG) {or antithymocyte globulin (ATG)}: suppresses T-cell-dependent autoimmune responses, (based on theory that aplastic anemia is due to an autoimmune response). It is given IV over 12 to 16 hours.

Androgens: may be used with ATG, it may stimulate erythropoiesis.

Cyclosporin A (CSA): (can be given PO or IV), an immunosuppressant (inhibits T-lymphocyte immune response), it is given to children, who fail to respond to ATG.

Solu-medrol (High-dose methylprednisolone): (IV), an anti-inflammatory and immunosuppressant); it is also sometimes given, it has been successful.

Immunoglobulin: (IV) has been successful in the acquired type of aplastic anemia (of infectious origin).

Bone marrow transplantation: it is the treatment of choice for severe aplastic anemia. It is the only mode of treatment which may result in a cure of this disease. Prognosis is highly correlated with the number of pre-transplant transfusions (better to consider early in the course of the disease).

Cyclophosphamide: (IV) a chemotherapy agent, used in patients who have received multiple transfusions prior to receiving a bone marrow transplantation.

NURSING CARE PLANS

Essential nursing diagnoses and plans associated with these conditions:

Altered tissue perfusion (6)

Related to: Impaired oxygen-carrying capacity of the blood associated with hemolysis of red blood cells and subsequent anemia; and hypervolemia

Defining characteristics: In iron deficiency anemia: irritability, anxiety, blood loss in the stool, hypochronic RBCs, normal or near normal RBC count, decreased serum ferritin and iron. In sickle cell anemia: pallor, weakness, anorexia, ease fatigability, jaundice and developmental delays. In aplastic anemia: pallor, fatigue, weakness, loss of appetite, normochromic, normocytic RBCs in reduced numbers, leukopenia, thrombocytopenia (risk of spontaneous bleeding or bleeding after mild to severe trauma)

Risk for fluid volume deficit (222)

Related to: Impaired kidney function to concentrate urine (in the sickle cell patient)

Defining characteristics: Dilute urine or low specific gravity; diuresis; enuresis; dehydration (dry mucous membranes; dry diapers and sunken fontanel in the infant); prone to dehydration from environmental factors (i.e., overheating)

Altered nutrition: Less than body requirements (168)

Related to: Inadequate ingestion of iron in food/feeding

Defining characteristics: In iron deficiency: underweight or may be overweight (because of excessive cow's milk ingestion); fecal loss of blood; pallor; poor muscle development; prone to infections; inadequate intake of iron rich foods; weakness

Risk for impaired skin integrity (397)

Related to: Allergic response to ATG therapy

Defining characteristics: Skin rash from ATG is common (i.e., itching, rash, urticaria, face and lymph node swelling); risk of sclerosing from extravasation at venous access when receiving ATG

SPECIFIC DIAGNOSES AND CARE PLANS

Pain

Related to: Biological injuring agents (tissue anoxia)

Defining characteristics: Communication of pain descriptors, guarding and protective behavior of area, soft tissue swelling, warmth over painful area, crying, clinging behavior

Outcome Criteria

Absence or control of pain

Interventions	Rationales
Assess for location, severity, and duration of pain	Provides information about pain caused by vaso-occlusive resulting from RBC sickling that leads to occlusion, ischemia, and necrosis in soft tissue, joints, abdomen, back, or wherever occlusion occurs
Administer analgesic as ordered; administer intermittently over 24-hour period before pain becomes severe rather than wait for request or complaint from child	Controls pain and promotes comfort
Provide rest periods, refrain from disturbing child unless necessary	Decreases stimuli that increase pain and promotes rest, decreases oxygen expenditure
Apply dry heat to area and note response of pain decrease	Promotes vasodilation and circulation to area to reduce pain
Maintain position of comfort, handle painful areas gently and support with pillows	Promotes comfort and prevents pain from movement

Information, Instruction, Demonstration

Interventions	Rationales
Inform parent(s) and child of cause of pain, methods to control it	Provides information and rationale for treatment
Inform parent(s) to avoid situations that cause stress for the child, and clothing or positions that restrict and impede blood flow	Provides measures to control sickling, which results in pain

Discharge or Maintenance Evaluation

- Controls or manages pain effectively
- Maintains comfort and rest with measures that prevent sickling and pain
- Administers analgesic with effective results
- Avoids pain-provoking situations

Activity intolerance

Related to: Generalized weakness, imbalance between oxygen supply and demand
Defining characteristics: Reduced oxygen delivery to tissues from reduced RBC or RBC sickling; fatigue; verbalization of weakness; changes in respiratory rate, depth, and ease; irritability; low tolerance to activity; increased pulse

Outcome Criteria

Maintenance of energy and endurance levels and tissue oxygenation
Management of fatigue with increasing activity level

Interventions	Rationales
Assess temperature, respirations, and pulse; changes in behavior (irritability, lightheadedness, short attention span); if easily fatigued, unable to sleep, or weak; ability to tolerate any activity or ADL	Provides information about VS changes caused by hypoxia and about behavior changes caused by reduced oxygenation of the brain
Assist with activities that require exertion and are beyond tolerance and ability	Minimizes physical exertion, which increases oxygen to tissues
Provides rest periods, plan care and activities around rest/sleep	Decreases oxygen expenditure to enhance tissue oxygenation
Provide appropriate quiet play and activities, and allow interaction with child of same age, if possible	Promotes diversionary activity and prevents withdrawal
Administer oxygen therapy as ordered	Provides supplemental oxygen, if needed, to treat hypoxia

Interventions	Rationales
Administer transfusion of blood, packed RBC, platelets as ordered	Replaces blood or blood components depending on type of anemia and need

Information, Instruction, Demonstration

Interventions	Rationales
Inform parent(s) and child of measures to take to conserve energy and increase endurance of child, including placing articles within reach, anticipating needs and assisting before child attempts activity, allowing for rest; remain with child as needed	Provides information to prevent fatigue by minimizing physical activity or exertion, which utilizes more oxygen
Inform parent(s) to avoid stressful situations	Promotes quiet environment for child

Discharge or Maintenance Evaluation

- Minimizes oxygen expenditure and hypoxia
- Reduces activity, intolerance, fatigue, weakness
- Promotes restful environment
- Provides oxygen, transfusion, other treatments and procedures without incident
- Provides play and diversionary activities with minimal exertion

Risk for infection

Related to: All three types of anemia: decreased Hgb and decreased immune system functions; in aplastic anemia: immunosuppressive therapy, ATG, and steroids; in sickle cell anemia: splenic dysfunction

Defining characteristics: Temperature elevation (greater than or equal to a temperature of 101° F or 38.5° C; elevated WBC counts; positive cultures for bacterial organisims; positive throat, urine or blood culture; changes in respirations and sputum characteristics; cloudy, foul-smelling urine

Outcome Criteria

Absence of infectious process at any site

Interventions	Rationales
Assess for signs, symptoms, and laboratory tests indicating infectious process irritability and malaise, swelling in soft tissue or lymph nodes	Provides information about infection in a child made susceptible by steroid and globulin therapy, particularly in aplastic anemia, or pneumococcal and salmonella infections in child with sickle cell anemia
If an infection is present, administer antibiotics as ordered, based on culture and sensitivity results	Prevents and/or treats infection; children with sickle cell anemia are prone to infections, which precipitate a crisis episode
Provide protective isolation if neutrophil count is less than 500/cu mm; use mask and gown and good handwashing when caring for child	Prevents transmission of pathogens to a susceptible child
Obtain culture of body fluid for examination	Identifies pathogens and sensitivity to antibiotic therapy if an infection is present

Information, Instruction, Demonstration

Interventions	Rationales
Inform parent(s) and child to limit contact with persons who are ill or have respiratory infections	Prevents exposure to those with infections or illness that may be transmitted to child with anemia
Instruct in handwashing technique and when to use it, including before meals, after using bathroom	Prevents exposure to infectious agents transmitted by hands or hard surfaces
Inform parent(s) of recommended childhood immunizations; and of acquiring the following vaccines when the child is two years of age or older: meningococcal and pneumococcal	Prevents infectious disease in the susceptible child
Inform parent(s) to report any temperature elevation, changes in respirations and pulse, pain or swelling in any area	Indicates possible infection that may be controlled with early intervention

Discharge or Maintenance Evaluation

- Absence of infection in any area
- Protects child from exposure to infectious agents
- Administers antibiotic therapy properly and correctly
- Reports signs and symptoms of infectious process

Risk for injury

Related to: Internal factor of abnormal blood profile (Thrombocytopenia) reaction to transfusion or ATG administration

Defining characteristics: Fever; restlessness; chills; shortness of breath; chest pain; tachycardia; hypotension; headache; thrombocytopenia at 20,000/cu mm level; bruising; petechiae; bleeding from mucous membranes; blood in urine, sputum, stool; nosebleed; blood in vomitus; stomatitis

Outcome Criteria

Absence of active bleeding from any site
Absence of allergic reaction to transfusion or medications

Interventions	Rationales
Assess for signs of bleeding from any site as manifested in skin changes; also, blood from nose, oral cavity, urinary or gastrointestinal tract, and factors that precipitate or increase bleeding	Provides information indicating blood loss as tendency increases with therapy for aplastic anemia
Assess blood in urine with dipsticks and hematests	Identifies occult blood in urine or stool
Protect child from trauma by padding bed and toys, using soft toothbrush and towels or swabs for cleaning mouth, avoiding rectal temperature and injections	Prevents bleeding in skin layers, deeper tissues, or mucous membranes
Discontinue transfusion if allergic reaction occurs, notify physician	Prevents irreversible reaction to blood or blood products
If ordered, perform skin test for ATG before dose, administer steroid daily 30 minutes before ATG, which is given in normal saline IV	Alerts to possible sensitivity to horse serum and protects from allergic reaction to ATG

Information, Instruction, Demonstration

Interventions	Rationales
Inform parent(s) and child of activities to avoid while on therapy, such as contact sports or activities that cause falls	Prevents trauma, which causes bleeding when tendency is present
Advise parent(s) to avoid aspirin and aspirin products	Encourages bleeding by its effect on platelet aggregation
Instruct parent(s) to report any bleeding from any site, nosebleed that won't stop, blood in urine or stool	Provides for early interventions to control bleeding

Discharge or Maintenance Evaluation

- Bleeding absent or controlled
- Absence of allergic reactions or complications to transfusion or medication
- Complies with correct administration of medications
- Provides protective measures to prevent trauma, bleeding, or allergic reaction
- Assesses tests, and reports bleeding from any site

Knowledge deficit of parent(s), child

Related to: Lack of information about anemia
Defining characteristics: Request for information about pathophysiology of anemia, changes that occur, preventative measures and treatments

Outcome Criteria

Adequate knowledge of condition, cause, prevention, and prognosis

Interventions	Rationales
Assess for knowledge level of type of anemia, cause, treatment, prevention	Provides information needed for appropriate teaching content for parent(s) and child
Inform of RBC physiology and the changes that occur in each of the anemias as pertain to the child	Promotes understanding of RBC function to provide a rationale for signs, symptoms, and treatments

Interventions	Rationales
Inform parent(s) of importance of genetic counseling for sickle cell anemia	Provides information about risk of offspring having the disease
Inform parent(s) and child of bone marrow transplant treatment if appropriate	Provides information of this therapy if child has aplastic anemia
Instruct child to carry or wear identification information, including condition, treatments, and physician's name and number	Provides information in the event of an emergency
Instruct parent(s) and child in dietary intake of iron, including foods such as iron-rich formula for infant, meats, whole grains, green leafy vegetables, dried fruits	Provides iron intake or replacement in iron-deficiency anemia
Administer oral iron replacement and instruct to take with orange juice to promote absorption; give iron preparation between meals, avoid administering with milk, use straw or dropper and have child rinse mouth after ingestion	Provides iron replacement therapy
Inform parent(s) and child to contact National Association for Sickle Cell Disease and other community agencies and groups for family, parent(s) or child	Provides information and support for child and family with sickle cell or aplastic anemia
Inform parent(s) of importance of child attending school and participating in family activities	Treats child as member of family and integrates him or her into social, mental, and physical activities, which will enhance growth and development needs
Reinforce risks to avoid, including signs and symptoms of infection, bleeding, hypoxia, malnutrition, immunizations, high altitudes, side effects of steroid therapy, emotional and physical stress	Prevents complications of disease

Discharge or Maintenance Evaluation

- Verbalizations of knowledge of disease, cause, implications and interventions for compliance of medical regimen
- Applies knowledge to care and measures to prevent complications
- Seeks out counseling (genetic) information and support from groups and agencies
- Complies with correct medication/replacement administration

Anemias

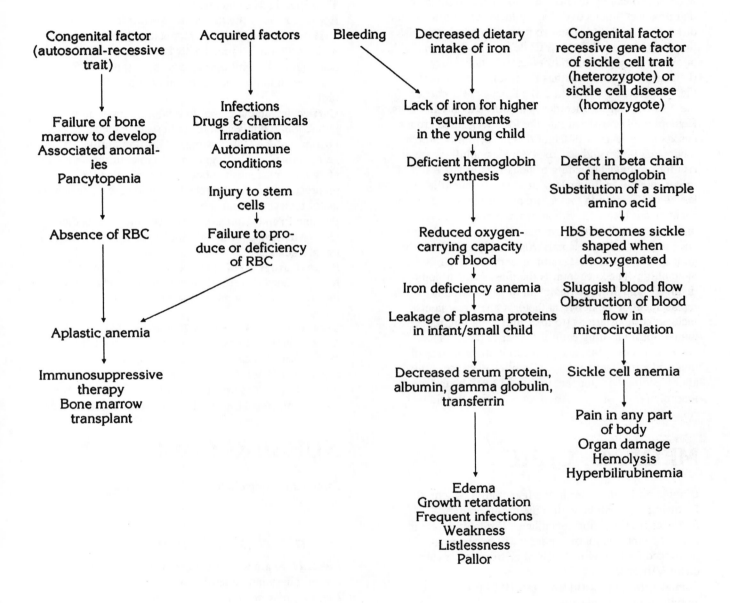

Congenital factor
(autosomal-recessive
trait)

↓

Failure of bone
marrow to develop
Associated anomal-
ies
Pancytopenia

↓

Absence of RBC

↓

Aplastic anemia

↓

Immunosuppressive
therapy
Bone marrow
transplant

Acquired factors

↓

Infections
Drugs & chemicals
Irradiation
Autoimmune
conditions

Injury to stem
cells
↓
Failure to pro-
duce or deficiency
of RBC

Bleeding

Decreased dietary
intake of iron

↓

Lack of iron for higher
requirements
in the young child

↓

Deficient hemoglobin
synthesis

↓

Reduced oxygen-
carrying capacity
of blood

↓

Iron deficiency anemia

↓

Leakage of plasma proteins
in infant/small child

↓

Decreased serum protein,
albumin, gamma globulin,
transferrin

↓

Edema
Growth retardation
Frequent infections
Weakness
Listlessness
Pallor

Congenital factor
recessive gene factor
of sickle cell trait
(heterozygote) or
sickle cell disease
(homozygote)

↓

Defect in beta chain
of hemoglobin
Substitution of a simple
amino acid

↓

HbS becomes sickle
shaped when
deoxygenated

↓

Sluggish blood flow
Obstruction of blood
flow in
microcirculation

↓

Sickle cell anemia

↓

Pain in any part
of body
Organ damage
Hemolysis
Hyperbilirubinemia

Hemophilia

Hemophilia, an X-linked disorder, is a congenital hereditary bleeding disorder due to an abnormal gene that produces a defective clotting factor protein with little or no clotting ability. The two most common forms of this disorder are: 1) factor VIII deficiency (hemophilia A, or classic hemophilia) and 2) factor IX deficiency (hemophilia B, or Christmas Disease). Because both of these disorders are X-linked, the female is the carrier of the disorder and the disorder is manifested only in males. Hemophilia is classified into the following three groups, based on the severity of factor deficiency, mild (5-50%), moderate (1-5%) and severe (1%). Hemophiliacs are at risk for prolonged bleeding or hemorrhage as a result of minor trauma. Individuals with severe hemophilia, or less than 1% clotting factor, are also at risk to suffer from spontaneous bleeding without trauma or more severe prolonged bleeding after trauma. Bleeding can occur at any part of the body. Hemarthrosis, or bleeding into the joint spaces, is the most common complication of severe hemophilia. The knee joint is the most frequent joint involved. The primary treatment of hemophilia is replacement of the deficient factor. Other treatments include: corticosteriods (to treat inflammation in the joints); local bleeding control measures (such as ice packs and elastic bandages); initial immobilization of involved joints; active range of motion exercises (only after bleeding has stopped, within 24 to 48 hours); and Ibuprofen (i.e., Motrin, Advil, or Nuprin) for pain control.

MEDICAL CARE

Diagnostic Evaluation: in the hemophilia patient, the following tests will be within the normal range: prothrombin time, fibrinogen level, thrombin level, and platelet count; the following tests will be abnormal: prolonged PTT and low levels of clotting factor (for factor VIII or IX).
Partial thromboplastin time test (PTT): measures activity of thromboplastin.
Thromboplastin generation test (TGT): measures blood's ability to generate thromboplastin. Specific for determination of specific factor deficiencies, especially factor VIII and IX.
Prothrombin test (PT): measures activity of prothrombin and detects deficiencies only for factor V, VII, X, fibrinogen, and prothrombin.
Platelet test: total number of circulating platelets.

Bleeding time: measures time interval for bleeding from small superficial wound to cease.
Factor VIII: antihemophilic factor A or antihemophilic globulin (AHG).
Factor IX: Antihemophilic factor B or plasma thromboplastin component (PTC).
Therapeutic Management:
Replacement of the deficient clotting factor: factor VIII and factor IX (IV): (monoclonal), (reconstituted with sterile water immediately before use); DDAVP: (1-deamino-8-D-arginine vasopressin), a synthetic form of vasopressin that is the treatment of choice for hemophilia.
Corticosteriods: are used to treat inflammation in the joints; Ibuprofen is used for pain management.
Oral use of EACA or Amicar (Epsilon aminocaproic acid): promotes clotting, it is used in children (> 1 year of age) for mucous membrane bleeding; also for preprocedural and postprocedural oral surgery (a dose of factor replacement must be given first).
Porcine Preparations: prevents inhibitor antibodies (30% will develop inhibitor antibodies against factor replacements).
Regular program of exercise: active range-of-motion is recommended to strengthen muscles around joints and may decrease the number of spontaneous bleeding episodes.
Treatments not Currently Recommended:
Cryoprecipitate: has not been recommended (since 1988) because it cannot be treated to safely eliminate hepatitis or HIV viruses.
NSAIDS: (such as aspirin, Indocin, or Butazolidin) are not recommended because they inhibit platelet function.

NURSING CARE PLANS

Essential nursing diagnoses and plans associated with this condition:

Impaired physical mobility (278)

Related to: Pain and discomfort with the onset of bleeding episodes; and hemarthrosis
Defining characteristics: Pain in affected joint, and decreased ability to move the joint; immobilized joints (first 24 to 48 hours after a bleeding episode), potential contractures in affected joints

Risk for impaired skin integrity (397)

Related to: Spontaneous bleeding episodes or bleeding episodes related to trauma
Defining characteristics: Bleeding into soft tissue, muscles, and, most frequently, joint capsules

SPECIFIC DIAGNOSES AND CARE PLANS

Pain

Related to: Hemarthrosis associated with trauma to a limb
Defining characteristics: A feeling of stiffness, tingling or ache in the affected joint, followed by a decrease in the ability to move a joint, verbal descriptors of pain, irritability, crying, restlessness

Outcome Criteria

Absence or control of pain

Interventions	Rationales
Assess for joint pain, swelling and limited ROM	Bleeding episodes should be treated at the onset of discomfort, which requires replacement of the deficient factor
Immobilization of joints and elastic bandages to the affected joint, if prescribed; elevate affected extremity/joint; avoid heat application; ice pack applications are used with caution in young children	Immobilization is mandatory for comfort and to avoid further bleeding; elastic bandage most often prevents muscle bleeding; elevation of affected extremity/joint will minimize swelling; heat application will promote vasodilatation and which may prolong bleeding time; ice packs promote vasoconstriction to active bleeding sites, but must be used cautiously to prevent skin damage in young children
Administer analgesics for pain	Administer ibuprofen for pain management; avoid NSAIDS (aspirin), since they may inhibit platelet function

Interventions	Rationales
Provide bed cradle over painful joints and/or other sites of bleeding	Prevents pressure of linens on affected sites, especially joints (i.e., hemarthrosis)
Maintain immobilization of the affected extremity during the acute phase (24 to 48 hours); apply a splint or sling to the affected extremity if prescribed	Prevents increase of pain and potential increased bleeding time caused by movement
Interventions which may also be used: casting, traction or aspiration of blood	All of these interventions may be necessary to preserve joint function

Discharge and Maintenance Evaluation

- Verbalizes that pain is reduced or absent
- Verbalizes understanding of appropriate pain assessment, management and medications
- Verbalizes understanding of signs of bleeding episodes and hemarthrosis
- Verbalizes understanding of immobilization principles for bleeding episodes which occur in the home
- Verbalizes understanding of principles of a home program of exercise and physical therapy in the home
- Verbalizes understanding of safety precautions related to ice pack applications

Risk for Injury

Related to: Decreased clotting factor (VIII or IX)
Defining characteristics: Prolonged bleeding anywhere from or in the body; spontaneous bleeding episodes; mild to severe bleeding episodes after trauma; hemarthrosis (bleeding to the joint and swelling of the joint); affected bleeding site will display warmth, redness, swelling, and pain with limited movement

Outcome Criteria

Recognition, prevention and management of bleeding episodes
Prevention and management of bleeding caused by trauma
Prevention of crippling effects of bleeding

Interventions	Rationales
Assess signs and symptoms of bleeding: hemarthrosis (stiffness, tingling, or pain); subcutaneous and intramuscular hemorrhage; oral bleeding; epistaxis (is not a frequent sign); petechiae (are uncommon)	Early detection of bleeding episodes will delay initiation of factor replacement therapy and will minimize complications; oral bleeding is often due to trauma to the gums; petechiae is due to low platelet function versus a deficient clotting factor
Provide appropriate oral hygiene (use of a water irrigating device; use of a soft toothbrush or softening the toothbrush with warm water before brushing; use of sponge-tipped toothbrush)	Implementation of appropriate oral hygiene will minimize trauma to the gums
Advise adolescents to use an electric shaver versus manual razor devices (with blades)	High risk of bleeding is related to use of razor blades; minimal risk of bleeding is associated with use of electric shaver
Substitute the subcutaneous route for intramuscular injections; utilize venipuncture blood drawing technique for all required blood testing samples versus use of a finger or heel puncture	Both of these measures are associated with less bleeding after implementing a subcutaneous injection or venipuncture blood sample
Utilize appropriate toys (soft, not pointed or small sharp objects); for infants, may need to use padded bed rail sides on crib; avoid rectal temperatures	All of these recommendations will minimize and/or prevent bleeding episodes due to trauma
Implement the following measures to control and stop all bleeding episodes: 1) apply pressure (10 to 15 mins)	To allow clot formation
2) immobilize and elevate affected extremity above the heart	To decrease blood flow to control bleeding
3) application of cold pack (if prescribed)	To promote vasoconstriction, but use caution with small children to avoid tissue damage

Interventions	Rationales
4) institute factor replacement therapy (based on medical protocol) 5) institute DDAVP (it can be given IV or intra-nasally)	To control and stop bleeding episode and to prevent crippling effects from joint bleeding
Other recommended adjunct measures: 1) complete bed rest for intramuscular hemorrhage of lower spine area and non-weight bearing support	To minimize hemorrhage in muscles of lower spine (i.e., attaching to trochanter or femur)
2) assess laboratory values for blood clotting factors (VIII or IX) and vital signs	These values determine current hemodynamic status and factor replacement therapy guidelines or protocols
3) stop passive range-of-motion exercises after an acute episode of bleeding	To avoid injury to the affected extremity or joint and to avoid recurrence of bleeding to these

Information, Instruction, Demonstration

Interventions	Rationales
Education of need to always wear appropriate medical identification and to notify medical personnel of diagnosis	To prepare medical personnel, family members and others of accurate information in the event of an emergency
Education to parent(s), family members and affected child: signs and symptoms of bleeding; and appropriate measures to control bleeding at home	Empowers others with accurate information to recognize and control bleeding episodes; to prevent bleeding; and to prevent crippling effects of bleeding
Limit use of helmets and padding of joints during participation in contact sports activities	Daily use of these measures may cause the child to feel ostracized or may create emotional discomfort
Recommend non-contact sports activities such as swimming, hiking, or bicycling	These activities are considered a safe activity by the Hemophilia Foundation

Interventions	Rationales
Avoid contact sports such as football, soccer, ice hockey, karate	Contact sports will predispose the child to injury and bleeding episodes
Education related to provision of a normal environment of the affected child; such as, maintain close supervision during play time to minimize injuries	To prevent bleeding related to trauma in the child's environment (i.e., school or park)
Education related to home health maintenance: 1) the affected child should receive all routine immunizations (use subcutaneous route, recommend pressure and elastic bandage after injections) 2) reinforce importance of appropriate dental hygiene program 3) reinforce the provision of a safe but normal home environment, such as safety measures that are employed for all children of different ages are recommended; example: for the toddler, gates over stairs but avoid restraining the toddler's attempt to master motor skills; for the older child, participating in sports activities (use helmets and padding) 4) provide a home environment free of hazards, including clear pathways, and supervise child during ambulation and play without being overprotective	To protect the child from childhood communicable diseases (but use subcutaneous route administration to prevent prolonged bleeding) To minimize oral trauma To minimize emotional distress during the child's progression through the different developmental stages To minimize risk of trauma in the home by falls, infants and toddlers frequently fall or sustain injuries
Instruct parent(s) and child, if age appropriate, to administer factor VIII via IV if signs and symptoms appear, or before dental visits or other possible invasive procedures; instruct in mixing the precipitate, drawing into syringe, venipuncture, and application of pressure following	Prevents or manages bleeding by factor replacement

Interventions	Rationales
IV, and allow for return demonstration	
Instruct parent(s) in dietary inclusions of iron-rich foods; provide list of foods and sample menus	Maintains iron level to prevent anemia
Inform parent(s) and child of possible reactions to IV concentrate administration and that blood is tested for AIDS	Reduces anxiety caused by risk of infections such as hepatitis and aids from replacement products

Discharge or Maintenance Evaluation

- Absence of excessive bleeding
- Complies with measures to prevent trauma, which results in bleeding
- Reports signs and symptoms of bleeding to physician
- Complies with protocol in administration of concentrates and measures to control bleeding
- Prevents joint degeneration from prolonged bleeding and repeated hemarthrosis
- Participates in acceptable activities and physical therapy to prevent trauma and joint damage

Ineffective family coping: Compromised

Related to: Inadequate or incorrect information or understanding, prolonged disease or disability progression that exhausts the physical and emotional supportive capacity of caretakers
Defining Characteristics: Expression and/or confirmation of concern and inadequate knowledge about long-term care needs, problems and complications, anxiety and guilt, overprotection of child

Outcome Criteria

Development of family coping skills, support, and long-term care
Adaptation of family to child's condition and disabilities
Adequate knowledge regarding long-term therapy and interdisciplinary approach to treatment

Interventions	Rationales
Assess family's coping methods and their effectiveness; family interactions and expectations related to long-term care, developmental level of family; response of siblings; knowledge and use of support systems and resources; presence of guilt and anxiety; overprotection and/or overindulgent behaviors	Identifies coping methods that work and the need to develop new coping skills and behaviors, family attitudes; child with special long-term needs may strengthen or strain family relationships and an undue degree of overprotection may be detrimental to child's growth and development (disallowing school attendance or peer activities, avoiding discipline of child, and disallowing child to assume responsibility for ADL
Encourage family members to express problem areas and explore solutions responsibly	Reduces anxiety and enhances understanding; provides family an opportunity to identify problems and develop problem solving strategies
Help family establish short- and long-term goals for child and integrate child into family activities, include participation of all family members in care routines	Promotes involvement and control over situations and maintains role of family members and parent(s)
Provide assistance of social worker, counselor, or other as needed	Gives support to the family faced with long-term care of child with a serious illness
Suggest community agencies and contact with the National Hemophilia Foundation or other families with a child with hemophilia	Provides information and support to child and family
Allow family members to express feelings, such as how they deal with the chronic needs of family member and coping patterns that help or hinder adjustment to the problems	Allows for venting of feelings, which relieves guilt and anxiety and helps determine need for information and support

Information, Instruction, Demonstration

Interventions	Rationales
Inform family of requested and needed information regarding long-term care and treatments	Enhances family understanding of medical regimen and responsibilities of family members
Inform family that overprotective behavior may hinder growth and development and that child should be treated as normally as possible	Promotes understanding of importance of making child one of the family and the adverse effects of overprotection of the child
Discuss importance of follow-up appointments for physical and occupational therapy, examinations, laboratory	Promotes positive outcome when family collaborates with the physician and health team to monitor disease

Discharge or Maintenance Evaluation

- Verbalizes and clarifies child's and family's knowledge about long-term needs and care
- Develops and uses coping skills and problem solving techniques effectively
- Family members support and care for child while meeting own needs
- Preserves family relationships, minimizes family stressors, resolves differences
- Family progressively adapts and accepts hemophilia condition and therapy by family
- Implements preventative measures of follow-up care to ensure optimal function and heart of child

Information, Instruction, Demonstration

Interventions	Rationales
Inform child of cause of pain and interventions to relieve it; how medications must be administered via mouth, while injections are avoided; to avoid taking aspirin or aspirin product for pain	Promotes understanding of pain responses and methods to reduce it
Instruct child to support and protect painful areas and in the importance of immobilization	Promotes comfort and prevents further bleeding into joints

Hemophilia A

Genetic factor (sex-linked recessive gene)

↓

deficiency of factor VIII
Inactive factor VIII

↓

Deficient coagulation process

↓

Prolonged bleeding

Spontaneous hemorrhage ← → Traumatic hemorrhage

Bleeding into subcutaneous tissue
Bleeding into muscle tissue
Bleeding into mouth, gums, lips, tongue
Bleeding into joints
Hematuria
Blood in stool

↓

Replacement of factor VIII via IV
Blood transfusion for severe blood loss

Idiopathic Thrombocytopenic Purpura

Idiopathic (immune) thrombocytopenic purpura (ITP) is referred to as an acquired blood disorder, (a hemorrhagic disorder). It is characterized by excessive destruction of platelets (thrombocytopenia) and purpura (a discoloration caused by petechiae beneath the skin). Etiology is unknown but it is believed to be an autoimmune response to disease-related antigens. ITP is classified into two forms: 1) acute form, which arises usually after an upper respiratory infection, measles, mumps or chickenpox; and 2) chronic form, which is unresponsive to treatment (with persistent thrombocytopenia) beyond 6 months of diagnosis. Classic signs and symptoms of ITP may include: easy bruising with petechiae, and/or ecchymosis over bony prominences; bleeding from mucous membranes (ie., epistaxis, bleeding gums); hematuria; hematemesis; hemarthrosis; hematomas over the lower extremities. ITP is seen most frequently between the ages of 2 and 10 years in children. It is rarely seen in infants less than 6 months of age. Treatment is primarily supportive since the course of this disease is self-limiting.

MEDICAL CARE

Diagnostic evaluation of ITP:
Platelet count (below 20,000 to 30,000); bone marrow aspiration (to rule out malignant infiltration of the marrow); abnormal platelet function (prolonged bleeding time, tourniquet test, and clot retraction); higher than normal levels of megakaryocytes; all other blood studies are typically normal. Also, lab studies are performed to rule out systemic lupus erythema, lymphoma and leukemia.
Medical Management of ITP: there is no standard treatment for ITP.
Gamma globulin (IVIG) (IV): is usually helpful in increasing the platelet count (within 24 hours). It can be given as a single dose or daily over 2 to 5 days. It is very expensive. It has few side effects.
Corticosteriods {Prednisone, (PO); or Methylprednisolone (IV)}: is sometimes helpful in increasing the platelet count. It is cheaper than IVIG but is associated with significant side effects.

Immunosuppressive therapy {Vincristine (IV) or Cyclophosphamide (PO or IV)}: are sometimes used for the chronic type of ITP.
Ascorbate supplements (PO): (a product of ascorbic acid or Vitamin C) may be helpful in sustaining an elevation in platelet counts.
Blood transfusions: packed red blood cells are given to replace blood lost in symptomatic children with ITP. Platelet transfusions are seldom administered.
Splenectomy: is reserved for symptomatic children with the chronic form of ITP or used as an emergency treatment when life-threatening hemorrhage occurs. Usually only performed in children older than 5 years.
Pain control: acetaminophen products (i.e., Tylenol) are substituted for salicylates.

NURSING CARE PLANS

Essential nursing diagnoses and plans associated with this condition:

Risk for injury (9)
Related to: Risk of bleeding episodes and/or hemorrhage; autoimmune destruction of platelets
Defining characteristics: Petechiae, ecchymoses, hematomas, damage from trauma

Hyperthermia (112)
Related to: Increased susceptibility to infection during immunsuppresive therapy
Defining characteristics: Elevated temperature (above 38.5° C); elevated WBC counts indicating infection; and/or the presence of a positive culture for a bacterial organism

SPECIFIC DIAGNOSES AND CARE PLANS
Altered protection
Related to: Abnormal blood profile (thrombocytopenia)
Defining characteristics: Platelet count below 20,000 cu mm/dl, petechiae, ecchymoses, bleeding from any mucous membrane area, hematomas on legs

Outcome Criteria
Absence of bleeding from any source
Maintenance of measures to prevent trauma or bleeding

Interventions	Rationales
Assess for bleeding from gums, hematemesis, hematuria, hemathrosis, hematomas, epistaxis or evidence of easy bruising, petechial rash	Provides information and data indicating low platelet level and increased tendency for bleeding
Avoid trauma to tissues by avoiding use of hard toothbrush or dental floss, taking rectal temperatures, performing unnecessary invasive procedures, and if administering an IM injection, applying pressure for 5 minutes to site	Prevents bleeding caused by trauma to sensitive areas
Administer anti-inflammatories PO, gamma globulin IV as ordered	Administered to children who are at highest risk for excessive bleeding
Administer packed RBCs as ordered and monitor for responses, expected and adverse reactions; platelets are rarely given	Administered to replace blood loss or increase platelets
Provide support in a warm, accepting environment for parent(s) and child	Promotes trust and comfort during periods of stress

Interventions	Rationales
Inform child to avoid those with upper respiratory infections or any illness	Prevents risk for infection in susceptible child
Instruct and allow return demonstration of urine and stool testing for blood using dipstick and hematest; inform to report other signs of bleeding including fatigue, pallor, headache, and blood in sputum or vomitus	Identifies presence of bleeding in gastrointestinal or urinary tract or any other area

Discharge or Maintenance Evaluation

- Absence of bleeding from any area
- Complies with measures to prevent bleeding or infection
- Reports signs and symptoms of bleeding to physician

Information, Instruction, Demonstration

Interventions	Rationales
Inform parent(s) and child of cause of disorder, reason for treatment and signs and symptoms indicating presence or relapse of disease	Provides information about the disease needed to understand treatments and care
Inform parent(s) and child to avoid rough contact play; blowing nose hard; straining at defecation; toys with sharp edges; using hard toothbrush; eating hard, rough foods	Prevents trauma that causes bleeding
Instruct parent(s) and child in medication administration and to avoid aspirin and aspirin over the counter products	Promotes compliance in drug therapy to prevent relapses in bleeding; aspirin prevents platelet aggregation

Idiopathic Thrombocytopenic Purpura

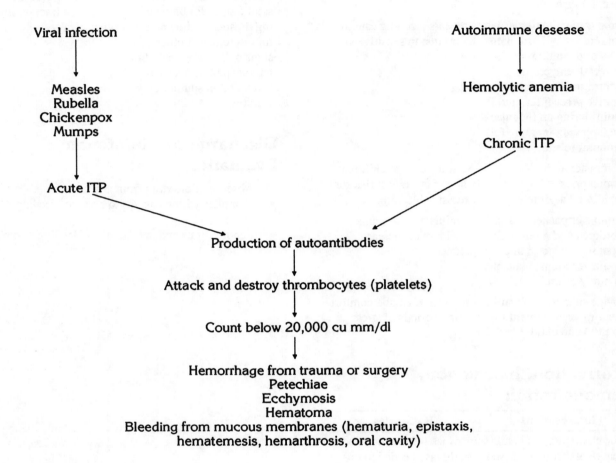

Viral infection

↓

Measles
Rubella
Chickenpox
Mumps

↓

Acute ITP

Autoimmune desease

↓

Hemolytic anemia

↓

Chronic ITP

Production of autoantibodies

↓

Attack and destroy thrombocytes (platelets)

↓

Count below 20,000 cu mm/dl

↓

Hemorrhage from trauma or surgery
Petechiae
Ecchymosis
Hematoma
Bleeding from mucous membranes (hematuria, epistaxis,
hematemesis, hemarthrosis, oral cavity)

Leukemia/ Lymphoma

Leukemia is a malignant hemopoietic disease which is characterized by an unrestricted proliferation of poorly differentiated lymphocytes called blast cells replace normal blood marrow elements. It occurs more frequently in male children, than in females after age 1 year, and the peak age of onset is the age range between 2 and 6 years. In children, the two most common forms of leukemia are recognized: acute lymphoid leukemia (ALL) and acute myelogenous leukemia (AML). Pathologic effects of leukemia include the replacement of normal bone marrow elements by leukemic cells which results in clinical manifestations of anemia, neutropenia and thrombocytopenia. Symptoms related to anemia may result in fatigue, weakness, pallor, and lethargy. Neutropenia predisposes the child to febrile episodes and infection. Symptoms related to thrombocytopenia may result in cutaneous bruises or purpura, petechiae, epistaxis, melena, and gingival bleeding. Other common symptoms related to leukemic infiltration include: hepatosplenomegaly and lymphadenopathy; bone and joint pain; anorexia; abdominal pain; weight loss. Other related symptoms, but are very rare, may include: hematuria, gastrointestinal bleeding, or central nervous system (CNS) bleeding. Prognosis is based on age and initial WBC at diagnosis, sex, histologic type of the disease, number of chromosomes, the DNA-index, morphology and cell-surface immunologic markers.

MEDICAL CARE

For Leukemia: Treatment of leukemia involves multimodal therapy, including the use of chemotherapeutic agents with or without cranial irradiation in 3 phases. These three phases are: (1) Remission Induction Therapy, includes corticosteriods (usually prednisone), vincristine (Oncovin), L-asparaginase, with or without doxorubicin; (2) CNS Prophylactic Therapy, includes cranial irradiation and intrathecal methotrexate (IT MTX); (3) Maintenance Therapy (or Consolidation) includes, weekly oral or intramuscular MTX and daily oral 6-mercaptopurine. Other chemotherapy agents, which may be given during this phase include: vincristine, prednisone, cyclophosphamide, cytosine arabinoside, and daunorubicin.

Supportive Therapies: for the treatment of side effects induced by the chemotherapy agents.
Prophylactic Antibiotic Therapy: PO trimethoprim/sulfamethoxazole (Bactrim, Septra) is utilized to reduce the incidence of infections. Infection is a frequent threat due to immunosuppression effects of chemotherapy agents.
Granulocyte Colony-Stimulating Factors (GCSF): filgrastim (Neupogen) IV or subcutaneously 24 hours after chemotherapy is discontinued and is given for 10 to 14 days. GCSF directs granulocyte development, which decreases the duration of the neutropenia.
Replacement of blood elements: for the treatment of anemia, agranulocytopenia and thrombocytopenia.
Prevention of hyperuricemia: is achieved by intravenous hydration, urinary alkalinization to a pH of 7 or 8, and administration of Allopurinol (a xanthineoxidase inhibitor) PO or IV, to prevent metabolic breakdown of xanthine to uric acid which will result in accumulation and precipitation in the renal tubules, causing tubular obstruction and acute renal failure.
Prevention and treatment of oral ulcers (stomatitis): Chlorhexidine gluconate (Peridex) PO is the most commonly used mouth rinse to prevent or treat Candida and bacterial infections. Other mouth rinses which can be used include normal saline or baking soda solutions. Procedure for all mouth rinses are to swish and spit the solution (before or after feedings) two to four times a day. Antifungal and antibacterial mouthwashes (nystatin) are used after mouth rinses (30 minutes after using Peridex) to treat or prevent infection. Also, use of a soft sponge toothbrush (Toothette).
Severe oral infections: Acyclovir (PO or IV) may be used to treat severe oral lesions.
Treatment of oral ulcer pain: utilization of analgesics such as Chloraseptic lozenges, Orabase or opiates. Also, reduce oral pain by massaging the mouth ulcer with an ice cube for 5 to 7 minutes until the area becomes numb.
Prevention and management of nausea and vomiting: administration of antiemetic before the chemotherapy begins (30 minutes to 1 hour) and every 2, 4, or 6 hours for at least 24 hours after chemotherapy. Commonly used antiemetic include: Ondansetron (Zofran), dexamethasone or metoclopramide (Reglan) (PO or IV). For mild to moderate vomiting, the following antiemetic agents may be effective: promethazine (Phenergan), chlorpromazine (Thorazine), prochlorperazine (Compozine), or trimethobenzamide (Tigan).
Diagnostic Evaluation of Leukemia (includes the following):
Complete blood count: decreased white blood cells, red blood cells, and platelets.

Physical examination: liver, spleen, lymph nodes and the mediastinal area; weight loss; bone or joint pain; petechiae; abdominal pain.

Bone marrow aspiration: reveals hypercellularity with 60% to 100% blast cells.

Lumbar puncture: evaluates the presence of central nervous system (CNS) leukemia.

Number of chromosomes: number of chromosomes (ploidy or the DNA index) in the lymphoblasts. Better prognosis: DNA index of more than 1.16 and more than 46 chromosomes.

Cytogenic abnormalities: presence of translocation of portions of one chromosome (ex. the Philadelphia chromosome). Presence of the Philadelphia chromosome is least favorable.

Enzymes: lactic dehydrogenase (LDH), serum glutamic oxaloacetic transaminase (SOOT) and serum glutamic pyruvic transaminase.

Monoclonal antibodies (MoAbs): used to detect the presence of the common ALL antigen (CALLA) on leukemic cells. A positive CALLA is associated with a good prognosis.

Cell-surface immunologic markers: B-cell (early pre B-cell, pre B-cell or B-cell) or T-cell.

Urine tests: blood urea nitrogen (BUN), creatinine and uric acid may be elevated.

Computerized tomography scans (CT): may reveal infiltrated sites with leukemic cells, such as the kidneys, testes, prostrate, ovaries, gastrointestinal tract and lungs.

Lymphomas: a group of neoplastic diseases that arise from the lymphoid and hemopoietic systems. There are two types: Hodgkin's disease and non-Hodgkin's disease (NHL). NHL occurs more frequently and is the third most common childhood malignancy. In both types, it is observed in children under 15 years of age, and boys are affected more than girls. The peak incidence of NHL is between the ages of 7 and 11 years. Characteristics of Hodgkin's disease: differentiated cells; pattern of infiltration is specific; subacute and a prolonged onset; and localized disease is present at the time of diagnosis. Characteristics of NHL: undifferentiated cells; pattern of infiltration is diffuse; rapid onset; wide spread involvement at the time of diagnosis. Clinical manifestations of Hodgkin's disease: 60% to 90% of cases will present with cervical or supraclavicular adenopathy; the enlarged lymph node will be painless, firm, and movable; 50% of cases will also have mediastinal involvement with symptoms of airway obstruction; anorexia; weight loss; malaise; lethargy and fever. Clinical manifestations of NHL: depend on site of involvement: 1/3 of cases, intra-abdominal site, with mediastinal, peripheral nodal, right quadrant pain, with or without fever; 1/4 of cases, mediastinal site, with respiratory symptoms.

Medical Care for Hodgkin's Disease and NHL:
Diagnostic Evaluation for Hodgkin's Disease:
I. Laboratory studies: CBC, erythrocyte sedimentation rate (ESR), serum copper and iron levels, serum ferritin and transferrin, renal and liver function tests, baseline thyroid function tests, T and B lymphocyte levels, PPD skin test.

II. Evaluation includes: chest x-ray; CT scan of the mediastinal, pulmonary and upper abdominal area; ultrasound of neck and abdomen; Isotope scanning; MRI; lymphangiogram (LAG); lymph node biopsy.

Diagnostic Evaluation for Non-Hodgkin's Disease:
I. Laboratory studies: CBC with differential, liver and renal function studies, electrolyte, calcium, phosphorus, magnesium, lactate dehydrogenase (LDH), uric acid, EBV titers and urinalysis.

II. Evaluation includes: bone marrow aspiration, lumbar puncture, lymph node biopsy, radiographic studies, CT scans of the lungs and gastrointestinal tract.

Supportive therapies for both types: are similar to the care discussed in the leukemia child.

Treatment for Hodgkin's Disease: radiation and chemotherapy.

Chemotherapy Agents for Hodgkin's Disease: (2 regimens)
1) **MOPP:** mechlorethamine [nitrogen mustard], vincristine, prednisone, and procarbazine;
2) **ABVD:** (for advanced disease) doxorubicin, bleomycin, vinblastine, and dacarbazine.

Treatment for Non-Hodgkin's Disease: chemotherapy, (radiation is not recommended), may include splenectomy.

Chemotherapy Agents for NHL: (2 regimens)
1) **lymphoblastic lymphoma:** ABO: cyclophosphamide, vincristine, daunomycin or doxorubcin, L-asparaginase, cytosine arabinoside, and methotrexate.
2) **small noncleaved lymphoma:** COMP: cyclophosphamide and methotrexate.

NURSING CARE PLANS

Essential nursing diagnosis and plans associated with these conditions:

Altered nutrition: Less than body requirements (168)

Related to: Loss of appetite; and/or pain in mouth; induced malabsorption or enteropathy (caused by abdominal radiation, chemotherapy, abdominal surgery, or frequent antibiotic use); and anorexia-inducing substances (secreted by tumor cells); Xerostomia (irreversible dryness of mouth), destruction of microvilli of taste buds and/or lining of salivary glands (all can be caused by radiation therapy)

Defining Characteristics: Anorexia, nausea, vomiting, stomatitis, mucositis, decreased salivation, cachexia, fatigue, diarrhea, alterations in taste, gustatory changes, weight loss, abdominal pain, psychologic and sociocultural factors

Risk for fluid volume deficit (222)

Related to: Altered intake and output (excessive losses related to the disease process and required chemotherapy/radiation treatments)

Defining characteristics: Vomiting and diarrhea; blood losses (i.e., hemorrhagic cystitis, epistaxis, hemoptysis)

Diarrhea (171)

Related to: Surgery, radiation, chemotherapy, increased emotional stress, use of nutritional supplements, lactose intolerance, fecal impaction, tumor growth, infection or antibiotics

Defining characteristics: Abnormal increase in quantity, frequency, and fluid content of stool

Risk for impaired skin integrity (397)

Related to: Delayed wound healing, immobility, external exposure to radiation, administration of chemotherapy and antibiotics

Defining characteristics: Radiation effects: erythema, dryness, itching, increased pigmentation, dry desquamation, necrotic tissue; chemotherapy and antibiotic induced side effects: local phlebitis, stomatitis, mucositis, maculopapular rash, hyperpigmentation, nail changes, pruritus, dermatitis, alopecia, photosensitivity, acne, erythema, poor wound healing

Risk for infection (36)

Related to: Disease process; immunosuppression due to required chemotherapy; prolonged antibiotic and prednisone therapy; skin breakdown, serious bacterial, viral fungal, and protozoan infections; surgery and/or splenectomy; invasive procedures; GI obstruction; malnutrition, inadequate serum protein level

Defining characteristics: Increase in body temperature above normal range (>38.3°C or 101°F), neutropenia; inadequate number of neutrophils: severe risk of infec-

tion (<500/mm3) or moderate risk of infection (< 1000 mm3); presence of pathogens may or may not be identified from blood cultures

SPECIFIC DIAGNOSES AND CARE PLANS

Fear

Related to: Diagnostic tests, procedures, treatments, diagnosis and prognosis

Defining characteristics: Child: crying, screaming, combative behaviors, anger, withdrawn behaviors, and verbalized fears; parent(s): fear, guilt, depression, anxiety

Outcome Criteria

Interventions	Rationales
Assess child and parent(s)' level	Provides information about fears and other psychosocial stressors related to various procedures, required treatments, and a serious illness; provide information on adaptive coping skills
Explain to the child what will take place and what the child will feel, see, and hear during various procedures	To increase the child's sense of control before and during procedures
Provide child and parent(s) with some means for involvement with procedure	To promote the child's and parent(s)' sense of control
Encourage parent(s) participation	Fosters child and parent(s)' coping skills
Remain nonjudgmental regarding the child's behaviors and fears	Encourages supportive relationship child's behavior

Information, Instruction, Demonstration

Interventions	Rationales
Inform parent(s) and child of the disease process and treatments, including radiation chemotherapy and its benefits and side effects	Provides information that will relieve fear and anxiety; understanding of treatments and effect on body image

Interventions	Rationales
(nausea, vomiting, diarrhea, stomatitis, alopecia are possibilities but are temporary)	
Explain all procedures, treatments, and care in simple, direct, honest terms and repeat as often as necessary; reinforce physician information if necessary and provide specific information as needed	Supplies information about diagnostic procedures and tests, such as CBC, platelets with chemotherapy; and scans and x-rays for diagnosis
Introduce child to another who has same disease	Provides information and support from a peer with the same condition and who has empathy

Discharge or Maintenance Evaluation

- Gains knowledge and understanding of child's illness and treatment needs
- Verbalizes fears and other psychosocial
- Gains self-awareness of psychosocial stressors about diagnosis, treatment and prognosis
- Utilizes existing and new support systems

Pain

Related to: Disease-related, treatment-related and procedure-related
Defining characteristics: Multidimensional aspects of the cancer pain experience in children with cancer include components of assessment of cognitive or self-report, physiologic responses, behavioral manifestations, and the child's developmental level

Outcome Criteria

Absence of pain or effective pain control

Interventions	Rationales
Assess the following three areas: (1) self-report responses of the child's pain (use words and pain assessment tools that help the child to describe pain; selection is dependent upon the child's develop-	Provides information about pain that varies with age, developmental level of child and is unique to a particular child's learned emotional responses; degree of pain and fatigue influence ability of child to

Interventions	Rationales
mental level); (2) behavioral manifestations (i.e., crying, facial expressions, muscle tension, screaming, pain verbalization, physical resistance, favors affected body parts, more common to observe during procedure-related pain or acute episodes); and (3) physiologic responses (evaluation of sweating palms, increased heart and respiratory rates, increased blood pressure, use along with self-report and behavioral assessments)	perceive and identify discomfort
Assess need for pain management	Ensures consistency of pain management strategies
Administer analgesics as prescribed, on a preventative pain schedule, and monitor side effects of analgesics	Ensures effective pain management; promotes comfort and rest; fosters a trusting and caring relationship between the child, family, and health care team
Apply EMLA cream to sites to be used for intrusive painful procedures (i.e. venipuncture, bone marrow aspiration, lumbar puncture, implanted port access, subcutaneous and intramuscular injections); it must be applied 1 hour before the procedure to be effective	Minimizes pain related to intrusive procedures; ensures child's safety during scheduled intrusive procedures
Evaluate effectiveness of pain relief from all pain medication used	Ensures effective pain control and management
Promote rest and avoid disturbing child unnecessarily	Decreases stimuli that increase pain, and promotes rest to conserve energy
Maintain body alignment and support, and immobilize limbs with pillows and sand bags	Promotes comfort and prevents contractures

Interventions	Rationales
Apply heat (moist or dry) to painful areas	Relieves pain by promoting circulation to the area
Provide toys and activities for quiet play appropriate for age; use music, relaxation techniques; remain with child when pain is most acute	Provides diversion and distraction from pain

Information, Instruction, Demonstration

Interventions	Rationales
Inform child of cause of pain and interventions to relieve it, of how medications are administered and actions to expect; to report pain before it becomes severe	Promotes understanding of pain response and methods to reduce it
Educate child and parent(s) on various distraction techniques (i.e., counting, music, imagery, deep breathing, self-talk, positioning, reassurance, prayer, massage, therapeutic touch, relaxation)	Enhances trust between the nurse, child and the family; also, may minimize the child's pain perceptions and foster a sense of control during intrusive procedures

Discharge or Maintenance Evaluation

- Accurate and successful assessment and management of the child's pain
- Pain control must be recognized as a priority of child's well-being
- Child rests quietly, reports and/or exhibits no evidence of discomfort
- Verbalizes no complaints of discomfort
- Utilizes various distraction techniques during intrusive procedures

Altered oral mucous membranes

Related to: Administration of chemotherapy agents, side effect of radiotherapy, long-term administration of antibiotics

Defining characteristics: (1) oral ulcers (stomatitis) are red, eroded, painful areas in the mouth and pharynx; and

(2) similar lesions (as stomatitis) which may extend along the esophagus and in the rectal area

Outcome Criteria

Mucous membrane remain intact
Oral ulcers show evidence of healing
Child reports and/or exhibits no evidence of discomfort

Interventions	Rationales
Assess mouth daily for oral ulcers, pain, ability to ingest foods; provide meticulous oral hygiene, to prevent oral breakdown and to promote healing (start as soon as a drug is used that causes oral ulcers): use a softsponge toothbrush or toothette, administer frequent mouth rinses, at least every 4 hours and after meals; mouth rinses commonly used include Peridex, normal saline with or without sodium bicarbonate solution	To effectively treat oral ulcers and to promote healing; to prevent bacterial and candida infections; to prevent trauma to oral mucosa
Administer nystatin mouthwashes after mouth rinses; restrict oral intake for 30 minutes after taking this mouthwash	To maintain oral integrity; to treat bacterial and fungal infections
Administer Acyclovir (topically or IV) for oral lesions	To prevent or treat herpetic infections
Apply local anesthetics to ulcerated areas before meals and as needed to relieve pain; topical agents include: Ora-base, dyclonine (Dyclone), diphen-hydramine (Benadryl), and Kaopectate; these agents can be applied directly to oral lesions or swished and spit; avoid using viscus lidocain (may cause a depressed gag reflex, increasing risk of aspiration, and may cause seizures	To relieve pain associated with oral ulcers

Interventions	Rationales
Administer IV narcotics (i.e., morphine) for severe stomatitis	
Apply lip balm (daily)	To prevent cracking and fissuring of lips; to maintain lip integrity
Encourage a bland, soft diet and selection of foods by child	To minimize oral discomfort and irritation; enhances sense of control, independence, decreases sense of helplessness; may increase child's level of nutrition
Avoid using lemon glycerin swabs	To prevent irritation of mouth ulcers decay of teeth
Avoid juices containing ascorbic acid, hot, cold, or spicy foods	To prevent discomfort to oral ulcers
Avoid use of hydrogen peroxide as a mouth rinse	It will delay healing of oral ulcers by breaking down protein
Avoid use of milk of magnesia	To prevent drying of oral mucosa

Information, Instruction, Demonstration

Interventions	Rationales
Provide education to parent(s) and child: 1) chemotherapy and radiation may cause oral ulcers; 2) effective oral hygiene strategies to prevent and treat oral ulcers; 3) child may require hospitalization (for hydration, parental nutrition, pain control of oral ulcers) if stomatitis interferes with food or fluid intake	Promotes understanding of oral stomatitis significance of daily oral hygiene, and pain control for oral ulcers

Discharge or Maintenance Evaluation

- Mucous membranes remain intact
- Child and family adhere to oral hygiene care
- Oral ulcers show evidence of healing

- Child reports and/or exhibits no evidence of discomfort

Risk for injury

Related to: Disease process; immunosuppression, thrombocytopenia and other side effects from chemotherapy and radiation treatments

Defining characteristics: Fever (>38.3°C or 101° F), secondary infections; fatigue; anemia (hemoglobin level <11 g); neutropenia (absolute neutrophil count <1000/mm^3); risk of hemorrhage or bleeding tendencies (platelet count of 20,000/mm 3); side effects of chemotherapy

Outcome Criteria

Child exhibits no evidence of fever, infections or bleeding
Child is not exposed to individuals with infection or communicable diseases
Child is not exposed to contact sports/activities

Interventions	Rationales
Assess for bleeding from any site, WBC, platelet count, Hct, absolute neutrophil count, and febrile episodes	Provides information about frank bleeding or blood profile abnormalities that predispose to bleeding caused by bone marrow suppression and immunosuppression resulting from chemotherapy or radiation therapy
Avoid trauma by not using hard toothbrush or dental floss, not taking rectal temperatures, not performing unnecessary invasive procedures	Prevents bleeding during chemotherapy regimen, which alters platelet and clotting factors
Carry out handwashing technique before giving care, use mask and gown when appropriate, provide a private room, monitor for any signs and symptoms of infection, especially pulmonary	Prevents transmission of pathogens to a compromised immune system during chemotherapy if neutrophil count is less than 1000/cu mm

Information, Instruction, Demonstration

Interventions	Rationales
Inform parent(s) and child to avoid rough play or sports, straining at defecation, blowing nose hard	Prevents trauma that causes bleeding
Instruct parent(s) and child to avoid those with upper respiratory infection or any illness	Prevents risk for infection in the highly susceptible child
Instruct parent(s) to report any fever, behavior changes, headache, dizziness, fatigue, pallor, slow oozing of blood from any area, exposure to a communicable disease	Indicate complications associated with an abnormal blood profile
Impress on parent(s) the need for compliance in laboratory testing and physician appointments	Monitors affect of chemotherapy on child and need for modification of therapy or care
Instruct and allow for return demonstration of urine and stool testing for blood using dipstick and hematest	Identifies presence of bleeding in gastrointestinal or urinary tract

Discharge or Maintenance Evaluation

- Absence of excessive bleeding or infection during chemotherapy
- Complies with measures based on blood profile that prevent excessive bleeding or infection
- Reports signs and symptoms of complications to physician
- Complies with laboratory blood testing and follow-up visits to physician

Body image disturbance

Related to: Side effects of chemotherapy and radiation therapy

Defining characteristics: Loss of hair; moon face; weight loss or gain; hyper-pigmentation; skin rash or erythema; acne; skin thickening; or peeling of skin

Outcome Criteria

Child verbalizes feelings regarding body image changes
Child resumes former activities and relationships within own capabilities
Family demonstrates understanding of body image changes
Body image improved, preserved, and maintained
Accommodations made for adaptation to long-term needs and limitations of chronic illness

Interventions	Rationales
Assess child for feelings about multiple restrictions in lifestyle, chronic illness, difficulty in school and social situations, inability to keep up with peers and participate in activities	Provides information about status of self-concept and body image, which may require special attention
Encourage expression of feelings and concerns and support communication with parent(s), teachers and peers	Provides opportunity to vent feelings and reduce negative feelings about changes in appearance
Avoid negative comment and stress positive activities and accomplishments	Enhances body image and confidence
Note withdrawal behavior and signs of depression	Reveals responses to body image changes and possible poor adjustment to chances
Show support and acceptance of changes in appearance of child; provide privacy as needed	Promotes trust and demonstrates respect for child

Information, Instruction, Demonstration

Interventions	Rationales
Inform parent(s) of importance of maintaining support for child regardless of their needs	Encourages acceptance of the child with special needs (must deal with long-term steroid therapy and its side effects, lifelong activity restrictions)

Interventions	Rationales
Inform parent(s) and child of impact of the disease on body systems and risk for hair loss; correct misinformation and inform of ways to cope with body changes	Provides correct information to assist in dealing with negative feelings about body
Instruct parent(s) of need for flexibility in care of child, need to integrate care and routines into family activities, and need to allow child to participate in peer activities	Promotes child's sense of well-being and of belonging and having control of life events by allowing participation in normal activities for age and enhancing developmental task achievement
Inform parent(s) and child about how to deal with peer and perceptions of appearance and how to tell others about change in appearance	Prevents stigmatization of child by those who are not apprised of the child's disease; attitude of others will affect child's body image
Suggest a cap, scarf, or other head covering	Preserves body image by covering head if alopecia is present
Suggest psychological counseling or child-life worker, and inform of functions performed by these professionals	Assists in improving self-esteem and in learning, coping and problem solving skills

Discharge or Maintenance Evaluation

- Verbalizes improved body image and sense of well-being
- Participates in family, school, and social activities as appropriate
- Verbalizes feelings about special long-term needs in positive terms
- Supports positive body image and promotes adjustment to illness
- Identifies need and seeks out social services and psychological counseling as appropriate

Ineffective individual coping and compromised, ineffective family coping

Related to: For the child: separation from family, friends, home, and school activities; loss of control, altered self-image, altered body image, altered self-esteem, and altered sense of self-confidence. For the parents: uncertainty of child's future, sense of helplessness and powerlessness, multiple family stressors and demands (related to child's health care needs)

Defining characteristics: For the child: depression, anxiety, withdrawn, excessive outbursts of temper, insecurity, sleep and/or eating disturbances, regressive behaviors, behavioral problems (acting out), denial, difficulties in interpersonal relationships, non-adherence with treatment. For parents: shock, disbelief, anger, guilt, numbness, denial, ambivalence, bargaining, overprotectiveness, grief for the loss of their healthy child, anticipatory grief for the potential loss of their child

Outcome Criteria

Use of adaptive coping skills for the child and parent(s) is observed and verbalized as the child and parent(s) gain understanding and knowledge about the health care management needs throughout the child's illness, treatments and prognosis

Interventions	Rationales
Assess effectiveness of family coping methods; family interactions and expectations related to long-term, developmental level of family; response of siblings; knowledge and use of support systems and resources; presence of guilt, anxiety, overprotective and/or overindulgent behaviors	Provides information identifying successful coping methods or the need to develop new coping skills, behaviors and family attitudes; child with over-protection (e.g., not allowing child to attend school, participate in activities with peers, or assume responsibilities for ADL; avoiding disciplining of child) may be at risk in growth and development
Encourage family members to express problem areas and explore solutions responsibly	Reduces anxiety and enhances understanding; allows family to identify problems and develop problem solving strategies
Assist family in establishing short- and long-term goals for child and in integrating child into family activities; include participation of all family members in care routines	Promotes involvement and control over situations, and maintains role of family members and parent(s)

Interventions	Rationales
Provide assistance of social worker, counselor, clergy, or other as needed	Provides support to the family faced with long-term care of child with a serious, life-threatening illness
Suggest community agencies and the American Cancer Society, which could provide contacts with families that have a child with leukemia or lymphoma	Provides information and support to child and family
Allow family members to express feelings on how they deal with the chronic needs of family member and on coping patterns that help or hinder adjustment to the problems	Allows for venting of feelings to determine need for information and support, and relieves guilt and anxiety

Information, Instruction, Demonstration

Interventions	Rationales
Inform family of requested and needed information regarding long-term care and treatments	Enhances family understanding of medical regimen and responsibilities of family members
Inform family that over-protective behavior may hinder growth and development and that child should be treated as normally as possible	Promotes understanding of importance of making child one of the family and the adverse effects of overprotection of the child
Discuss importance of follow-up appointments for physical and occupational therapy, examinations, laboratory tests	Promotes positive outcome when family collaborates with the physician and health team to monitor disease

Discharge or Maintenance Evaluation

- Observe adaptive coping skills for the child and parent(s) as information and explanations are given
- Verbalizes psychosocial stressors and discusses application of adaptive coping skills
- Gains self-awareness of psychosocial stressors about diagnosis, treatment and prognosis
- Utilizes existing and new support systems
- Verbalizes and clarifies knowledge about child's long-term need and care
- Develops and uses coping skill and problem solving techniques effectively
- Family members support and care for child while meeting own needs
- Family relationships preserves family relationships and family stressors, minimize with differences resolved
- Progressive adaptation and acceptance of condition and therapy by family
- Implements preventative measures of follow-up care to ensure optimal function and health of child

Leukemia/Lymphoma

Unknown factors

↓

Diffuse and uncontrolled growth of leukocyte precursors in bone marrow

Reversal of RBC and WBC ratio and crowding out RBC and platelets

↓

Abnormal immature WBC in circulation
Infiltration of liver, spleen, lymph nodes and all tissue in the body with WBC

↓

Acute lymphocytic leukemia

↓

Hepatosplenomegaly
Anemia, fatigue, pallor, weight loss (reduced RBC)
Infection with fever, pain (neutropenia)
Bleeding tendency (thrombocytopenia)

Viral infection   Deficient immune state

↘   ↙

Proliferation of abnormal lymphocytes

↓

Hypogammaglobilinemia

↓

Reduced humoral antibody response

↓

Lymphoid tissue involvement
Spleen, liver involvement

↓

Staging from one node involvement to regional or distant tissue involvement

↓

Weight loss, anorexia
Fatigue
Fever, night sweats
Skin, bone marrow, neurologic, gastrointestinal involvement

Endocrine System

Endocrine System

The endocrine system includes the cells of certain glands that produce hormones; the organ or tissue sites that receive the hormone; and the transport system of the blood, lymph, and extracellular fluids that move the hormones from the point of origin to the point of utilization. Hormones may regulate general cell physiologic activities or may affect specific cells of the body. Glands included in this system are the pituitary, thyroid, parathyroid, adrenal, isles of Langerhans, ovaries, and testes. The system regulates and integrates functions with the neurologic system that assist the body to adjust behavior, growth, development, and sexual reproduction. In children, abnormal conditions involving these glands are caused by oversecretion or undersecretion of hormones or by a problem in the response to these hormones by the receiving organ or tissue. These abnormalities may result from congenital or acquired factors. They are usually treated by partial or complete surgical removal of the gland and/or drug therapy to replace deficiencies.

GENERAL ENDOCRINE GLAND CHANGES ASSOCIATED WITH PHYSICAL GROWTH AND DEVELOPMENT

- Endocrine glands are well developed at birth, but their functions are immature
- Secondary sex characteristics usually develop between 10 and 18 years of age in girls and between 12 and 20 years of age in boys; menarche usually occurs between 12 and 13 years of age

Insulin Dependent Diabetes Mellitus

Insulin Dependent Diabetes Mellitus (lDDM) is a metabolic disorder caused by a deficiency of insulin. The deficiency is thought to occur in those individuals who are genetically predisposed to the disease and who have experienced a precipitating event, commonly a viral infection or environmental change, causing an autoimmune condition affecting the beta cells of the pancreas. It is treated by injection of insulin and regulation of diet and activity that maintain body functions. Complications that occur from improper coordination of these include hypoglycemia and hyperglycemia which, if untreated, lead to insulin shock or ketoacidosis. Long-term effects of the disease include neuropathy, nephropathy, retinopathy, atherosclerosis, and microangiopathy.

MEDICAL CARE

Antidiabetics: regular insulin, using U 500 given SC alone or in combination with intermediate and long-acting insulins using U100 given SC to control blood glucose concentrations by converting glucose to glycogen; administered two or more times/day individually prescribed for child.
Blood glucose: reveals levels greater than 120mg/dl in a fasting specimen and 200 mg/dl or greater in a random specimen; 300mg/dl level in ketoacidosis.
Ketones: reveals increase in the blood and urine.
Urine glucose: reveals glycosuria.

NURSING CARE PLANS

Essential nursing diagnoses and plans associated with this condition:

Altered nutrition: less than body requirements (168)

Related to: Inability to ingest, digest food
Defining characteristics: Loss of weight with adequate food intake, lack of interest in food, inadequate intake, insufficient insulin, too much insulin

Risk for impaired skin integrity (397)

Related to: External factor of SC injections and blood glucose monitoring, internal factor of altered metabolic state, sensation, nutritional state
Defining characteristics: Disruption of skin surfaces with daily injections (lipodystrophy), failure to rotate sites, weight loss, poor wound healing, dry skin

Risk for fluid volume deficit (222)

Related to: Active loss (osmotic diuresis)
Defining characteristics: Output greater than intake, decreased urine output, dry skin and mucous membranes, poor skin turgor, dehydration with electrolyte depletion (K, Na, Cl, Mg, PO4) with ketoacidosis, polyuria, polydipsia

SPECIFIC DIAGNOSES AND CARE PLANS

Risk for injury

Related to: Internal biochemical factors of hyperglycemia or hypoglycemia
Defining characteristics: Hyperglycemia — fatigue, irritability, headache, abdominal discomfort, weight loss, polyuria, polydipsia, polyphagia, dehydration, blurred vision
Hypoglycemia — nervousness, sweating, hunger, palpitations, weakness, dizziness, pallor, behavior changes, uncoordinated gait

Outcome Criteria

Absence of signs and symptoms of hyperglycemia or hypoglycemia
Blood glucose levels maintained within normal levels

Interventions	Rationales
Assess for signs and symptoms of hyperglycemia, blood glucose level, urinary glucose and ketones, pH and electrolyte levels	Provides information about complication caused by increased glucose levels resulting from improper diet, an illness, or omission of insulin administration; glucose is unable to enter the cells, and protein is broken down and converted to glucose by the liver, causing the hyperglycemia; fat and protein stores are depleted to provide energy for the body when carbohydrates are not able to be used for energy
Administer insulin SC as ordered, rotate sites, increase dosage as indicated by glucose levels; decrease food intake during an infection or illness and adjust insulin dosage during an illness	Provides insulin replacement to maintain normal blood glucose levels without causing hypoglycemia; two or more injections may be given daily SC with a portable syringe pump or by intermittent bolus injections with a syringe and needle
Provide diet with calories that balance expenditure for energy and correspond to type and action of insulin, and snacks between meals and at bedtime as appropriate	Provides child's nutritional needs for proper growth and development using the exchange system developed and approved by the American Diabetic Association (ADA), or by carbohydrate counting — monitoring carbohydrate intake only, maintaining consistent level at meals and snacks, and adjusting insulin as needed (requires close collaboration with physician)
Promote exercise program consistent with dietary and insulin regimen; increase carbohydrate intake before vigorous activities	Aids in the utilization of dietary intake, regular activity may reduce amount of insulin required; a decrease in insulin and increased carbohydrate intake before vigorous exercise or activity may prevent hypoglycemia

Interventions	Rationales
Assess for signs and symptoms of hypoglycemia, blood glucose level	Provides information about episodes of hypoglycemia resulting from increased activity without additional food intake or omission or incomplete ingestion of meals, incorrect insulin administration, illness
Provide rest and immediate source of a simple carbohydrate such as honey, milk, or fruit juice followed by a complex carbohydrate such as bread in amounts of 15 Gm; repeat intake in 10 minutes for expected response of a reduced pulse rate; administer IV 50 percent glucose or glucagon IM if hypoglycemia is severe	Alleviates the symptoms of hypoglycemia as soon as symptoms are noted; glucagon releases the glycogen stored in the liver to assist in restoring glucose levels; IV glucose is administered when condition is severe and child is unable to take glucose source PO. Glucagon, a hormone, releases stored glycogen from the liver and raises blood glucose in 5-15 minutes

Information, Instruction, Demonstration

Interventions	Rationales
Inform parent(s) and child of signs and symptoms to note, reasons why they occur, and importance of interventions to correct the complication	Provides information about abnormal blood glucose levels causing complications of hyperglycemia, hypoglycemia, and the consequences
Inform parent(s) and child of regulating insulin, dietary intake, and exercising to accommodate needs of individual child	Maintains child's growth and development needs while preventing complications
Instruct parent(s) and child to adjust insulin administration based on blood glucose testing and glycosuria, during an illness or after changes in food intake or activities	Prevents and/or treats hyperglycemia; avoids serious complication of ketoacidosis
Instruct parent(s) and child to administer a quick-acting carbohydrate followed by a longer-acting	Prevents and/or treats hypoglycemia

Interventions	Rationales
carbohydrate and to have Lifesavers, sugar cubes, Insta-glucose on hand at all times; instruct parent(s) that, in the case of severe hypoglycemia, if the child is unconscious or unable to take oral fluids, to rub honey or syrup on the child's buccal glucose until alert enough to take fluids/foods by mouth	
Inform parent(s) and child to report erratic blood and urine test results, difficulty in controlling blood glucose levels, presence of an infection or illness	Prevents more serious complications and long-term effects of the disease; poor control leads to serious and severe consequences in a few hours

Discharge or Maintenance Evaluation

- Maintains blood glucose level of less than 120 mg/dl or more than 60 mg/dl
- Absence of blood ketones and urine acetone
- Absence of signs and symptoms of hyperglycemia or hypoglycemia
- Provides and complies with medical regimen to maintain growth and development and to control severe blood glucose fluctuations
- Verbalizes causes and measures to take to prevent complications

Knowledge deficit of parent(s), child

Related to: Lack of information about disease
Defining characteristics: New diagnosis of IDDM; request for information about pathology, insulin therapy, dietary requirements, activity/exercise needs, blood and urine testing, personal hygiene and health promotion

Outcome Criteria

Demonstration of procedures included in medical regimen for diabetes
Progressive management of the disease by the child if appropriate

Interventions	Rationales
Assess parent(s) and child for knowledge of disease and reliability in performing procedures and care, for educational level and learning capacity, and for developmental level	Provides information needed to plan teaching program; children 8-10 years of age may be able to take responsibility for some of the care
Inform of cause of disease, disease process and pathology; use pamphlets and other aids appropriate for age of child and level of comprehension of parent(s)	Provides basic information that may be used as a rationale for treatments and care and allows for different teaching strategies
Provide a quiet, comfortable environment; allow time for teaching small amounts at a time and for reinforcement, demonstrations and return demonstrations; start teaching 1 day following diagnosis and limit sessions to 30-60 minutes	Prevents distractions and facilitates learning
Include as many family members in teaching sessions as possible	Promotes understanding and support of family and feeling of security for child
Instruct parent(s) and child in insulin administration including storing insulin, drawing up insulin into syringe, rotating vial instead of shaking, drawing clear insulin first if mixing 2 types in same syringe, injecting SC, rotating sites, adjusting dosages, reusing syringe and needle, and disposing of them	Promotes accurate administration of insulin, which prevents complications
Instruct in use of syringe-loaded injector	Provides temporary method of insulin administration if child is afraid to puncture skin
Instruct parent(s) and child in operation and use of a portable insulin pump to adjust insulin delivery	Provides continuous subcutaneous insulin infusion

Interventions	Rationales
Instruct parent(s) and child in collection and testing of blood for glucose done 4 times a day (before meals and before bed), with a lancet and blood-testing meter or a reagent strip compared to a color chart; collection and testing of urine with ketostix or Clinitest	Monitors glucose and ketone levels in blood and urine
Instruct parent(s) and child in dietary planning with emphasis on proper meal times and adequate caloric intake according to age; offer food lists for free foods and exchanges according to the basic four groups and assist in preparing sample menus; inform that food intake depends on activity, and describe methods to judge amounts of foods; provide list of acceptable food items from "fast food" restaurants, published by the ADA	Provides information about an important aspect of total care of the child with diabetes according to the American Diabetic Association guidelines
Inform parent(s) and child of role of exercise and alterations needed in food and insulin intake with increased or decreased activity	Provides information about usual activity pattern and effect on dietary intake and insulin needs
Inform parent(s) and child of skin problems associated with diabetes, need for regular dental examinations, foot care, protection of and proper care of nails, prevention of infections and exposure to infections, eye examinations, immunizations	Provides information about common problems resulting from long-term effects of the disease
Instruct parent(s) and child of record keeping for insulin, test results, responses to diet and exercise, noncompliance in medical regimen and effects	Provides a method to enhance self-care and demonstrates the need to notify physician for treatment evaluation and possible change

Interventions	Rationales
Inform parent(s) and child to wear or carry identification and information about the disease, treatment, and physician	Provides information in event of emergency

Discharge or Maintenance Evaluation

- Complies with medical regimen to control diabetes
- Prevents complications of diabetes
- Demonstrates correct insulin, dietary, and exercise procedures and interventions
- Promotes personal hygiene and health
- Verbalizes understanding of information and instructions to manage total care
- Facilitates self-care by maintaining accurate daily record
- Recognizes importance of compliance with medical regimen
- Maintains identification information at all times
- Utilizes the American Diabetic Association and other community agencies for information and support

Ineffective family coping: Compromised

Related to: Inadequate or incorrect information or understanding, prolonged disease or disability progression that exhausts the physical and emotional supportive capacity of caretakers
Defining characteristics: Expression and/or confirmation of concern and inadequate knowledge about long-term care needs, problems and complications, anxiety and guilty, overprotection of child

Outcome Criteria

Adequate knowledge regarding long-term therapy and interdisciplinary approach to treatment

Interventions	Rationales
Assess family coping methods and effectiveness, family interactions and expectations related to long-term care, developmental level of family, response of siblings, knowl-	Identifies coping methods that work and the need to develop new coping skills and behaviors, family attitudes; child with special long-term needs may strengthen or strain family

Interventions	Rationales
edge and use of support systems and resources, presence of guilt and anxiety, overprotection and/or overindulgence behaviors	relationships, and that overprotection may be detrimental to child's growth and development (e.g., not allowing child to attend school or participate in peer activities; avoiding discipline of child; and not allowing child to assume responsibilities for care)
Encourage family members and child to express problem areas, anxiety and explore solutions responsibly	Reduces anxiety and enhances understanding; provides family an opportunity to identify problems and develop problem-solving strategies
Assist family to establish short- and long-term goals for child and to integrate child into family activities, include participation of all family members in care routines	Promotes involvement in and control over situations and maintains role of family members and parent(s)
Provide assistance of social worker, counselor, clergy, or other as needed	Provides support to the family faced with long-term care of child with a chronic illness
Suggest community agencies and contact with the American Diabetic Association or other families with a diabetic child	Provides information and support to child and family
Allow family members to express feelings, to tell how they deal with the chronic needs of family member, and to describe coping patterns that help or hinder adjustment to the problems	Allows for venting of feelings to determine need for information and support and to relieve guilt and anxiety

Information, Instruction, Demonstration

Interventions	Rationales
Inform family of requested and needed information regarding long-term care and treatments	Enhances family understanding of medical regimen and responsibilities of family

Interventions	Rationales
Inform family that overprotective behavior may hinder growth and development so they should treat child as normally as possible	Promotes understanding of importance of making child one of the family and demonstrates the adverse effects of overprotection of the child
Discuss importance of follow-up appointments for physical examinations, laboratory tests	Promotes positive outcome when family collaborates with the physician and health team to monitor disease

Discharge or Maintenance Evaluation

- Verbalizes and clarifies child's and family's knowledge about long-term needs and care
- Develops and uses coping skills and problem solving techniques effectively
- Family members provide support and care for child while meeting own needs
- Family relationships preserved and family stressors minimized; with differences resolved
- Progressive adaptation and acceptance by family of chronic condition and therapy
- Implements preventative measures of follow-up care to ensure optimal function and health of child

Diabetes Mellitus (IDDM)

Viral infection
↓
Mumps
Varicella
Measles
Rubella
Viral and bacterial pneumonia

Genetic factor
(Autosomal recessive)
↓

Autoimmune factors
↓
Thyroiditis
Addison's disease
Humoral antibody response
or
lymphocyte response

Reduction in beta cells of pancreas
Reduction and fibrosis of islets
Lymphocytic infiltration
↓
Absolute lack or deficiency of insulin
↓
Inability of glucose to enter muscle and fat cells
Inability to store glucose as glycogen
in the liver and muscle
Inability to metabolize glucose to produce energy
↓
Depletion of fat and protein stores
↓

Complications

Commons manifestations

Long-term effects
↓
Renal changes
↓
Retinopathy
Microangiopathy
Atherosclerosis
Polyneuropathy

Hypoglycemia
↓
Reaction to
insulin
↓
Increased act-
ivity without
enough food
intake
↓
Weakness
Nervousness
Sweating
Hunger
Palpitations

Carbohydrate
source
(milk or fruit
juice, candy or
sugar cube)

Ketoacidosis
↓
Inadequate
insulin
↓
Metabolism
of fats
↓
Ketone
production
increased by liver
with decreased
renal excretion
↓
Hyperglycemia
Lethargy
Vomiting

Abdominal pain
Metabolic acidosis
↓
Insulin
administration

Polyuria
Polyphagia
Polydipsia
Hyperglycemia
Glycosuria
Weight loss

Hypothyroidism

Hypothyroidism is the result of thyroid hormone production which is inadequate to maintain body processes. It may be the result of congenital thyroid abnormality and therefore present in infancy or it may become notable during the first two years of life. It appears later when production is inadequate to maintain body processes as rapid growth increases the need for hormones. Acquired causes of the condition may be thyrotoxicosis, thyroidectomy, irradiation, infections, and dietary deficiency of iodine. Secretions of the thyroid gland include thyroid hormone (thyroxine, T4 and triiodothyronine, T3) and thyrocalcitonin, which are bound to proteins in the blood (thyroxine-binding globulin, TBG) and thyrocalcitonin (maintains calcium levels in blood). The hormones are controlled by the thyroid-stimulating hormone (TSH) which is secreted by the anterior pituitary gland. Treatment of the deficiency is thyroid hormone replacement, which involves prompt intervention in the infant and gradual by increasing amounts of hormone administration in the child. Treatment is maintained throughout life to ensure restoration of thyroid deficiency. Hypothyroidism in infants accounts for one-third of diagnosed cases and, in children, accounts for two-thirds of cases.

MEDICAL CARE

Hormones: levothyroxine sodium (Synthroid) given PO as replacement therapy for diminished or absent thyroid function; may be given IV for rapid replacement as in an infant with severe symptoms.
Vitamins: calcitriol (Recaltrol) given PO as vitamin D to ensure calcium levels during growth periods of growth requiring increased demands.
Thyroid hormones: T3 (triodothyronine), T4 (thyroxine), TBG (thyroxine-binding globulin), TSH (thyroid-stimulating hormone) by RIA (radioimmunoassay testing) reveals decreases indicating hormone deficiency.
Protein-bound iodine: reveals increases after 2 months of age.
Bone x-ray: reveals bone age and effect of thyroid deficiency or treatment.
Scan: reveals presence of gland with location, size, and shape of the organ; radioactive iodine uptake by thyroid gland is scanned and displayed on a screen for examination.

NURSING CARE PLANS
Essential nursing diagnoses and plans associated with this condition:

Risk for impaired skin integrity (397)
Related to: Internal factor of altered metabolic state (hypothyroidism)
Defining characteristics: Skin pale, cool, dry, and scaly

Altered nutrition: Less than body requirements (168)
Related to: Inability to ingest or digest food; decreased body processes
Defining characteristics: Poor feeding, choking, thick tongue in infant; lethargy, reduced metabolic process, anorexia in child

Constipation (173)
Related to: Less than adequate physical activity, decreased body process
Defining characteristics: Lethargy, decreased peristalsis, fatigue, reduced activity level

SPECIFIC DIAGNOSES AND CARE PLANS
Knowledge deficit of parent(s), child
Related to: Lack of information about disorder
Defining characteristics: Request for information about cause and treatment of the disorder, thyroid replacement

Outcome Criteria
Adequate knowledge of disease and compliance with medication regimen
Absence of signs and symptoms of hypothyroidism

Interventions	Rationales
Assess knowledge of disorder, signs and symptoms for infant or child as appropriate, replacement therapy	Provides information needed to develop plan of instruction to ensure compliance with medical regimen

Interventions	Rationales
Inform parent(s) and child of cause of thyroid deficiency and need for prompt treatment in infants and for gradual increases in thyroxine in children to achieve euthyroidism	Provides thyroid replacement over 4-8 weeks in the child without causing hyperthyroidism
Instruct parent(s) and child in thyroid replacement including administering daily for life without missing doses, crushing and mixing with food, giving at breakfast time	Ensures compliance with correct administration of thyroid via oral route
Inform parent(s) and child to report nervousness, irritability, tachycardia, diarrhea	Indicates an excess of thyroid hormone and need for and adjustment in dosage
Inform parent(s) and child that improvement will be gradual as hormone levels are achieved and sleep, elimination, appetite, growth, and activity levels will improve	Promotes comfort and reduces anxiety caused by physical and mental changes brought about by the disorder; maintains realistic expectations from the treatment
Inform parent(s) that periodic laboratory tests are needed to monitor therapy	Inform physician of thyroid levels maintained at a therapeutic level

Discharge or Maintenance Evaluation

- Euthyroidism achieved
- Absence of signs and symptoms of hyperthyroidism
- Complies with daily thyroid replacement regimen
- Complies with periodic monitoring and follow-up care

Hypothyroidism

Congenital factor   Acquired factor

Deficiency of thyroid hormone
Deficiency of thyroid stimulating hormone

Decreased body processes
Decreased energy metabolism
Decreased growth rate if acquired at young age
Mental sluggishness, sleepiness
Skin changes (dry, puffy)

Thyroid hormone replacement
(thyroxine)

Resolution

Eye, Ear, Nose, Throat

Eye, Ear, Nose, Throat

The eye, ear, nose, and throat is a group affecting special organs that include eye, (vision), ear (hearing), nose, throat. Common disorders of these organs in children include chronic infections and the surgical procedures to correct them. Other conditions affecting these organs are included in the Neurologic System.

GENERAL EYE/EAR/NOSE/THROAT CHANGES ASSOCIATED WITH PHYSICAL GROWTH AND DEVELOPMENT

EENT changes in structure and function are found in the Neurologic and Respiratory Systems

Allergic Rhinitis

Allergic rhinitis is an episodic or perennial upper respiratory tract condition characterized by sneezing, itching nose and eyes, and discharge from the nose and throat. Chronic nasal stuffiness and obstruction to air flow cause mouth breathing, otitis media, and eustachian tube abnormalities. Allergic rhinitis may manifest itself at any age in childhood.

MEDICAL CARE

Antihistamines (H1 receptor antagonist): trimeprazine tartrate (Temaril) given PO alone or in combination with a decongestant for nasal congestion and cough.
Antihistamines (phenothiazine derivatives): promethazine hydrochloride (Phenergan) given PO to prevent action of histamine, which provides relief from allergic conditions.
Decongestants: phenylephrine (Neo-Synephrine) as nose drops or spray for older infants (over 6 months) and children; pseudoephedrine (PediaCare, Sudafed) given PO for children over 2 years of age to relieve nasal congestion and clear passages; nose drops reduce swelling by vasoconstriction resulting from topical application.
Antiasthmatics: cromolyn sodium (Intel) given by inhalation to inhibit release of histamine, thereby suppressing allergic response; used as prophylaxis to allergic response during sensitive seasons.
Topical nasal corticosteroids: (fluticasone propionate) by inhalation is an alternative to cromolyn sodium to decrease reactivity on a short-term basis during exacerbation.
Skin tests: identifies allergic responses and sensitivities to antigens as a basis for desensitization therapy.
Nasal culture: reveals presence of eosinophils.
Biopsy of nasal mucous membrane: reveals eosinophils and abnormal mucosa.
RAST test: reveals and measures the immunoglobulin.

NURSING CARE PLANS

Essential nursing diagnoses and plans associated with this condition:

Ineffective breathing pattern (45)

Related to: Inflammatory process, obstruction
Defining characteristics: Nasal stuffiness and obstruction, mouth breathing, mucus secretion and drainage, respiratory changes, breathing difficulty

Sleep pattern disturbance (114)

Related to: Internal factors of illness
Defining characteristics: Interrupted sleep, irritability, restlessness, inability to breathe through nose

SPECIFIC DIAGNOSES AND CARE PLANS

Risk for infection

Related to: Chronic disease (allergy), insufficient knowledge to avoid exposure to pathogens
Defining characteristics: Nasal discharge; red, itchy conjunctive; purulent discharge from nose or eyes; allergic shiners (dark areas under eyes), frequent colds, otitis media with pain and temperature elevation; pharyngitis

Outcome Criteria

Absence of infectious process in eyes, ears, or upper respiratory tract
Precautions taken to prevent infectious process

Interventions	Rationales
Assess for rubbing of nose, nasal discharge and its characteristics (clear, amount, purulent), dark areas around eye, nose itching and pushing hand up and back of nose, frequent sneezing, red and itchy eyes and drainage or watering	Provides information about physical and behavioral effects of allergic rhinitis; chronic nasal obstruction causes edema and discoloration of the eyes and mouth breathing, wrinkling of face is caused by attempt to avoid rubbing or scratching of nose
Inspect nasal passages and throat with penlight for redness, swelling, and presence of mucus and/or exudate; check skin around nares for redness, irritation	Reveals inflammation and risk of infection spread
Assess for knowledge and use of preventative measures needed to avoid spread of microorganisms	Provides basis for information needed for health maintenance

Interventions	Rationales
Assess for knowledge and use of preventative measures needed to avoid spread of microorganisms	Provides basis for information needed for health maintenance
Assess for frequency of upper respiratory infections among family members; attendance at school, day-care, nursery school	Persistent reinfection usually the result of repeated exposures to microorganisms
Assess use of over-the-counter medications and type used	Combination products are not particularly useful; symptomatic treatment more effective in controlling upper respiratory responses; over-use of some medications may cause undesirable side effects (drowsiness) or rebound effects (return of symptoms)
Provide vaporizer or humidifier if nasal and oral mucous membranes are dry	Maintains moist mucous membranes to prevent breaks and soreness
Administer antihistamines and immunotherapy if ordered alone or in combination with decongestants	Provides control of the symptoms when exposed to allergens

Information, Instruction, Demonstration

Interventions	Rationales
Handwashing technique after exposure to nasopharyngeal secretions (sneezing, blowing nose)	Hands found to be most common carrier of microorganisms
Instruct in disposal of tissues used for cough or nose wiping	Prevents transmission of microorganisms
Inform to avoid contact with infected people or family members, although transmission commonly occurs in families, schools, nursery schools, recreational gatherings	Prevents exposure to the infectious agent, although isolation is not realistic within a family

Interventions	Rationales
Instruct parent(s) in administration of medications via oral and inhalation routes	Ensures compliance with medication regimen to control symptoms and prevent infection
Instruct to administer all of the antibiotic prescribed for infection (if present), and explain consequences of incorrect administration	Ensures effective treatment of bacterial infection for prompt response within 24 hours after antibiotic administration
Instruct in desensitization injection schedule, and inform child that the treatments will make him/her feel better	Allays child's anxiety and fear caused by injections
Instruct parent(s) in measures to control environment (air conditioning; removal of dust, pets, smoke)	Supports environment free of allergens or irritants that cause attacks
Inform to notify physician if the temperature increases, ear hurts, throat is sore or nose has purulent drainage	Allows for immediate interventions to treat at complications

Discharge or Maintenance Evaluation

- Demonstrates proper disposal of materials contaminated with respiratory secretions
- Demonstrates proper handwashing technique
- Protects from exposure to upper respiratory infections
- Correctly administers full course of antibiotic
- Complies with desensitization schedule
- Maintains an allergen-free environment
- Reports signs and symptoms of impending or existing infectious process
- Relieves allergic rhinitis symptoms with prescribed antihistamines, decongestants, steroid administration by oral spray or inhalation route

Allergic Rhinitis

Allergic reactions

↓

Environmental inhalants

↓

Pets
Dust
Pollens
Mold
Cold air

↓

Enters respiratory tract

↓

IgE antibody production

↓

Antigen-antibody reaction

↓

Mast cell mediators released

↓

Inflammation

↓

Sneezing, nasal stuffiness, and polyps
Secretion, mucus, and postnasal drainage
Pale, boggy nasal mucosa
Itchy eyes, nose, pharynx
Red, swollen conjunctiva with drainage
Desensitization
Removal of allergens from environment

Otitis Media/ Myringotomy and Insertion of Tube

Otitis media, the most common disease of childhood, is a viral or bacterial infection of the middle ear. It is primarily due to a dysfunction of one or both eustachian tubes. The eustachian tube, located between the nasopharynx and the middle ear, drains, ventilates and protects the middle ear. Obstruction of the eustachian tube (usually from inflammation due to a pharyngitis or allergy) causes accumulation of secretions in the middle ear and negative pressure from lack of ventilation. The negative pressure pulls fluid into the middle ear from surrounding tissues. This results in otitis media with effusion (OME). Contamination of the middle ear occurs when reflex, aspiration or insufflation (by crying, sneezing or nose blowing) forces organisms into the middle ear through the eustachian tube. Organisms frequently responsible for middle ear infections are Streptococcus pneumoniae, Haemophilus influenzae, Staphylococcus aureus, and Moraxella catarrhalis. Middle ear infections can be acute (AOM) or chronic. Complications of OM include hearing loss (from effusion and/or scarring of the tympanic membrane), mastoiditis and meningitis. Myringotomy is a surgical procedure performed to equalize middle ear pressure by inserting tubes into the tympanic membrane to facilitate drainage. The tympanostomy tubes remain in place about 6 months, at which time they spontaneously fall out. The procedure prevents fluid retention in the middle ear, promotes healing of the membrane, and prevents scarring of the membrane.

MEDICAL CARE

Antipyretics/Analgesics: acetaminophen (Tylenol tablets, Pedric wafers or elixir, Liquiprin solution drops) given PO to reduce fever and/or for ear pain.

Antibiotics: Amoxicillin PO or erythromycin (Ilosone tablets, chewables, suspension or drops) PO if allergic to penicillin; sulfonamides, trimethoprim-sulfamethoxazole (Bactrim, Septra) PO; erythromycin-sulfisoxazole (Pediazole) PO; cephalosporins (Suprax, Ceclor) PO; or single-dose drugs such as cephalosporin ceftriaxone (Rocephin) IM.

Decongestants: Phenylephrine (Neo-Synephrine) as nose drops or spray for older infants (over 6 months and children), pseudoephedrine (PediaCare, Sudafed) PO for children over 2 years of age to relieve nasal congestion and clear passages; topical application of nose drops reduce swelling by vasoconstriction.

Acoustic reflectometry: reveals canal length measurement and presence of effusion.

Tympanometry: reveals compliance of the tympanic membrane or stiffness in the presence of effusion.

Audiometry: reveals hearing loss and severity if present; may be an air or bone conduction audiogram.

NURSING CARE PLANS

Essential nursing diagnoses and plans associated with the conditions:

Hyperthermia (112)

Related to: Illness (inflammation)
Defining characteristics: Increase in body temperature above normal range; flushed skin, warm to touch; increased pulse and respiration rate

Altered nutrition: Less than body requirements (168)

Related to: Inability to ingest food
Defining characteristics: Anorexia, vomiting

Risk for fluid volume deficit (222)

Related to: Excessive losses through normal routes
Defining characteristics: Vomiting, diarrhea, diaphoresis, elevated temperature, altered intake

SPECIFIC DIAGNOSES AND CARE PLANS

Pain

Related to: Biological injuring agents (infection)
Defining characteristics: Communication of pain descriptors: red tympanic membrane, irritability, pulling on ear, earache, tilting of the head, cough, drainage from ear

Outcome Criteria

Absence of relief of ear pain

Interventions	Rationales
Assess verbal and nonverbal behavior, type and location and severity; use a pain scale and include irritability, fever, pulling at ear, red, bulging tympanic membrane, in the infant; as for child; anorexia and earache, fever, cough, congestion, drainage from ear, temporary change in auditory acuity, red, bulging tympanic membrane	Provides information about pain and manifestations that vary with age
Administer analgesic, antipyretic, and antibiotic as ordered	Reduces pain and fever; destroys cell and wall of bacterial agents to decrease infectious process; usually given for 10 days
Promote rest and avoid disturbing unnecessarily	Promotes rest and reduces stimuli that increase pain
Apply dry heat or cold to affected ear based on pain relief and comfort achievement	Facilitates drainage if heat is applied; reduces edema and pressure if cold is applied
Cleanse external canal with cotton ball and hydrogen peroxide if needed	Provides drainage removal from ear without introducing pathogens
Place child in lying position on side with affected ear	Promotes drainage from the affected ear

Information, Instruction, Demonstration

Interventions	Rationales
Instruct parent(s) in an a analgesic/antipyretic medication administration and antibiotic therapy; inform to maintain regularity of antibiotic and to complete administration of all of the medication; explain form, route, dosage, and side effects of medications	Promotes compliance with medication regimen even though child feels better after 1-2 days of antibiotic administration

Interventions	Rationales
Instruct parent(s) to clean external canal of drainage with cotton ball and not to allow water to enter ear canal; gently pat dry	Prevents introduction of contaminated water or swabs

Discharge or Maintenance Evaluation

- Complies with medication administration regimen
- Maintains comfort and rest needs for child
- Controls ear pain

Knowledge deficit of parent(s), child

Related to: Lack of information about condition
Defining characteristics: Request for information about cause of condition, prevention of reinfection, postoperative care for myringotomy and tube insertion

Outcome Criteria

Verbalization of knowledge and understanding of follow-up care with tubes in place and how to prevent recurrent infections

Interventions	Rationales
Assess past infections, knowledge of ear condition and treatments to prevent complications, and knowledge of surgical procedure to insert tubes that provide drainage of middle ear	Provides information needed by parent(s) about infection
Inform parent(s) of causes of otitis media in infant and child and of tendency for repeated infections depending on age group	Provides information about physiological aspects of the ear canal and frequent upper respiratory infections that lead to ear obstruction and infection
Inform parent(s) to feed infant in upright position, to discourage forceful blowing of nose in child, and to encourage gum chewing and blowing games	Preventative measures to control ear infections and promote aeration of the middle ear

Interventions	Rationales
Reinforce teaching of antibiotic therapy for 10 days to 2 weeks	Ensures that infection has been eradicated
Inform parent(s) that hearing acuity is diminished temporarily during acute stage, and to face child and speak clearly at close proximity to communicate with child	Reduces anxiety of parent(s) when child does not respond to words spoken to them
Inform of surgical procedure to place tubes in the middle ear that drain area in back of tympanic membrane and equalize pressure; that tubes remain for 6 months to 1 year, eventually falling out without further interventions	Informs parent(s) of procedure to promote continuous drainage ventilation of ear and prevent further infections if condition is chronic or does not respond to traditional therapy
Instruct parent(s) and child in care of tubes following surgery, including keeping water (bath, swimming, etc.) and shampoo out of ear; maintaining dry ear wick that is placed in ear; cleansing area and applying zinc oxide or Vaseline to the area if draining and excoriating skin	Prevents entry of water or contaminated substances into ear canal or via tubes, and maintains skin integrity of the area by removing normal drainage for 1-2 days following surgery
Report any hearing impairment, pain behind ear, lethargy, increasing temperature, purulent drainage	Allows for immediate interventions to prevent hearing loss, mastoid infection, or reinfection
Instruct child to avoid noseblowing, swimming, diving, or any activities that allow water to enter ear for 10 days; use ear plug if practical for bathing or swimming	Informs child of actions to take to prevent disruption

Discharge or Maintenance Evaluation

- Prevents reinfection of middle ear with compliance with medical regimen
- Avoids activities that expose infected middle ear or ear with tube placement to risk of infection

- Complies with postoperative care for tube insertion as instructed
- Takes measures to prevent reinfection
- Verbalizes surgical procedure and postoperative care for tube insertion (myringotomy)

Otitis Media/Myringotomy

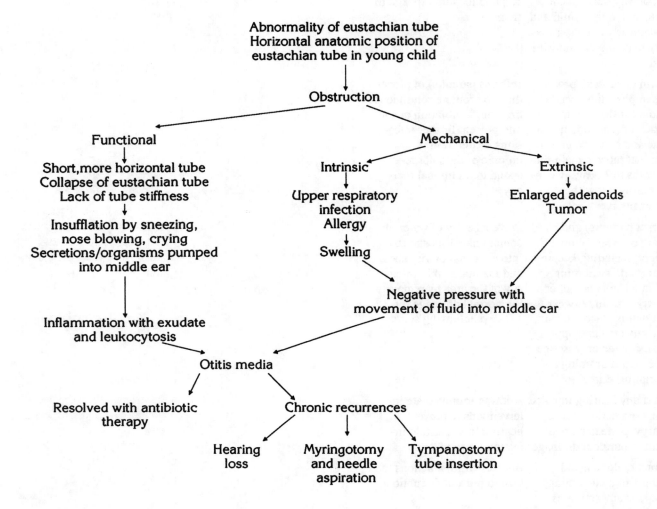

Abnormality of eustachian tube
Horizontal anatomic position of
eustachian tube in young child

Obstruction

Functional

Short, more horizontal tube
Collapse of eustachian tube
Lack of tube stiffness

Insufflation by sneezing,
nose blowing, crying
Secretions/organisms pumped
into middle ear

Inflammation with exudate
and leukocytosis

Mechanical

Intrinsic

Upper respiratory
infection
Allergy

Swelling

Extrinsic

Enlarged adenoids
Tumor

Negative pressure with
movement of fluid into middle car

Otitis media

Resolved with antibiotic
therapy

Chronic recurrences

Hearing
loss

Myringotomy
and needle
aspiration

Tympanostomy
tube insertion

Strabismus

Strabismus, sometimes known as "cross eye," is non-binocular vision in which one eye deviates from the point of fixation. The weaker eye becomes lazy, and the brain eventually suppresses the image in the eye. Strabismus is caused by muscle paralysis or imbalance, poor vision, or congenital factors. Correction may be nonsurgical, or if that is unsuccessful, surgical, to align the eyes. Left undiagnosed and untreated, strabismus may lead to amblyopia and vision loss.

MEDICAL CARE

Corneal light reflex test: reveals malalignment of eyes if present.
Cover test: reveals movement of the uncovered eye, indicating malalignment.

NURSING CARE PLANS

Essential nursing diagnoses and plans associated with this condition:

Altered growth and development (423)

Related to: Perceptual impairment (vision)
Defining characteristics: Reported, measured, or observed impairment of visual acuity; change in behavior pattern; change in response to stimuli; visual distortions

SPECIFIC DIAGNOSES AND CARE PLANS

Knowledge deficit

Related to: Lack of information about condition and treatment
Defining characteristics: Request for information about abnormal eye deviation and treatments to prevent complication and preserve vision

Outcome Criteria

Adequate knowledge of condition, cause, measures to prevent complication

Maintenance of treatment interventions to preserve vision as instructed

Interventions	Rationales
Assess visual acuity using Snellen chart, cover test, or Hirschberg test depending on age of child; note obvious deviations and direction of deviation	Provides screening for visual deficit and muscle balance or deviation
Inform child to note diplopia, headache, photophobia, inability to see clearly or focus from one distance to another; parent(s) to note frowning or squinting eyes together, tilting head to one side, closing one eye to see	Indicates strabismus and behavior changes associated with it
Inform parent(s) that the condition results from a weakness or paralysis of the eye muscle(s) or that the child may have been born with the defect; that condition is treated with prescription glasses, occlusion patching of the good eye, or surgery to prevent amblyopia, which leads to vision loss	Identifies cause of the disorder for the parent(s) and suggests possible treatments to correct the condition
Instruct parent(s) and child in eye-patching treatment to improve use and function of the affected eye: apply patch to good eye for 8 weeks, or 1 week for each year of child's age, and do not remove it except to stimulate good eye	Promotes use of the deviated eye by patching good eye
Instruct parent(s) and child about wearing glasses and caring for the glasses, including cleansing with soft cloth or tissue, keeping the glasses in a case when not wearing them, handling the glasses on the frame part when putting on or taking off and cleaning, using straps to keep glasses	Promotes correction with proper use of glasses

Interventions	Rationales
from falling off; allow child to assist in the selection of the glasses	
Instruct the child in eye exercises if ordered	Promotes muscle use and corrects deviation
Inform parent(s) and child of surgical procedure to preserve vision and improve appearance of the deviated eye, that medication will be given for pain, that eyes will be patched following surgery and restraints may be needed temporarily to prevent touching or rubbing eye, that some eye drainage will be present for 24 to 48 hours; use a doll and allow the child to play the situation to expect before and after surgery	Provides information if surgery is proposed to correct deviation rather than restore vision; therapeutic play informs the child of procedures to expect from surgery
Instruct parent(s) in administration of eye drops and/or application of ophthalmic ointment as ordered	Provides information and procedure for correct administration of medications
Inform parent(s) and child of importance of performing procedures and therapies as instructed and of making follow-up visits to ophthalmologist	Promotes compliance of corrective therapy

Discharge or Maintenance Evaluation

- Complies with prescribed therapy and procedures
- Administers medications correctly
- Performs proper use and care of glasses, patching of eye
- Verbalizes surgical procedure and responsibilities for cooperation
- Prevents complication from strabismus
- Adapts to body image change caused by eye appearance until eye is corrected
- Complies with ongoing follow-up physician visits and eye examinations

Strabismus

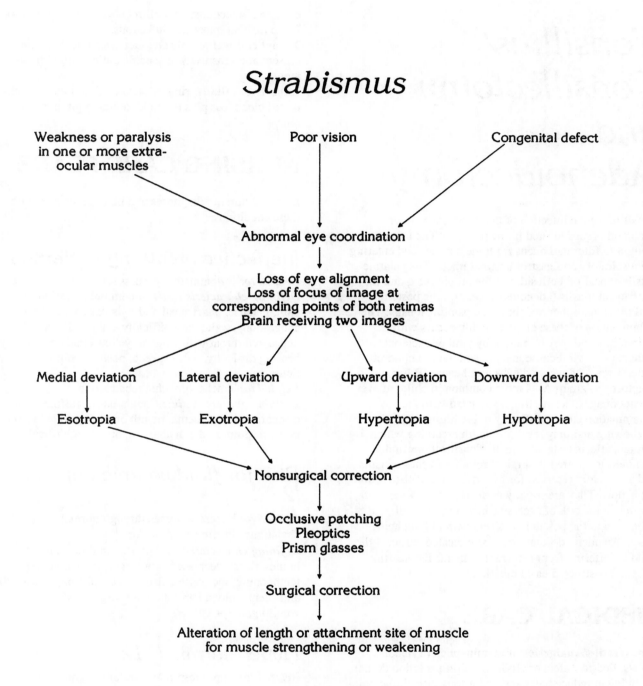

Weakness or paralysis in one or more extra-ocular muscles

Poor vision

Congenital defect

Abnormal eye coordination

Loss of eye alignment
Loss of focus of image at corresponding points of both retinas
Brain receiving two images

Medial deviation

Lateral deviation

Upward deviation

Downward deviation

Esotropia

Exotropia

Hypertropia

Hypotropia

Nonsurgical correction

Occlusive patching
Pleoptics
Prism glasses

Surgical correction

Alteration of length or attachment site of muscle
for muscle strengthening or weakening

Tonsillitis/ Tonsillectomy and Adenoidectomy

Tonsillitis is the infection of the tonsils, which are lymphoid organs located in the pharynx. The tonsils are thought to filter pathogens from the air and food entering the respiratory and gastrointestinal tracts. The palatine tonsils appear on both sides of the oropharynx, and the pharyugeal tonsils (adenoids) appear on the posterior wall of the nasopharynx above the palatine tonsils. The inflammation of these organs usually occurs with pharyngitis and may be caused by viral or bacterial pathogens. A viral cause is more common in children under 3 years of age, and a bacterial cause (B hemolytic streptococci, group A) is more common in children over 6 years of age. The swelling associated with the inflammation causes difficulty in breathing and swallowing and may result in mouth breathing which, if chronic, affects taste and smell. Tonsillectomy and adenoidectomy are the surgical removal of these organs and are usually reserved for hypertrophy and obstruction of air flow. They are usually performed after 4 years of age due to the risk of excessive bleeding in small children and the possibility of regrowth of lymphoid tissue. An adenoidectomy may be indicated earlier if the child is suffering from recurrent otitis media, hearing loss, and obstructed nasal breathing.

MEDICAL CARE

Antipyretics/Analgesics: acetaminophen (Tylenol tablets, Pedric wafers or elixir, Liquiprin solution drops) given PO to reduce fever and/or for tonsillitis throat pain; IV morphine in first 2 hours post-operative and acetaminophen with codeine, either liquid PO or rectal suppository after tonsillectomy.
Antibiotics: penicillin G potassium (Pentids solution) or ampicillin (Amcill suspension or pediatric drops) given PO; [erythromycin (Ilosone tablets, chewables, suspension, or drops) given PO if allergic to penicillins] or cefaclor (Ceclor suspension) given PO to treat streptococ-cal throat infections; penicillin G benzathine (Bicillin) IM to treat streptococcal infections.
Throat culture: reveals and identifies infectious agent if present and sensitivity to specific antimicrobial treatment.
Intravenous fluids: ringers lactate IV; 3 times the estimated blood loss plus the fluid deficit, after tonsillectomy.

NURSING CARE PLANS

Essential nursing diagnoses and plans associated with these conditions:

Ineffective breathing pattern (45)

Related to: Inflammatory process
Defining characteristics: Temperature elevation, throat pain, malaise, pharyngeal and tonsillar edema, head congestion, swallowing difficulty, enlarged cervical nodes, red throat with white or yellow exudate, lethargy, hearing difficulty, nasal speech, positive culture of infectious agent
Related to: Tracheobronchial obstruction
Defining characteristics: Cough, nasal stuffiness and discharge, throat edema, mouth breathing, rapid respirations, respiratory depth changes, breathing difficulty

Risk for fluid volume deficit (222)

Related to: Excessive losses through normal routes; deviations affecting fluid intake
Defining characteristics: Dry skin and mucous membranes, thirst, decreased skin turgor, increased body temperature, increased pulse rate, dysphagia, throat pain and edema, blood loss following surgery, NPO status, vomiting, dysphasia

Hyperthermia (112)

Related to: Upper respiratory inflammation/infection illness
Defining characteristics: Increase of body temperature above normal range, increased respiratory and pulse rates, flushed, hot skin, low grade fever in nasopharyngitis, higher temperature of 100°F or more in streptococcal pharyogitis and tonsillitis

SPECIFIC DIAGNOSES AND CARE PLANS

Risk for injury

Related to: Excessive bleeding at surgical site; airway obstruction from bleeding and/or swelling
Defining characteristics: Stridor, drooling, restlessness, agitation, increased respiratory rate, progressive cyanosis, pallor, frequent clearing of the throat, coughing, continuous swallowing, fresh blood in mouth or throat, and vomiting of bright red blood

Outcome Criteria

No excessive bleeding or airway obstruction occurs, or, if present, signs and symptoms are recognized early and treatment prevents any injury

Interventions	Rationales
Inspect throat for bleeding using a flashlight/penlight; inspect emesis for bright red blood, assess vital signs for increased pulse and respiratory rate and decreased BP; assess child for continuous swallowing or frequent coughing; notify physician immediately if signs of hemorrhage	Post-operative hemorrhage, although uncommon, is a serious complication; frequent assessment for the signs of hemorrhage in the first 24 hours post-op allows early intervention if necessary
Assess child for signs of respiratory distress (stridor, cyanosis, agitation, increased respiratory rate); suction mouth to remove excess secretions if necessary (avoid oropharynx); administer O$_2$ if in respiratory distress; notify physician	Bleeding and/or swelling may obstruct the airway; assessing for signs of respiratory distress allows early intervention; suctioning the oropharynx may cause further bleeding, so use caution
Place child on side or abdomen for first 24 hours	Promotes drainage of secretions and prevents pooling in oropharynx which may cause obstruction
Discourage child from clearing their throat or coughing	Coughing/throat clearing is irritating to the throat and may cause bleeding

Information, Instruction, Demonstration

Interventions	Rationales
Inform parent(s) and child that coughing, clearing the throat, placing hard objects in mouth (straws), vigorous tooth brushing or gargling should be avoided for two weeks and that drainage should be expectorated and not swallowed	Prevents irritation of operative site and reduces risk of bleeding
Inform parent(s) to assess child for bleeding 24-48 hours after surgery and again 72 hours later; instruct parent(s) to notify physician of any bleeding or difficulty breathing	Provides information parent(s) need to assess child for recovery; bleeding 7-14 days after surgery would be from tissue sloughing

Discharge or Maintenance Evaluation

- No fresh bleeding
- Airway is patent
- Vital signs are stable
- Parent(s) verbalize signs and symptoms of bleeding to report to physician after discharge

Pain

Related to: Injuring biological agent (inflammation/infection) and surgical intervention
Defining characteristics: Complaints of throat soreness, difficulty in swallowing, headache and muscle aches; crying; restlessness; listless; drooling; edema; bright red pus on tonsillar tissue; enlarged cervical nodes; postoperative pain in throat

Outcome Criteria

Pain reduced and controlled as throat inflammation subsides or as surgical site heals

Interventions	Rationales
Assess site of pain, verbal or nonverbal responses of holding or rubbing site of pain, irritability, pointing to site, restlessness, de-	Expression of pain varies with age, developmental level, and is unique to particular child and learned emotional responses;

Interventions	Rationales
pendent behaviors, crying, groaning, whining, stating of general location and severity of pain	degree of pain, fatigue influences ability of child to perceive and identify discomfort
Inspect throat for redness; swelling; presence of mucus or pus; examine dry, irritated oropharynx with a pen-light; note mouth breathing, lethargy halitosis, nasal speech, or hearing difficulty	Provides clues to source of pain and manifestations of tonsils and adenoids inflammation causing changes in breathing, taste, and smell perception as the enlarged adenoids block the air from passing behind the nares; this results in mouth breathing, dry mouth, and changes in voice sounds as the air unable to be trapped for speech results in a nasal or muffled sound
Assess postoperative pain in throat for severity, associated bleeding, and difficulty in swallowing	Provides information which forms basis for analgesic therapy, about pain caused by raw surfaces left by tonsillectomy
Assess effect on food and fluid intake, and effect on rest and sleep patterns as a result of throat pain and/or obstruction of passage of food, fluids, and air	Provides information about pain resulting from tonsillitis or tonsillectomy and associated manifestations of impaired swallowing and restlessness
Administer analgesic and/or antibiotic; for tonsillitis, inject IM antibiotic deeply into large muscle (vastus lateralis in young child, and gluteus in older child)	Analgesic relieves pain, and antibiotic destroys streptococcus by interfering with cell wall synthesis
Provide analgesic for postoperative pain: administer acetaminophen with codeine q4 hours PRN; liquid analgesic PO or suppository PR for young children or for those not tolerating the oral medication; nonpharmacologic pain-reduction interventions including ice collar, relaxation techniques, music therapy	Promotes continuous comfort and pain relief PO, IV, or rectally for about 24-48 hours postoperatively, and provides diversion from pain stimuli; ice promotes vasoconstriction, which reduces edema and pain

Interventions	Rationales
For tonsillitis, provide cool, mild fluids to drink, ice chips q2h, and soft foods to eat if child accepts food; hard candies to suck on or gum to chew; warm gargle for older child or throat irrigation for younger child; throat lozenges, if appropriate, for tonsillitis	Promotes comfort and maintain fluids, moistens and soothes throat by increasing saliva production; warm throat irrigation reduces inflammation in the younger child, and the older child may be able to gargle
Postoperatively provide cool, bland fluids 30-60 cc q hour, for 24 hours, followed by soft, bland foods; avoid irritating, highly seasoned, rough, solid foods or acidic or irritating fluids	Provides fluids and nutrients that do not irritate sore throat or aggravate surgical site and cause bleeding
Place on abdomen or side in position of comfort	Promotes comfort and rest, which reduce pain and allow for drainage

Information, Instruction, Demonstration

Interventions	Rationales
Inform parent(s) and child of cause of pain and length of time pain may persist (usually 24-48 hours after surgery or oral antibiotic administration, 2-3 days with an antibiotic IM injection)	Promotes understanding of pain response to gradual reduction as condition is resolved
Instruct parent(s) and child to ingest cool, mild fluids and avoid citrus juices; to ingest soft, bland foods and avoid raw, rough, seasoned foods; following surgery, to avoid milk, puddings, and ice cream, but to include gelatin, sherbet, soup, mashed potato	Prevents irritating throat and causing pain; milk products coat the throat and promote coughing which irritates the throat
Inform parent(s) that cool mist vaporizer may be used, gargle with warm water or use lozenges to relieve pain from tonsillitis	Prevents drying of mucous membranes and promotes comfort

Interventions	Rationales
(but to avoid these post-operatively as they may cause bleeding)	

Discharge or Maintenance Evaluation

- Verbalizes that pain is reduced or controlled
- Swallows allowed fluids and foods without discomfort
- Ingests sufficient fluid to prevent dehydration
- Provides both pharmacologic and nonpharmacologic relief measures to reduce pain
- Promotes rest and diversionary activities
- Avoids fluids and foods that increase throat pain

Knowledge deficit of parent(s), child

Related to: Lack of information about condition
Defining characteristics: Request for information about prevention and treatment for tonsillitis, and about pre- and post-operative care for tonsillectomy/adenoidectomy

Outcome Criteria

Verbalization of knowledge and understanding surgical procedure, care, and measures to prevent recurrent throat infections

Interventions	Rationales
Assess frequency of tonsillitis, knowledge of treatment; knowledge of surgical procedure to remove tonsils and adenoids and prognosis	Provides information about infection and surgery if contemplated
Inform parent(s) of causes of recurrent infections, need for surgery, procedure performed, and pre-operative preparation	Reduces anxiety caused by lack of information and not knowing what to expect
Explain importance of having throat culture done if sore throat and temperature present; instruct in administration of analgesic, antipyretic, and antibiotic as prescribed, all of medication should be taken, even though child feels better in 24-48 hours	Identifies bacterial infection of throat that will respond to antibiotic therapy

Interventions	Rationales
Inform parent(s) and child that medication will be given for pain; that IV will be given for pain fluid maintenance, as needed, for 24 hours; that throat will be observed for bleeding; and that some secretions, bleeding, and possibly vomiting is not uncommon	Provides information about postoperative treatments
Reinforce instruction in which type of foods and fluid to take and which to avoid, and to position on side when asleep and upright when eating or drinking; instruct in diet progression as pain and discomfort subside	Prevents irritation to throat and aspiration of drainage, food or fluids
Inform parent(s) and child that ear pain, slight temperature, and mouth odor may occur postoperatively; and to report persistent temperature	Assures parent(s) that these occur as a result of surgery and only need reporting if they persist
Inform parent(s) and child that limited activities and school attendance are usually resumed 2 weeks after surgery but that child should be kept quiet and indoors for 2 days following surgery	Provides information about return to normal parameters by 3 weeks postoperatively

Discharge or Maintenance Evaluation

- Prevents reinfection of throat with correct compliance with medication regimen
- Avoids activities that irritate or cause risk of complication following surgery
- Complies with postoperative care for fluid, food, rest, activity regimen
- Verbalizes surgical procedure and postoperative measures
- Reports severe and/or persistent symptoms of tonsillitis or postoperative complications
- Secures throat culture if ordered

Tonsillitis/Tonsillectomy

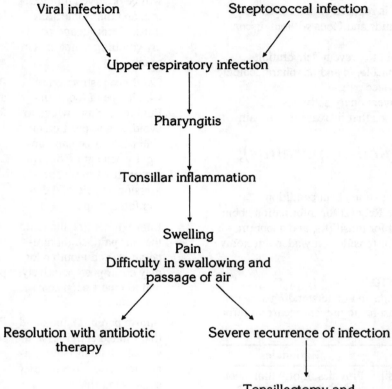

Viral infection   Streptococcal infection

Upper respiratory infection

Pharyngitis

Tonsillar inflammation

Swelling
Pain
Difficulty in swallowing and
passage of air

Resolution with antibiotic
therapy

Severe recurrence of infection

Tonsillectomy and
adenoidectomy

Integumentary System

Integumentary System

The integumentary system includes the skin and associated structures or appendages, which are hair, nails, and sensory skin receptors. Skin acts as a barrier to retain body fluids and electrolytes, a regulator of body heat, and a receptor of sensory stimuli (tactile, pain, heat and cold). It is made up of three layers including the epidermis (outer layer), and the dermis (thicker layer directly under the epidermis), and the subcutaneous (fat and connective tissue under the dermis). Its appearance reflects the general health of an infant or child. Changes in the skin that alter appearance are a source of psychological stress and embarrassment to children. Common integumentary conditions of childhood are infections, lesions, wounds, and dermatitis disorders.

GENERAL INTEGUMENTARY CHANGES ASSOCIATED WITH PHYSICAL GROWTH AND DEVELOPMENT

Integumentary component structure and function

- Skin is 1 mm thick at birth and increases to twice this thickness by maturity
- Perspiration is present in the child over 1 month of age
- Lanugo disappears by 3 months of age
- Hair is soft and fine in texture in the young child and takes on adult characteristics with growth
- Nails are soft in infant and young child and become hardened with growth and development
- Pubic and axillary hair appear between 8-12 years of age, with axillary hair occurring 6 months later than pubic hair and facial hair in males occurring 6 months later than pubic hair; texture becomes coarse and curly with growth and development

ESSENTIAL NURSING DIAGNOSES AND CARE PLANS

Risk for impaired skin integrity

Related to: External mechanical factors of shearing, pressure, restraint forces
External factor of radiation
External factor of immobilization
External factors of excretions, secretions, humidity, infection
Defining characteristics: Redness; edema; irritation of skin, perianal area, buttocks; excoriation or maceration of skin; enforced bedrest; induration or fissure in skin; scratching; rash; scales; crusting disruption of skin surface; destruction of skin layers with or without necrosis; open wound with drainage; pressure from cast, splint, brace, or other appliance/device; prolonged placement in one position
Related to: Internal factors of altered nutrition, circulation, sensation, skin turgor, metabolic rate, pigmentation and internal factors of medications, skeletal prominence, immunosuppression, developmental status, communicable disease
Defining characteristics: Thin, fragile skin; temperature elevation; dryness; flakiness; pruritus; pallor; cyanosis; redness; jaundice; allergic response to food, medication; dermatitis; rash; muscle tissue wasting; weakness; decreased muscle strength; edema; disruption of skin surface; eruptions (papule, macule, vesicle); loss of tactile perception in extremities

Outcome Criteria

Skin remains intact and free from trauma and effects of factors that result in alteration of integrity
Alterations in skin or mucous membranes minimized
Progressive healing of impaired skin or mucous membranes

Interventions	Rationales
Assess skin and mucous membranes for color changes, warmth, dryness, firmness, swelling or edema, lesions or breaks, and infection or inflammation of the oral cavity, nose, eyes, ears, and scalp	Provides information about potential for disruption of skin integrity in any part of the body to ensure identification and intervention before impairment becomes too severe or extensive

Interventions	Rationales
Assess mobility status, ability to move in bed, use of restraints and length of time restraint used, enforced bedrest as part of medical regimen, presence of any immobilization device	Reveals ability for movement, external factors that produce pressure leading to skin breakdown as circulation of oxygen and nutrients is reduced
Assess for any skin rashes, dermatitis, pruritis and scratching	Reveals skin conditions that lead to impairment
Assess for open wounds and type of drainage (serosanguineous or purulent), peristomal skin, diarrhea and effect on perianal area, diaper rash from prolonged exposure to ammonia from urine decomposition	Reveals presence of secretions and excretions that lead to skin impairment especially in infants and young children who have thinner, more sensitive skin
Assess skin under cast edges, tightness of cast, color and sensation in toes or fingers, redness and fit discomfort under any immobilization or assistive (prosthetic) device	Reveals skin impairment causes and neuro-circulatory effects of cast, splint, brace application
Assess nutritional and hydration status including dehydration or fluid imbalances and obesity or emaciation with muscle wasting and weakness	Reveals information regarding ability to maintain healthy skin and mucous membranes with proper nutrition and circulation to tissues and the preservation of muscle mass and strength needed to pad bony prominences and allow movement and position change
Assess effect of radiation therapy, presence and extent of burns, chemotherapy on skin and mucous membranes and areas of vulnerability	Provides rationale for preventative measures to treat risk for burns, stomatitis, impairment, and infection caused by immunosuppression
Assess skin cleanliness and examine bony prominences for changes, condition of hair and nails, use of cleansing products, and skin response; include	Provides information about removal of dirt, irritants, bacteria, sweat, urine, feces to promote skin integrity and offers an assessment opportunity

Interventions	Rationales
assessment of effect of contact allergens that cause skin changes	
Provide bathing in bed, tub, or shower; use warm water and mild soap and rinse well, with a soft towel pat dry and (avoid rubbing) including all folds, crevices, and creases	Promotes health and cleanliness of skin, reduces accumulation of body secretions and excretions, and reduces bacteria in skin folds where bacterial growth is enhanced
Provide careful cleansing of eyes with either warm, sterile water or saline and soft cloth from inner to outer aspect of eye; nasal mucosa with warm water and application of a protective lubricant; oral mucosa with a peroxide solution mouthwash	Promotes intact mucous membranes from irritation and breakdown caused by pressure or inflammation from tubes or by suctioning, chemotherapy, or NPO status; rapidly dividing epithelial tissue of oral and nasal mucosa leads to breakdown when receiving chemo-therapeutic agents
Provide hair shampooing, nail trimming as needed; cut nails straight across with round-tipped scissors; dry hair well with hair dryer, rubbing gently with soft towel	Promotes cleanliness and prevents skin irritation or break caused by scratching with long nails
Apply emollients, lotions to skin, bony prominences with gentle massage using fingers and/or hands	Protects and softens skin and promotes circulation to vulnerable parts
Apply skin adhesive barrier to peristomal area including tracheostomy, urinary or bowel diversion and over bony prominences if immobilized or too weak or ill to move in bed	Protects skin that is exposed to secretions and excretion or pressure
Provide position change q1-2h as indicated with prone, supine, side or elevated position utilized; if child is able, encourage to change positions on own	Prevents prolonged pressure on any one area leading to skin and tissue breakdown
Maintain body alignment and encourage to maintain correct posture when sitting, lying, and walking	Promotes even pressure on body parts

Interventions	Rationales
Pad bony prominences and susceptible parts with sheepskin, foam rubber, pillows, alternating pads and mattress, special apparatus such as Stryker frame	Protects vulnerable parts from pressure and redistribution weight and improves circulation
Maintain tight, wrinkle-free linens and bed free of crumbs, sharp toys, and dampness from urine or feces	Prevents irritation and excoriation of skin
Correct tight dressings by loosening tape, correct dry and sticking dressings with saline solution before removing, secure tubing away from skin contact, correct fit of any prosthesis or immobilization device, petal edges of cast with soft adhesive material	Reduces external sources of pressure that decrease circulation or irritate skin
Apply topical skin medications (ointments, solutions) as ordered; bathe or soak area or extremity	Promotes healing and prevents infection
Provide bath with oatmeal or other emollients, mitts on hands, temporary soft restraints as needed	Soothes pruritis and prevents scratching
Provide nutritional diet that is high in protein and calories and includes vitamins A and C	Promotes tissue healing with synthesis of protein to meet metabolic needs and formation of collagen and connective tissue by vitamins A and C
If wound present, provide dressing change, irrigations, debridement, wet or dry dressing, Op-site as indicated specific to wound	Promotes healing and prevents infection and further skin breakdown

Information, Instruction, Demonstration

Interventions	Rationales
Inform parent(s) to remove all environmental irritants, chemical agents, and allergens that have an outward	Prevents or controls skin rashes or eruptions caused by contact with offending substances

Interventions	Rationales
effect on the child's skin (fabrics, soaps, lotions, toys, dust, pollens, plants, animals, others)	
Instruct parent(s) and child in bathing and personal hygiene measures regarding toileting, mouth and teeth care, nail and hair care, and to avoid wearing tight-fitting clothing	Promotes cleanliness and removes infectious agents from the skin
Instruct parent(s) and child in nutritional diet and fluids to provide or replenish needed intake if skin disruption is present	Promotes healing of any skin wound or breakdown
Instruct parent(s) in dressing change using sterile technique, allow for return demonstration	Promotes wound cleanliness and healing
Inform parent(s) to maintain mobility of child, avoid allowing child to remain in same position over 1 hour	Promotes circulation to skin and tissues
Inform parent(s) to report any changes in skin color, irritation, pain or absence of sensations, breaks in skin	Allows for adjustment of device prosthesis or appliance
Inform parent(s) to report any redness, swelling, pain, purulent drainage from skin or mucous membrane, lesions or open wounds	Provides early interventions if skin infection present
Instruct in application of lotions or ointments (antiseptic, antibiotic, or palliative) to skin and irritated areas	Protects skin and promotes comfort
Advise child to avoid scratching or picking at skin or squeezing eruptions	Prevents further damage to skin and risk for infection
Instruct parent(s) in safety issues to prevent burn injuries	Provides information for protective measures

Interventions	Rationales
Instruct parent(s) on first aid measures for skin insults (e.g., burns, insect bites)	Provides information for early intervention

Discharge or Maintenance Evaluation

- Absence of skin impairment with intactness maintained
- Skin and mucous membranes free of inflammation, irritation, infection
- Skin breakdown or wound healing in progress
- Prevents or reduces pressure on skin
- Maintains appliances, devices, prosthesis, cast within parameters to safeguard skin integrity
- Provides nutritional, fluid requirements for skin healing and integrity
- Maintains skin, hair, nail cleanliness
- Provides protective measures, devices and topical applications to ensure skin and mucous membrane integrity
- Maintains body alignment and body posture conducive to preventing skin breakdown
- Provides effective wound care and dressing change without contamination of site
- Complies with medical regimen to treat any skin eruption or destruction to tissues

Burns/Skin Graft

Burns, which are injuries to the skin and underlying tissues caused by flames, electricity, contact with hot articles or water, or radiation therapy, affect children of all ages. They are classified according to severity, source, and extent of surface involved. Most burn injuries occur in children under 5 years of age. Severe burns affect all systems with local responses that include edema, circulatory stasis, and fluid loss. Systemic responses include circulation alteration, anemia, fluid loss, metabolic alteration, acidosis, and stress response. Burns that involve over 10% of body surface require hospitalization with management of ventilation, fluid and electrolyte imbalance, pain control, nutrition, wound care, infection prevention, skin grafting, and rehabilitation.

MEDICAL CARE

Analgesics: acetaminophen (Tylenol tablets, Pedric wafers or elixir, Liquiprin solution or drops) given PO for mild to moderate pain relief, oxycodone (Percodan) given PO for moderate pain relief, morphine sulfate, (MS) given IV for severe pain relief.

Antimicrobials: gentamicin sulfate (Garamycing 0.1%), silver sulfadiazine (Silvadene 1%), mafenide acetate (Sulfamylon 10%) silver nitrate (AgNO3 0.5%), povidone-iodine (Betadine) applied topically as ointment to affected areas, Bacitracin.

Vitamins/Minerals: tretinoin (Vitamin A Acid), Zinc sulfate given PO to facilitate growth and replace depleted stores.

Complete blood count (CBC): reveals decreased RBC, Hgb, HCT.

Electrolyte panel: reveals decreases because of loss from burned areas.

Proteins: reveals decreases with protein breakdown and losses.

Blood urea nitrogen/creatinine: reveals increases as tissue is destroyed and in presence of oliguria.

Wound culture: reveals and identifies infectious organism if present and sensitivity to anti-infective treatment.

NURSING CARE PLANS

Essential nursing diagnoses and plans associated with this condition:

Risk for impaired skin integrity (397)

Related to: External factor of burn
Defining characteristics: Disruption of skin surface or layers, destruction of skin layers, edema, altered circulation, altered nutritional state, altered metabolic state

Altered nutrition: Less than body requirements (168)

Related to: Inability to ingest, metabolize nutrients
Defining characteristics: Catabolism, protein and fat wasting, anorexia, diarrhea, weight loss

Impaired physical mobility (278)

Related to: Pain and discomfort, musculoskeletal impairment
Defining characteristics: Limited range of motion, impaired joint flexibility, scar formation, reluctance to attempt movement

Ineffective breathing pattern (45)

Related to: Musculoskeletal impairment
Defining characteristics: Trauma/edema of airway, oral or nasal membranes, restlessness, tachypnea, dyspnea

Risk for fluid volume deficit (222)

Related to: Excessive losses through normal routes (wound)
Defining characteristics: Loss of protective skin, blood loss from stress ulcer, electrolyte imbalance, reduced cardiac output with reduced plasma and blood volume

Altered growth and development (419)

Related to: Effects of long-term disability
Defining characteristics: Altered physical growth, inability to perform self-care of self-control activities appropriate for age

SPECIFIC DIAGNOSES AND CARE PLANS

Pain

Related to: Injuring biological, chemical, physical agents (burn injury)

Defining characteristics: Communication (verbal or nonverbal) of pain descriptors depending on severity and type of burn, moaning, crying, restlessness, guarding of injured area

Outcome Criteria

Pain minimized or controlled

Interventions	Rationales
Assess pain in burned area for severity and degree of burn	Provides information about pain that varies in severity with extent and depth of burn, cause of burn injury (chemical, thermal)
Administer analgesic PO or IV as ordered depending on severity of pain and status of other systems; administer before procedures and care are performed; anticipate need before pain becomes severe	Relieves and controls pain response caused by injury to superficial nerve endings
Provide relaxation, diversionary activities	Provides nonpharmacologic relief of pain
Place in position of comfort, change q2h, and handle injured parts gently	Promotes comfort and prevents additional pain caused by rough handling or pressure on injured body parts
Avoid touching painful parts, use bed cradle over injured, painful parts	Prevents contact with linens or hard surfaces that cause pain
Apply ointment to healing skin that is itchy and flaking	Provides relief from discomfort of itching with use of an antihistamine cream

Information, Instruction, Demonstration

Interventions	Rationales
Inform parent(s) of methods to relieve pain including quiet play, reading to child, television, music, games, soft toys, other activities of interest to child	Provides information about interventions that may distract child from any discomfort experienced
Inform parent(s) of reason for pain medication during acute phase of injury	Promotes understanding of treatment from pain relief
Instruct parent(s) and child to protect injured areas from contact with pain including stimuli	Prevents further injury and pain

Discharge or Maintenance Evaluation

- Pain absent or controlled
- Utilizes nonpharmacologic measures to control pain
- Protects injured and healing areas from stimuli that cause pain
- Absence of complaints of pain or discomfort

Risk for infection

Related to: Inadequate primary defenses

Defining characteristics: Broken skin, traumatized tissue, new skin graft, fever, purulent drainage from open wound or under eschar, positive wound culture

Outcome Criteria

Wound healing without presence of infectious process

Interventions	Rationales
Assess healing wounds for changes in color, odor and drainage, changes in VS, and temperature elevation	Provides information indicating infection of wound or skin graft area
Administer antibiotics PO or IV based on positive culture results and physician's order	Prevents or treats infection with antibiotic specific to microorganism; destroys infectious agent by preventing cell wall synthesis

Interventions	Rationales
Perform protective isolation as appropriate including mask, gown, gloves; perform handwash before giving any care; discourage visits from those who are suffering from an infection or who are ill	Protects child from exposure to infectious organisms
Apply antimicrobial wet dressings to wound or antimicrobial ointment as ordered when performing a dressing change	Destroys infectious agents and protects wound from infection
Use sterile technique to perform all dressing changes and wound care	Protects wound from pathogens and reduces risk of infection

Information, Instruction, Demonstration

Interventions	Rationales
Instruct parent(s) in handwashing technique and importance of procedure in caring for child	Provides method of controlling exposure to infectious agents
Instruct parent(s) in healing process and expected changes in skin during healing; how to assess wound and graft for signs of infection that should be reported	Provides information about process of healing and changes to note that should be reported
Instruct parent(s) to avoid any contact with family, friends, visitors that are ill with an infection	Prevents transmission of infectious agents to the child
Instruct parent(s) in administration of antimicrobial therapy via PO or topical application	Promotes compliance with medication regimen to prevent or treat infection

Discharge or Maintenance Evaluation

- Controls contact with infectious agents
- Protects wound site(s) from infectious agents
- Absence of evidence of signs and symptoms of wound infection
- Administers antibiotic therapy via appropriate route

- Eliminates sources of transmission of microorganisms to the child

Body image disturbance

Related to: Biophysical and psychosocial factors
Defining characteristics: Verbal and nonverbal responses to change in body appearance (scarring, deformity), loss of control, dependence, negative feelings about body, multiple stressors and change in daily living limitations and social relationships

Outcome Criteria

Body image improved, preserved, and maintained
Accommodations made for adaptation to long-term needs and limitations, during periods of healing and rehabilitation

Interventions	Rationales
Assess child for feelings about multiple restrictions in lifestyle, change in appearance, difficulty in school and social situations, inability to keep up with peers and participate in activities	Provides information about status of self-concept and body image that require special attention
Encourage expression of feelings and concerns and support communications with parent(s), teachers, and peers	Provides opportunity to vent feelings and reduce negative feelings about changes in appearance
Avoid negative comments and stress positive aspect of activities and accomplishments	Enhances body image and confidence
Note withdrawal behavior and signs of depression	Reveals responses to body image changes and possible poor adjustment to changes
Show support and acceptance of changes in appearance of child; provide privacy as needed	Promotes trust and demonstrates respect for child
Allow as much control and decision making by child as possible	Promotes independence and gives child some control over the situation
Allow and encourage parental and peer visits when possible	Promotes social acceptance by peers and support by parents

Information, Instruction, Demonstration

Interventions	Rationales
Inform parent(s) of importance of maintaining support for child regardless of their needs	Encourages acceptance of the child with special needs, long-term rehabilitation needs, lifelong activity restrictions
Inform parent(s) and child of impact of the disease on body systems and risk of scarring, physical disability; correct any misinformation and inform of ways to cope with body changes	Provides correct information to assist in dealing with negative feelings about body
Instruct parent(s) of need for flexibility in care of child and need to integrate care and routines into family activities; to allow child to participate in peer activities	Promotes well-being of child and sense of belonging and control of life events by participating in normal activities for age and enhancing developmental task achievement
Inform parent(s) and child about how to deal with peer and school perceptions of appearance and how to tell others about change in appearance	Prevents stigmatization of child by those who are not apprised of the child's disease; attitude of others will affect child's body image
Inform of clothing, wigs, scarves, makeup that may assist in preserving body image	Provides suggestions for aids that will camouflage scarring or disfigurement
Suggest psychological counseling or child life worker and inform of functions performed by these professionals	Assists to improve self-esteem and to learn coping and problem solving skills

Discharge or Maintenance Evaluation

- Verbalizes improved body image and sense of well-being
- Participates in family, school, and social activities as appropriate
- Verbalizes feelings about special long-term needs in positive terms
- Supports positive body image and promotes adjustment to change in appearance
- Identifies need for and seeks out social services, psychological counseling as appropriate

Burns/Skin Graft

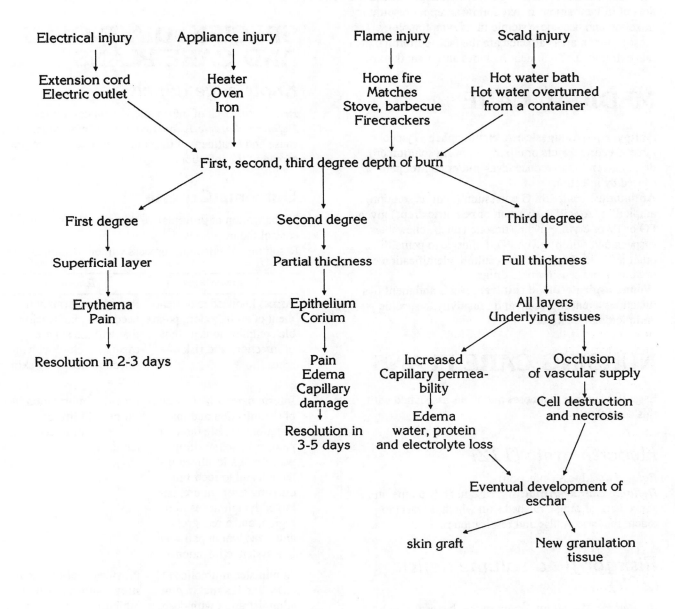

Electrical injury

Appliance injury

Flame injury

Scald injury

Extension cord
Electric outlet

Heater
Oven
Iron

Home fire
Matches
Stove, barbecue
Firecrackers

Hot water bath
Hot water overturned
from a container

First, second, third degree depth of burn

First degree

Second degree

Third degree

Superficial layer

Partial thickness

Full thickness

Erythema
Pain

Epithelium
Corium

All layers
Underlying tissues

Resolution in 2-3 days

Pain
Edema
Capillary
damage

Increased
Capillary permea-
bility

Occlusion
of vascular supply

Resolution in
3-5 days

Edema
water, protein
and electrolyte loss

Cell destruction
and necrosis

Eventual development of
eschar

skin graft

New granulation
tissue

Cellulitis

Cellulitis is an infection of the skin and underlying subcutaneous tissue affecting the lymph nodes within the area of inflammation. It may follow an upper respiratory infection and become systemic in its symptomology. The most common areas affected are the face, periorbital area and extremities. Treatment includes antibiotic therapy.

MEDICAL CARE

Antipyretics/Analgesics: Acetaminophen (Tylenol tablets, Pedric wafers or elixir, Liquiprin solution or drops) given PO to reduce fever and/or control pain caused by infection.

Antibiotics: penicillin G potassium (Pentids solution), ampicillin (Amcill suspension or pediatric drops) given PO or IV or erythromycin (Ilosone tablets, chewables, suspension or drop) given PO if allergic to penicillins; other antimicrobials based on culture identification of organism and sensitivity to drugs.

Wound aspirate/Blood culture: reveals and identifies infectious agent if present and sensitivity to specific antimicrobial treatment.

NURSING CARE PLANS

Essential nursing diagnoses and plans associated with this condition:

Hyperthermia (112)

Related to: Illness (infection)
Defining characteristics: Increase in body temperature above normal range, flushed skin which is warm to touch, increased pulse and respiration rate

Risk for fluid volume deficit (222)

Related to: Altered intake; excessive losses through normal routes
Defining characteristics: Temperature elevation, diaphoresis, insensible losses, dry, hot skin and mucous membranes

Risk for impaired skin integrity (397)

Related to: Internal factor of infection of skin layers
Defining characteristics: Redness, swelling, induration, warmth, pain at affected areas, destruction of skin layers

SPECIFIC DIAGNOSES AND CARE PLANS

Knowledge deficit

Related to: Lack of information about condition
Defining characteristics: Request for information about cause and treatment of the condition, measures to prevent spread of the infection

Outcome Criteria

Verbalization of preventative and curative measures to control the infections
Resolution of infectious process without complications

Interventions	Rationales
Assess knowledge of treatment of an infection, possible complications, extent of infection, and risk of spread	Provides information needed to plan teaching that will assist parent(s) in caring for child with an infection involving skin layers
Inform parent(s) of cause of the infection and manifestations to note including pain, redness, swelling, warmth of a localized infection and to report increasing temperature, enlarged lymph nodes in the region, and a red streak along the lymph pathway in a systemic infection	Provides information indicating cellulitis and spreading of infection systemically
Administer antibiotics PO or IV and instruct in oral administration with dose, time, frequency, side effects, and instruct to take until entire prescription is ingested	Provides treatment to destroy causative agent by inhibiting cell wall synthesis; route is dependent upon site and severity of the infection

Interventions	Rationales
Inform parent(s) that culture is done to determine treatment	Provides identification of microorganism and sensitivity to specific antibiotics
Instruct parent(s) to apply warm compresses or soaks to affected area or limb	Promotes vasodilation and circulation to the area to promote healing
Instruct parent(s) in dressing change using sterile technique if an incision and drainage has been done at infection site, and instruct in proper disposal of soiled dressing	Promotes wound cleanliness and prevents introduction of additional pathogens
Instruct parent(s) and child in handwashing technique and instruct them to perform this before and after giving care to the child	Prevents transmission of infectious agents
Inform parent(s) to immobilize limb and maintain bedrest for the child	Promotes healing and reduces pain caused by movement if an extremity is involved

Discharge or Maintenance Evaluation

- Progressive resolution of the infectious process
- Administers antibiotic therapy correctly
- Reports persistent signs and symptoms and those indicating spread of infection
- Promotes comfort and measures to enhance healing
- Performs treatments to resolve infection
- Implements universal precautions and positive hygienic habits

Cellulitis

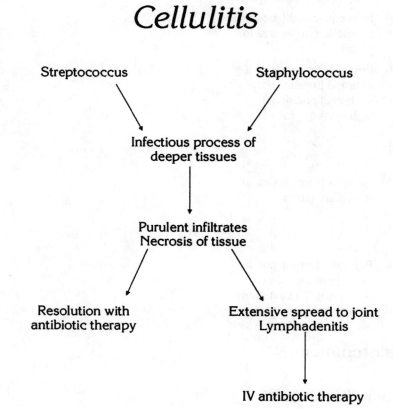

Streptococcus   Staphylococcus

Infectious process of
deeper tissues

Purulent infiltrates
Necrosis of tissue

Resolution with   Extensive spread to joint
antibiotic therapy   Lymphadenitis

IV antibiotic therapy

Dermatitis (Contact)

Dermatitis is an inflammatory condition of the superficial layer of the skin. It may be caused by contact with an allergen, urine, or feces, and it may cause irritation characterized by erythema, papules, or vesicles. Treatment includes actions to prevent infection and skin breakdown.

MEDICAL CARE

Anti-inflammatories: hydrocortisone (DermaCort), hydrocortisone valerate (Westcort) in cream, lotion, ointment forms to apply topically to suppress inflammatory process and modify immune response to hypersensitivities.

Antihistamines: diphenhydramine hydrochloride (Benadryl) given PO to relieve allergic response and promote rest.

Antipruritics: Aluminum acetate solution (Burrow's) applied topically as compresses, calamine lotion applied topically, Aveeno bath for bathing to allay itching.

Skin protectors: Vaseline, Desitin, Borofax A&D ointments applied topically to protect skin against contact with irritants.

NURSING CARE PLANS

Essential nursing diagnoses and plans associated with these conditions:

Risk for impaired skin integrity (397)

Related to: External factors of excretions and secretions, contact with allergens or irritants
Defining characteristics: Rash, erythema, papule, vesicle, lesions, disruptions of skin surface, itching

SPECIFIC DIAGNOSES AND CARE PLANS

Knowledge deficit

Related to: Lack of information about disorder
Defining characteristics: Request for information about cause and treatments of dermatitis and measures to prevent recurrence

Outcome Criteria

Verbalization of preventative and curative measures to control dermatitis
Resolution of dermatitis condition

Interventions	Rationales
Assess type and extent of dermatitis including site and offending irritant, presence of redness, papules, vesicles, breaks in skin, excoriation, itching	Provides information about rash resulting from contact which may be chemical or physical and most commonly is caused by ammonia from diaper, plant, animal, cloth, soap, or sun exposure
Inform of potential violators causing eruptions/dermatitis and how to avoid contact with offending agents (clothing covering all parts of body, to wash after contact with substance, to use hypoallergic soaps, proper use of skin applications, and proper changing and laundering of diapers)	Provides information to assist in avoiding contact with substances that cause dermatitis
Instruct in application of ointment or lotion (Vaseline, Desitin) to treat diaper rash, to cleanse and dry area well during diaper change, to expose irritated area to the air; laundering diapers by soaking, using mild soap, and double rinsing and drying well in clothes dryer or in sun	Promotes healing of skin irritation caused by ammonia in diapers
Instruct parent(s) in palliative treatments, such as application of warm, wet compresses and lotion or paste to the affected areas, and baths; discourage child from scratching the areas	Promotes comfort and healing, allays pruritis, and prevents infection if skin is broken down

Interventions	Rationales
Instruct parent(s) in administration of antibiotics, anti-inflammatories, antihistamines as ordered	Reduces allergic reactions and prevents complications associated with dermatitis
Inform parent(s) to avoid dressing child in tight clothing, to wash new clothing before wearing, to rinse clothing well during laundering	Promotes comfort and prevents risk of contact with substance that may cause rash
Inform parent(s) to use sun protection with a minimum sun protection factor of 15 such as PABA	Protects skin from sunburn by blocking or absorbing ultraviolet rays
Suggest toys, games, television, and activities preferred by child; maintain short, smooth nails	Provides diversion to prevent scratching

Discharge or Maintenance Evaluation

- Resolves dermatitis condition
- Prevents recurrence of contact dermatitis by removing or controlling offending agents
- Promotes comfort with palliative measures
- Administers medications correctly with desired effects

Dermatitis

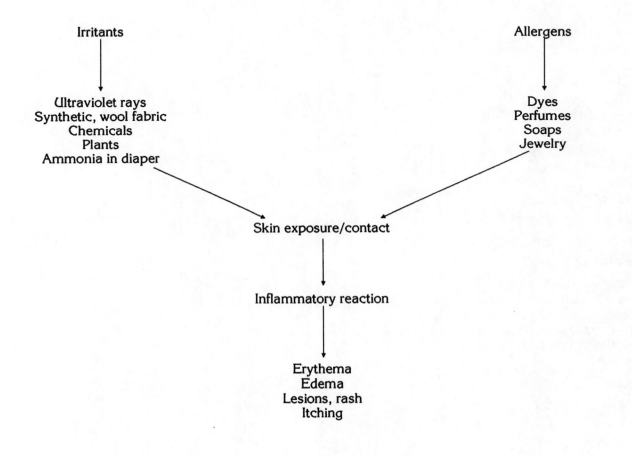

Irritants

Allergens

Ultraviolet rays
Synthetic, wool fabric
Chemicals
Plants
Ammonia in diaper

Dyes
Perfumes
Soaps
Jewelry

Skin exposure/contact

Inflammatory reaction

Erythema
Edema
Lesions, rash
Itching

Physiopsychosocial Considerations

Physiopsychosocial Considerations

The physical, mental, and social considerations of children's health problems do not lend themselves to specific conditions. These considerations include the child's ability to deal with hospitalization, abuse, and death. They require special empathy and sensitivity to the needs and feelings of children based on age and related growth and development parameters.

GENERAL CHANGES ASSOCIATED WITH PHYSICAL, MENTAL, SOCIAL GROWTH AND DEVELOPMENT

- Psychosocial Development (Erickson):

    Trust vs Mistrust, Infant (birth to 1 year): Characterized by taking through all the senses; loving care of a mothering person is essential to develop trust; need to have basic needs met, attachment to primary caretaker, oral stage, limited ability to communicate.
    The favorable outcome is faith and optimism.

    Autonomy vs Shame and Doubt, Toddler (1 to 3 years): Characterized by increasing ability to control bodies, themselves and their environment; seeks independence, negativism, threatened by changes in routine, curious explorer, sensorimotor cognition, limited ability to communicate reason, and understand time; learning is acquired through imitation of others.
    The favorable outcome is self-control and will power.

    Initiative vs Guilt, Preschool (3 to 6 years): Characterized by vigorous, intrusive behavior, enterprise, and a strong imagination; develops conscience; feelings of being punished, preoperational cognition, egocentric, inquisitive, acquiring better language skills, rich fantasy life and magical thinking.
    The favorable outcome is direction and purpose.

    Industry vs Inferiority, School age (6 to 12 years): Characterized by concrete cognition, active learners, well-developed language skills and con-

cept of time, concerns about body image, understands concept of death.
    The favorable outcome is competence.

    Identity vs Role Confusion, Adolescent (13-18): Characterized by the ability to deal with reality, abstract cognition, rapid mood swings, rapidly changing body image; preoccupied with the way they appear in the eyes of others as compared to their own self-concept.
    The favorable outcome is devotion and fidelity to others and to values and ideologists.

- Psychosexual Development (Freud):

    Oral Stage (birth to 1 year): Characterized by infant seeking pleasure via oral activities such as biting, sucking, chewing, and vocalizing; preferred method of oral gratification can provide some indication of personality development.

    Anal Stage (1 to 3 years): Characterized by interest in the anal region and sphincter muscles (child is able to withhold or expel feces); toilet training is a major milestone (method of parent discipline, may have lasting effects on child's personality development).

    Phallic Stage (3 to 6 years): Characterized by interest and recognition in differences between the sexes and becomes very curious about these differences; often described as interest by females as penis envy and by males as castration anxiety.

    Latency period (6 to 12 years): Characterized by gaining increased skill on newly acquired traits and skills; very interested in acquiring knowledge and vigorous play.

    Genital stage (12 and over): Characterized by maturation of the reproductive system and production of sex hormones; genital organs become a source of tension and pleasure; interested in forming friendships and preparation for marriage as an adult.

- Interpersonal Development (Sullivan)

    Infant (0-1 year): Receives gratification and comfort from loving, tender care; develops trust and ability to count on others.

    Childhood (2-5 years): Engages in peer, family, neighborhood activities; needs adult participation; learns to delay gratification and accept interference with wishes; gradually seeks attention and approval from peers.

    Juvenile (5-12 years): Engages in socialization, competition, cooperation, and compromise; develops shared interests and genuine friendships with peers of same sex, and later with opposite sex; gives more allegiance to peers than to family; promotes personal identity

- Cognitive Development (Piaget):

  Sensorimotor (birth to 2 years): Characterized by progression from reflex activity through simple repetitive behaviors to imitate behaviors; develop a sense of "cause and effect"; problem solving is by trial and error; high level of curiosity, experimentation, and enjoyment in novelty; begin to separate self from others; develop sense of "object permanence"; begin language development.

  Pre-operational (2 to 7 years): Characterized by egocentrism (inability to put oneself in the place of others); interpret objects and events in terms of their relationships or use of them; they cannot see another's point of view; thinking is concrete tangible; inability to make deductions or generalizations; display high level of imagination and questioning; their reasoning is intuitive.

  Concrete Operations (7 to 11 years): Characterized by thoughts; become increasingly logical and coherent; able to classify, sort, organize facts, and begin to problem solve; develop conservation (realize volume, weight, and number remain the same even though outward appearances are changed); unable to develop inductive thinking (ability to solve problems in a concrete, systematic fashion, based on their visual perceptions).

  Formal Operations (11 to 13 years): Characterized by thoughts which are adaptable and flexible; possess abstract thinking; able to make logical conclusions; able to make hypotheses and test them; they can consider abstract, theoretical, philosophical issues.

- Moral Development (Kohlberg): (based on cognitive developmental theory and consists of 3 major levels):

  Preconventional level (2 to 7 years): Parallels Erickson's preoperational level of cognitive development and intuitive thinking. Characterized by development of: cultural values; sense of right and wrong; integrate things in terms of physical or pleasurable consequences of their actions. Initially, the child determines the goodness or badness in terms of its consequences (attempt to avoid punishment). Later, the child determines the right behavior consists of what satisfies their own needs (and sometimes those of others).

  Conventional level (7 to 11 years): Parallels Erickson's stage of concrete operations of cognitive development. Characterized by a concern with conformity and loyalty; they value a specific group (i.e.,

their family, group or national expectations); behavior which conforms to this specific group (is considered good and earns approval). Values such as fairness; give and take; and sharing are interpreted in a practical manner without loyalty, gratitude or justice.

Postconventional, autonomous, or principled level (11 to 15 years): Parallels Erickson's stage of formal operations. Characterized by tendency/desire to display correct behavior (in terms of individual rights and standards); begins to question the possibility of changing existing laws/rules in terms of societal needs.

- Spiritual Development (Fowler) (5 stages of development of faith, four are closely associated with parallel cognitive (Erickson) and psychosocial (Erickson) development in childhood.

  Stage 0, (Undifferentiated): Characterized by infant period of development, in which the infant is unable to determine concept of right or wrong. Development of basic trust lays the foundation for beginning faith.

  Stage 1, (Intuitive-projectile): Characterized by toddler period of development, in which the primary behavior is referred to as imitating religious gestures and behaviors of others. Unable to comprehend meaning or significance of religious practices; begin to assimilate religious values and beliefs held by their parents; imitate religious behaviors of parents; do not attempt to understand basic concepts of religion.

  Stage 2, (Mythical-literal): Characterized by school age period of development, in which the child's spiritual development parallels cognitive development. Belief is that spiritual development is associated with previous experiences and societal interactions. Their newly-acquired conscience influences their actions (good versus bad; bad actions create guilt); petitions to an omnipotent being are important; are able to articulate their faith.

  Stage 3: (Synthetic-convention): Characterized by early phase of adolescent period of development, in which they become aware of spiritual disappointments (i.e., prayers are not always answered); may begin to abandon or modify previous religious practices, and those established by their parents.

  Stage 4: (Individuating-reflexive): Characterized by middle phase of adolescent period of development, in which the adolescent may become skeptical and begin to compare religious standards of their parents and significant others. The adolescent will begin to compare religious beliefs with scientific facts, described as a period of searching for answers; and to be uncertain about their religious ideas. Typically, they will obtain concrete insights during the late adolescence or early adult stage of development.

SELECTED GENERAL GROWTH AND DEVELOPMENT NORMS

- Gross Motor:

    0-4 months: Lifts head if in prone position; with head erect or bobbing and back rounded; raises chest with support of arms; position of arms and legs less flexed; arm and leg movements with swimming action in prone position; 0-1 month, startle and rooting reflex are very strong; moro reflex begins to fade at 2 months; rolls from side to back and then return; 2-4 months, decrease in head lag when pulled up to sitting position.

    4-8 months: Holds head up and erect without support, lifts head and shoulders to 90 degree angle and rolls from back to side, turns over both ways, supports weight on legs and may pull self into sitting position; beginning at 4 months, able to sit with support; head lag disappears; by 7 months, able to sit alone without support; likes to bounce on legs when held in standing position; newborn reflexes have disappeared.

    8-12 months: Sits alone, creeps, crawls, cruises, sits from standing position without assistance, prefers being up instead of lying down; at 9 months, stand while holding onto furniture and able to pull themselves to standing position; at 11 months they walk while holding onto furniture or with both hands held; at 12 months they may be able to walk with one hand held; 10 months, pincer grasp present, able to pick up small objects like a raisin; 11 months, able to put objects into a container and enjoys removing them; 12 months, displays interest in building a tower of two blocks, but they often fall down.

    12-15 months: Walks alone with side-based gait, creeps up stairs, throws things.

    15-24 months: Walks alone with improvement, runs, pulls toys when walking, walks on toes, walks backwards, climbs up steps, climbs on furniture, sits on small chair, stands on one foot.

    2 years: Walks with steady gait, runs with few falls, walks on toes, stands on one foot, walks up and down stairs, jumps, kicks ball, rides tricycle, throws ball overhand.

    3 and 4 years: Pedals tricycle, climbs and jumps well, walks up and down stairs with alternating feet, gains increased coordination and balance, dresses and undresses self, hops on one foot, throws ball overhand proficiently.

    5 and 6 years: Hops; skips well; jumps rope; has improved coordination and control of muscles; always active; throws and catches ball; runs without difficulty, hits nail on head; draws figure with body, arms and legs, mouth, eyes, nose and hair; begins to ride bicycle.

    7, 8 and 9 years: Repeats activities for mastery; always active; rhythm, smoothness, and control of muscular movements increases; cautious in play and motor activities; displays motor skills; strength and endurance increase.

    10, 11 and 12 years: Has control of timing, likes rough activities, has high level of energy, takes walks and explores environment, participates in team sports, builds or constructs things, interested in physical skills.

- Fine Motor:

    0-4 months: Attempts to grab object but misses, brings object to mouth, holds hands in front and plays with hands and feet, grasps object with both hands; 1 month displays grasp reflex; 3 months, hands are usually open; 2 - 4 months, looks and plays with own fingers; 3 months, when object is placed in hands, will retain briefly; 4 months, reaches for objects and picks them up with a raking action of fingers.

    4-8 months: Grasps with thumb and fingers, explores objects, moves arms at sight of toy, reaches for object, picks up object with cupped hands, holds objects in both hands at same time, holds own bottle, puts nipple in mouth, feeds self a cookie; 5 months, able to voluntarily grasp an object; 6-7 months, able to transfer objects from one hand to another, enjoys banging objects together.

    8-12 months: Releases toy or object, locates hands for play, eats with fingers, uses spoon with assistance, drinks from cup with assistance, holds crayon and makes marks on paper; 10 months, pincer grasp is present, able to pick up small objects like a raisin; 11 months, able to put objects into a container and enjoys removing them; 12 months, displays interest in building a tower of two blocks, but they often fall down.

    12-15 months: Builds tower of 2-4 blocks, opens boxes, pokes finger in hole, turns pages of book, uses spoon with spilling.

15-24 months: Drinks from cup with one hand, uses spoon without spilling, empties jar of contents, draws vertical line, scribbles, builds tower of 4 blocks.

2 years: Builds tower of 5 to 8 blocks, turns knob to open door, drinks from glass held in one hand, makes train of cubes by manipulating play materials.

3 and 4 years: Strings beads, builds tower of blocks, learns to use and masters use of scissors, copies a circle-and-cross figure, hold crayon with fingers, unbuttons buttons on side or front, laces shoes, brushes teeth, cuts out simple pictures.

5 and 6 years: Copies letters of alphabet and prints name, dresses self with assistance, uses hammer and nails, knows right from left hand, cuts and pastes well, may tie shoes, uses fork for eating.

7, 8 and 9 years: Hand-eye coordination improves; writes rather than prints words; may play musical instruments, sew, build models, work jigsaw puzzles; adds details to drawings and uses perspective in drawing, uses both hands independently.

10, 11 and 12 years: Uses increased detail in work, handwriting skill improves, more refinement to motor activities, gradual improvement to adult level.

- Language

0-4 months: Cries, whimpers; responds to sounds or activity; coos, gurgles, and babbles; smiles in response to adult sounds and makes sounds.

4-8 months: Laughs out loud, vocalizes, uses two syllable sounds like da da without meaning, imitates expressions, cries if scolded.

8-12 months: Responds to adult emotional tone, says one or two words, uses sounds to identify objects or persons, uses wide range of sounds, understands use of no, knows own name, communicates with others and self

12-24 months: Uses jargon, names for familiar pictures or objects; points to desired object or vocalizes wants, knows at least 10 words or more; uses short phrases; points to body parts.

2 years: Uses about 300 words, uses pronouns, speaks 3-4 word sentences, enjoys stories, does not ask for help.

3 and 4 years: Uses about 900 to 1500 words; talks in sentences; asks questions consistently; states own name; talks whether someone present or not; omits w from speech; uses d, b, t, k, and y; uses plural form of words; repeats words and sentences at will; omits prepositions, adverbs, adjectives in speech;

asks how and why; boasts and tattles; tells a story; counts to at least 3, understands simple questions.

5 and 6 years: Identifies colors, uses 2100 words, talks constantly, knows names of days of week, asks thoughtful questions, uses prepositions and conjunctions, uses complete sentences, shares experiences with others through language, expands vocabulary with exposure and stimulation, errors in sound disappear, begins to have a concept of abstract words.

7, 8 and 9 years: Increases use of words to express self, increases use of words for exchange and communication, considers what others say, uses all parts of speech.

10, 11 and 12 years: Uses 50,000 words, uses compound and complex sentences, understands abstract words.

- Sensory (or Social)

0-4 months: Stares at environment, smiles indiscriminately or responsively, enjoys having others around, recognizes familiar faces, determines that face is unfamiliar and freezes gaze, establishes cycle for sleep and awake periods; 0-1 month, prefers to look at faces, at black and white geometric designs, able to follow objects in line of vision; 2-4 months, follows objects 180°, turns head to look for voices and sounds.

4-8 months: Self-centered, begins to be fearful of strangers, tolerates some delay, thrashes arms and legs when irritated, begins to play; 4-6 months, watches the course of a falling object, responds readily to sounds, examines complex visual images); 6-8 months, recognizes own name and responds by smiling when it is heard.

8-12 months: Plays simple peek-a-boo, prefers mother, cries when upset, becomes anxious if separated from mother, recognizes family members' requests if one at a time, displays various emotions, feeds self with fingers, helps to dress self; understands words such as "no" and "cracker."

12-24 months: Plays pat-a-cake, is curious and gets into everything, has short attention span, enjoys solitary play or watching others play, has a favorite toy or object.

2 years: Views and treats other children as objects, unable to distinguish right from wrong, imitates parents and others, likes to take favorite toy to bed, enjoys parallel play, wants things own way, refuses to share possessions and is possessive, sees self as a separate person.

3 and 4 years: Decreases temper displays, able to share with peers and adults, interested in new activities and learning from them, plays with an imaginary playmate, participates in imaginative play, believes parents are most important people, has friends of same sex, argues and is more aggressive.

5 and 6 years: Likes achieving, wants to accept responsibilities, has strong feeling for family and home, identifies with parent of same sex, participates in fair play and cooperation, prefers friends to family, is self-centered, shows off, has rigid thinking, lives in here and now.

7, 8 and 9 years: Independently plays, able to reason and has a concept of right or wrong, likes rewards and praise, peer group gains in importance, likes peer group but has short-lived interests, completes tasks, rebels at parental control.

10, 11 and 12 years: Feels positive about self; is more tolerant; interested in rules and money; relates well with peers, friends, relatives; likes conversation, change, and variety in activities; avoids doing tasks; develops conscience.

ESSENTIAL NURSING DIAGNOSIS AND CARE PLAN

Altered growth and development

Related to: Separation from significant others (i.e., parent(s), siblings, peers and/or primary caretaker)

Defining characteristics: Ages 6-30 months (i.e., crying, screaming, withdraws from others, inactive, sad, detachment behaviors, regressive behaviors); 3-6 yrs (i.e., temper tantrums, refusal to comply with hospital routine/treatments, crying, refusal to eat); 6-12 yrs. (i.e., express feelings of loneliness, boredom, isolation, depression, worry about absence from school); 13-18 yrs. (i.e., may react with dependency, uncooperativeness, withdrawal behaviors, fear of loss of peer status/acceptance at school)

Related to: Decreased or increased environmental stimulation

Defining characteristics: Inability to perform self-care or self-control activities appropriate for age decreased responses, listlessness, flat affect; delay or difficulty in performing developmental tasks/skills (i.e., motor, social or language) typical for age group

Related to: Chronic illness or disability, parental reactions (over-benevolence), repeated hospitalizations

Defining characteristics: Inability to perform gross and fine motor tasks appropriate to age, altered physical growth

Outcome Criteria

Age-appropriate growth; development activities promoted with normal parameters achieved
Absence of growth and development deficits for age within limits imposed by illness

Interventions	Rationales
Provide or arrange for growth and development assessment with the administration of tools such as Washington Guide, Denver Developmental Screening Test (DDST), Denver Developmental Screening Test Revised (DDST-R), Denver II, Revised Denver Prescreening Developmental Questionnaire (R-PDQ), Denver Articulation Screening Exam (DASE)	Identifies developmental level or any lag in development to assist in plan of care or therapy; information should include age-expected gross and fine motor development, language and social development, psychosocial and psychosexual development, interpersonal skills, cognitive and moral and spiritual development
Reassess developmental levels at intervals appropriate for illness or other problem	Provides evidence of progress to evaluate program to correct any growth and developmental deficit
Provide consistent caretaker and care	Promotes trust and progress in development
Depending on age and abilities, encourage to participate in goal setting decision making, participation in care	Promotes independence needed for control and development
Provide visual, auditory, tactile stimulation, including mobiles with or without color, music, toys, books, television, games or other age-related activities; hold child and rock or pat on back, talk to child	Promotes stimulation needed to maintain developmental status
Provide time for child, either quiet or talking, to play with other children, time for parent(s) that remain in hospital to interact with child	Promotes independence and development or maintenance of motor skills to prevent regression

Interventions	Rationales
Initiate referral to child development expert if appropriate	Provides source of assistance to ensure proper age-related development
Provide developmentally appropriate activities based on child's age-related abilities	To enhance child's adjustment to hospitalization and treatment and to enhance child's maximum growth and developmental abilities
Explore the family's and child's feelings regarding child's health status and required treatments	Promotes family communication and attitude of acceptance and adaptation to child's health status and abilities
Encourage independence and choices in as many areas as possible (i.e., dressing, feeding, type of foods/drinks, or BandAids)	Fosters child's sense of control, adaptation, and developmental growth during their altered health state and hospitalization
Encourage socialization (i.e., in the play room, with siblings, peers, phone calls, if possible)	To foster child's ability to develop and maintain peer relationships
Recognize and support ritualistic behaviors (especially in the young child)	Fosters child's need for autonomy
Encourage mastery of self-care activities, required health care equipment, if appropriate	Fosters child's need for initiative and purpose; fosters child's self-esteem

Information, Instruction, Demonstration

Interventions	Rationales
Instruct parent(s) on normal growth and development for child's age	Provides information about age-related growth and development to ensure realistic expectations
Inform of age-related play and other activities that enhance growth and development and provide needed stimulation; include those that encourage gross and fine motor development, sensory and cognitive development, others as determined by testing and needs	Provides guidance for proper, safe activities and stimulation to prevent frustration of child and to promote normal development

Interventions	Rationales
Inform parent(s) whether developmental and growth lag is the result of the child's illness (acute or chronic) or some other reason	Promotes understanding and relief from anxiety and guilt
Discuss with child and parent(s) test results with child and parent(s) and possible plan to resolve any deficits, both short-term during hospitalization and long-term during convalescence	Promotes understanding of special needs and formulation of goals and actions based on findings

Discharge or Maintenance Evaluation

- Demonstrates growth and developmental advances appropriate for age and condition
- Resolves growth and developmental deficits for optimal cognitive, psychomotor, psychosocial functioning
- Complies with activities that enhance stimulation, independence, and developmental progression
- Secures appropriate testing for diagnosis and treatment of growth and development problems

Abused Child

The term child abuse is defined as any maltreatment to a child, including the following: infliction of injuries, sexual exploitation, infliction of emotional pain, or neglect of a child. Child abuse is usually caused or inflicted by the biologic parents. However, others who have been reported as causing child abuse upon a child has included: foster parents, other relatives, boyfriends, friends, day care workers, and babysitters. The "shaken child syndrome" is defined as inflicted injuries to the infant resulting from the combination of vigorous shaking with the application of force (the prognosis is usually poor, or fatal). Signs of "shaken child syndrome" include retinal hemorrhages and subarachnoid hemorrhage. The most common form of child abuse is neglect, which may include deprivation of physical and/or emotional needs (food, clothing, shelter, medical care, education, affection, love, nurture) or agressive emotional abuse (isolation, terrorizing, rejection). Physical abuse may include burns, bruises, fractures, lacerations, poisoning of the child. Sexual abuse may be indicated by bruising and bleeding of anus or genitals; discharge and pain in genitals; sexually transmitted disease; or odor, swelling, and itching of genitalia. Regardless of the type of abuse, the nurse's responsibilities are to identify the maltreatment and to protect the child from further abuse.

MEDICAL CARE

Complete blood count (CBC): reveals changes resulting from infection (increased WBC), blood loss (decreased RBC, Hgb).
Urinalysis: reveals blood, pus in urinary tract.
Vaginal/anal cultures: reveal sexually-transmitted disease.
X-ray: child abuse long bone series of x-rays are required to detect evidence of or to rule out healed fractures/current fractures.
C-scan: to rule out central nervous system damage due to shaken child syndrome.

NURSING CARE PLANS

Essential nursing diagnoses and plans associated with these conditions:

Altered nutrition: less than body requirements (168)

Related to: Inability to ingest food
Defining characteristics: Withholding of food by parent/caretaker, weight loss, malnutrition, lack of subcutaneous fat, failure to thrive, provides inadequate amount of food; knowledge of deficit regarding appropriate food preparations (i.e., cleaning bottles)

Risk for impaired skin integrity (397)

Related to: External factor of trauma
Defining characteristics: Disruption of skin surface (lacerations, burns, abrasions), various skin trauma in different stages of healing, lack of bathing causing unclean skin, teeth, hair

Altered growth and development (419)

Related to: Inadequate caretaking, indifference, environmental and stimulation deficiencies
Defining characteristics: Delay or difficulty in performing skills (motor, social, or expressive) typical of age group, altered physical growth, inability to perform self-care or self-control activities appropriate for age, flat affect, decreased responses, withdrawal, antisocial behavior, fearfulness, poor relationships with peers, regressive behavior, acting out behavior

SPECIFIC DIAGNOSES AND CARE PLANS

Anxiety

Related to: Threat to self-concept, change in health status, change in interaction patterns, situational crisis
Defining characteristics: Increased apprehension and uncertainty, fearfulness, feeling of powerlessness, fear of consequences, repeated episodes of maltreatment, mistrust, trembling, quivering voice, poor eye contact, lacks appropriate pain response, frozen watchfulness, developmental delays/regressive behaviors

Outcome Criteria

Reduced anxiety and fear, trust established between child and staff, and signs and symptoms decreased to manageable level

Interventions	Rationales
Assess level of anxiety and fear in child and how it is manifested; needs of child that are the source of anxiety and reactions to staff and parent(s)	Provides information about the source and level of anxiety and what might relieve it and basis to judge improvement
Demonstrate affection and acceptance of the child even if not returned or ignored; avoid reinforcing any negative behavior	Promotes trust of staff and positive behavior of the child
Provide a play program with other children; set aside time to be alone with child or quiet time for child as well; praise child or reward with a special treat when appropriate	Modifies negative behavior by promoting interactions with others and rewarding desired behaviors; promotes self-esteem
Provide consistent staffing for child, preferably those who seem to relate well to child	Promotes familiarity and trusting relationship with staff
Allow expression of concerns and fears of child about treatments, environment; allow questions and provide honest explanations and communication at child's age level	Provides opportunity to vent feelings, which reduces anxiety
Provide treatment of injuries; avoid treating child as a victim, asking too many questions, or forcing any discussion	Prevents increased anxiety and stress in child by discussion of abuse
Assess possible need for counseling services for the child	Reduces anxiety and supports child in dealing with abuse and negative behavior

Information, Instruction, Demonstration

Interventions	Rationales
Inform child of all treatments and procedures to be done and the purpose for them and that someone will accompany them to a different department if needed	Provides preparation and information that will assist in preventing fear or anxiety
Use therapeutic play kit to instruct child in any procedure to be done (dolls, syringe, tubing, dressing, other articles)	Reduces anxiety by familiarizing child with what to expect to reduce anxiety

Discharge or Maintenance Evaluation

- Reduces anxiety by establishing accepting, safe environment
- Participates in play with others
- Establishes relationships with staff member(s)
- Exhibits reduction in negative behavior, signs and symptoms of anxiety and fear

Altered parenting

Related to: Unmet social and emotional maturation needs of parental figures, ineffective role modeling, lack of knowledge, situational crisis or incident

Defining characteristics: Lack of parental attachment behaviors, verbalization of resentment toward child and of role inadequacy, inattention to needs of child, noncompliance with health practices and medical care, inappropriate discipline practices, frequent accidents and illness of child, growth and development lag in child, history of child abuse or abandonment, multiple caretakers without regard for needs of child, evidence of physical and psychological trauma, actual abandonment of child

Outcome Criteria

Demonstration of appropriate parenting behaviors
Maintenance of safe environment for child
Establishment of positive relationship with child and realistic expectations for self and child
Acceptance of support for achievement of desirable parenting skills

Interventions	Rationales
Assess parent(s) for achievement of developmental tasks of self and understanding of child's growth and development; how they are bonded and attached to child; how they interpret and respond to child; how they accept and support child; how they meet child's social, psychological and physical needs	Provides information about parent-child relationship and parenting styles that may lead to child abuse; identifies parents at risk for violence or other abusive behavior
Provide a child nurturing role model for parent(s) to emulate, and suggest what they might do to develop parenting skills	Promotes development of parenting skills by imitation
Praise parent(s) for their participation in child's care, tell them that they are giving good care to child	Reinforces positive parenting behaviors and increases feeling of adequacy
Include parent(s) in planning care and set goals	Promotes participation of parent(s) in meeting child's needs
Provide an opportunity for parent(s) to express their feelings, personal needs, and goals; avoid making judgmental remarks or comparing them to other parent(s)	Supports parent(s) in meeting their own needs
Initiate referrals to social services, parenting classes, or counseling as appropriate	Provides options if parenting is unsatisfactory or inadequate
Inform parent(s) that child protection services have been contacted to investigate the child's health status and safety; keep the parent(s) informed of the child's health status (unless or until custody of the child is removed from the parent(s))	

Information, Instruction, Demonstration

Interventions	Rationales
Inform parent(s) of developmental tasks for child and parent(s), difference in developmental level between child and parent(s), and appropriate tasks for age levels	Provides information that assists parent(s) in responding realistically and appropriately to child's needs at different age levels
Inform parent(s) of methods to reduce conflict by type of parenting (democratic or authoritarian), to be consistent in approach to child's behavior and needs, to avoid siding with child or other parent	Promotes a more positive child-parent relationship
Inform parent(s)to maintain their own health by getting adequate rest, nutrition, and exercise; and to participate in leisure activities and make social contacts	Provides information on importance of parents meeting their own needs to enable them to better care for and cope with their children
Inform of community agencies that offer parenting classes and support groups	Provides education in parenting skills

Discharge or Maintenance Evaluation

- Participate in child care with increased understanding of child's needs for age and developmental level
- Reduce behaviors that are harmful to child and to relationship between parent and child
- Demonstrate proper parenting behaviors
- Demonstrate improved and positive interaction with child
- Attend parenting classes and support group activities
- Meet own needs for health and optimal functioning
- Secure assistance to solve problems that lead to abusive behavior

Risk for Trauma

Related to: Characteristics of child, care giver(s), environment

Defining characteristics: Sexual assault of child, evidence of physical abuse of child, history of abuse of abuser, social isolation of family, low self-esteem of caretaker, inadequate support systems, violence against other members of the family

Outcome Criteria

Absence of violence or maltreatment of the child by parent(s) or other offenders
Protection of child from continued abuse

Interventions	Rationales
Assess the abuser for violent behavior or other abusive patterns, use of alcohol or drugs, or other psychosocial problems	Provides information to determine warning signs of child abuse
Assess behavior of parent(s) toward child, including responses to the child's behavior, ability to comfort the child, feelings and perceptions toward the child, expectations for the child, overprotective or concern for the child	Reveals characteristics that may indicate risk for abuse
Protect child and parental privacy by not discussing events with others and preventing others from discussing events with the abused child	Protects the rights of the child and parent(s)
Review laws governing child abuse	Provides information about legal aspects of child abuse and actions to take on behalf of all concerned
Communicate information and needs of child to those on the abuse team or to new caretakers if child being placed with a foster parent or someone other than parents; provide written instruction for care and child's needs	Provides care plan for child based on court decision to caretakers working with the family based on court decision for child's care

Interventions	Rationales
Maintain factual and objective documentation of all observations, including: child's physical condition, child's behavioral response to parents, health care workers, other visitors, parent's response to child, and interviews with family members	Provides information that may be used in legal action regarding abuse
Initiate referral to social worker, public health nurse, psychological counselor before discharge to home	Provides support to child and family, and monitors behaviors following discharge

Information, Instruction, Demonstration

Interventions	Rationales
Inform parent(s) of follow-up care and needs of child, need to evaluate child's progress	Promotes emphasis on child's care and prevention of recurrence of abuse
Instruct parent(s) in identifying events that lead to child abuse and in methods to deal with behavior without harming the child	Prevents further abusive behavior directed at the child
Inform of Parents Anonymous and other child protective groups to contact for assistance	Provides self-help group activities, information, and support based on type of abuse and parental needs
Inform parent(s) of child's placement in a foster home, allow them to meet and speak to new caretaker	Prepares parent(s) for court order of alternate placement to ensure a safe environment

Discharge or Maintenance Evaluation

- Protects child from recurrence of or continuance of abuse
- Protects privacy of child and family
- Complies with laws governing child abuse
- Records all events associated with suspected or actual child abuse
- Supports post-hospitalization placement of child by court decision

- Absence of trauma or injury to the child
- Identifies abusive behavior and acts to remove child from the abusive environment
- Assists parent(s) in seeking support and self-help groups
- Referral to social worker, nurse, or counselor for economic, social, psychological and physical needs of child and family

Abused Child

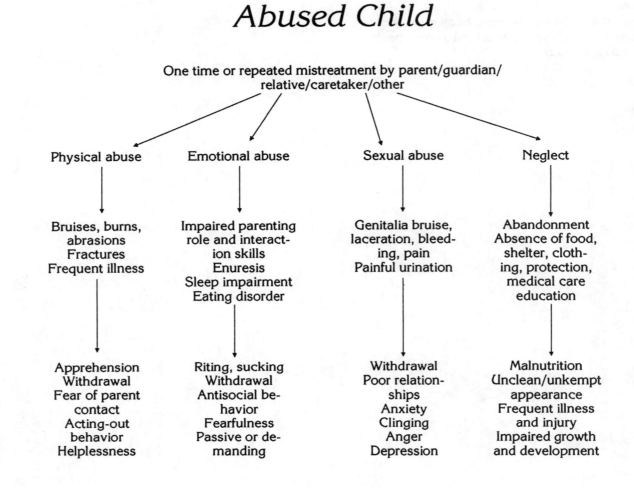

One time or repeated mistreatment by parent/guardian/
relative/caretaker/other

Physical abuse	Emotional abuse	Sexual abuse	Neglect
Bruises, burns, abrasions Fractures Frequent illness	Impaired parenting role and interaction skills Enuresis Sleep impairment Eating disorder	Genitalia bruise, laceration, bleeding, pain Painful urination	Abandonment Absence of food, shelter, clothing, protection, medical care education
Apprehension Withdrawal Fear of parent contact Acting-out behavior Helplessness	Riting, sucking Withdrawal Antisocial behavior Fearfulness Passive or demanding	Withdrawal Poor relationships Anxiety Clinging Anger Depression	Malnutrition Unclean/unkempt appearance Frequent illness and injury Impaired growth and development

Dying Child

Care of the dying child includes the physical and emotional interventions necessary to support the totally dependent child and grieving family. Nursing considerations involve the dissemination of information to the child, whose perceptions of death and responses to death and dying are age-related, and parent(s) with sensitivity, caring, and honesty. The nurse also helps the child move through the stages of awareness and acceptance, and helps the parent(s) and family move through the stages of grieving. An additional role of the pediatric nurse, when caring for dying children, is to direct the child and family to appropriate age-related reading materials about death and dying.

MEDICAL CARE

Medications that promote comfort, pain prevention/management, rest and proper body functions specific to the child's needs.

NURSING CARE PLANS

Essential nursing diagnoses and plans associated with this condition:

Sleep pattern disturbance (114)

Related to: Internal factors of illness and stressors, side effects of medications
Defining characteristics: Fatigue, lethargy, irritability, restlessness, pain, psychological stress (anxiety, fear), nausea and vomiting, increased voiding patterns

Impaired physical mobility (278)

Related to: Pain and discomfort, side effects of medications
Defining characteristics: Weakness, inability to purposefully move, fatigue, limited strength, changes in consciousness, neuropathy, foot drop, amputation, gait disturbances; muscle wasting; contractures

Altered nutrition: less than body requirements (168)

Related to: Loss of appetite, fatigue, oral ulcers, disinterest in food
Defining characteristics: Weakness, anorexia, poor feeding, lack of interest in food, anorexia-cachexia syndrome, nausea and vomiting, chronic constipation or diarrhea; dryness and cracking of lips; alterations in taste

Risk for impaired skin integrity (397)

Related to: External factors of immobilization, side effects of medications; invasive procedures/IV infiltration; radiation treatments
Defining characteristics: Redness, disruption of skin surface, prolonged pressure on skin and bony prominences

Altered thought processes (116)

Related to: Physiological changes, side effects of medication
Defining characteristics: Disorientation, changes in consciousness, fatigue, hallucinations, mood changes

Ineffective airway clearances (42)

Related to: Decreased energy and fatigue, tracheobronchial secretions, oral ulcers; decreased gag reflex
Defining characteristics: Increasing secretions, changes in respiratory rate or depth (stridor, irregularity), inability to cough and remove secretions, shortness of breath

Constipation (173)

Related to: Less than adequate physical activity and intake, side effects of medications, food allergy, secondary to disease process
Defining characteristics: Frequency less than usual pattern, hard-formed stool, decreased bowel sounds, abdominal pain, firm/hard abdomen; fecal impaction

SPECIFIC DIAGNOSES AND CARE PLANS

Pain

Related to: Biological, physical, psychological injuring agents

Defining characteristics: Communication (verbal or coded) of pain descriptors, guarding, protective behavior, facial mask of pain, crying, moaning, withdrawal, changes in VS, irritability, restlessness, age-related expression of pain behaviors, facial grimacing, tension or flexion of muscles

Outcome Criteria

Comfort maintained with absence of pain during terminal period of illness or dying

Interventions	Rationales
Assess severity of pain, fear of receiving pain medication, anxiety and coping mechanisms associated with pain, ability to rest and sleep	Provides information as a basis for analgesic administration
Administer analgesic intermittently or continuously depending on pain severity over 24 hours via PO, IV, using narcotic and non-narcotic medications; administer before any painful procedure or care is performed	Provides 24-hour coverage of pain medications to ensure freedom from any type of pain and discomfort including administration of analgesic for prompt relief if given intermittently
Provide position changes as tolerated, use pillows to support position, move slowly with gentle handling, give backrub	Reduces pain by nonpharmacologic measures
Provide companionship (family member or customary support person) for child, familiar toys	Reduces fear and supports comfort of child
Support coping mechanisms of child and family and adjust analgesic accordingly, with input from child, parent(s), and physician	Promotes child's comfort, supports coping abilities, and includes parent(s) and child in decision making regarding care

Interventions	Rationales
Dim lights, avoid noise, maintain clean, comfortable bed with loose sheets and clothing, disturb for care only when needed to promote comfort	Provides environment free of stimuli that increases anxiety and pain
Provide non-pharmacological pain management strategies: soothing baths; massage therapy to painful areas; education on possible (and encourage parent/child to use) distraction techniques, (i.e., music, aroma, humor, reading, journal writing, art work, pets, prayer, hypnosis, relaxation techniques)	Reduces pain perceptions and may foster a sense of control
Assess child's pain with developmentally based pain scales	Enhances accurate assessment and treatment of child's pain

Information, Instruction, Demonstration

Interventions	Rationales
Inform child and parent(s) of route of medication administration and effect to expect; that pain will be assessed continuously and medication adjusted as needed to control pain	Provides assurance that pain will be controlled continuously whether or not child is able to express pain
Inform child and parent(s) that fear of pain is common and that it is all right to express fear and feelings about pain and its control	Reduces anxiety by recognizing fear of pain and encouraging to vent feelings and concerns about methods of control
Inform parent(s) and child of all procedures that cause pain and that only palliative care and treatments will be administered	Reduces anxiety and stress caused by anticipation of painful interventions

Discharge or Maintenance Evaluation

- Controls pain and maintains comfort
- Reduces fear of pain and its consequences

- Administers correct analgesic by correct route based on continuous assessment of pain control
- Administers nonpharmacologic measures to maintain comfort
- Reduces stimuli that trigger or increase pain

Anticipatory grieving

Related to: Potential loss of a child

Defining characteristics: Expression of distress at potential loss of child, denial of loss, guilt, anger, sorrow, choked feelings, change in need fulfillment, crying, self-blame, shock and disbelief, overprotectiveness, loss of hope and depression, withdrawal and avoidance of ill child

Outcome Criteria

Family and parent(s) progress through grief process towards acceptance of potential loss

Interventions	Rationales
Assess stage of grief process, problems encountered, feelings regarding terminal nature of illness and potential loss of child	Provides information about need for grieving, which varies with individual members of a family when child's death is expected
Provide emotional and spiritual comfort in an accepting environment, and avoid conversations that cause guilt or anger	Provides for emotional need of parent(s) and family and helps them to cope with dying child without adding stressors that are difficult to resolve
Provide opportunities for family to express feelings and respond to child commensurate with stage of grieving	Promotes progression through grieving and ability to express desires for themselves and their child
Allow parent(s) and family members to be with child as much as they feel a need to, and help them understand the child's behavior and needs	Promotes feeling that they are helping and supporting their child
Assist family in identifying and use effective coping mechanisms and in understanding situation over which they have no control	Promotes effective coping that is positive for the family
Provide privacy when needed, while being available to the family	Promotes a helping relationship with the family

Interventions	Rationales
Arrange for clergy, social services, hospice care, or return to home for dying as appropriate; support choices made by the family	Provides for and assists with alternative care and preferences for that care
Encourage parent(s) to express their thoughts, feelings, and about the possible death of their child; to share memories of their child's life; to create memories (now, if possible); to take family pictures, and create a memory box of their child's memory	Promotes parent coping, acceptance of grief process, and may minimize sense of guilt
Encourage parent(s) to be involved with child's care (i.e., procedures, how to help with nausea, pain control)	Reduces parent feelings of powerlessness and helplessness
Inform parent(s) that their grief response is normal	Promotes parent understanding of their grief reaction and may enhance parent coping abilities
Educate parent(s) regarding child's developmental understanding of death; educate and encourage parent(s) to utilize children's books to aid in a discussion about the child's understanding/fears of death	Promotes family communication; promotes family coping abilities

Information, Instruction, Demonstration

Interventions	Rationales
Inform parent(s) and family of stages of grieving and acceptable behaviors during the grief process	Promotes understanding of feeling and behaviors manifested by the grieving process
Provide information about child's condition, including appearance of the child, and reactions to expect	Allows parent(s) to follow course of terminal condition and change to expect
Instruct parent(s) in care and procedures they want to participate in and in	Involves parent(s) involvement in child's care and allows them to share their

Interventions	Rationales
those they will carry out if the child is taken home to die; suggest resources to contact for assistance	sadness with child
Inform family to ask questions and to be honest about their feelings and acceptance of information about death and dying	Promotes honest and realistic view of situation to enhance grieving
Inform family to maintain own needs and health during this difficult time	Allows family to better cope with child's needs if own needs are fulfilled, since terminal period may be prolonged

Discharge or Maintenance Evaluation

- Verbalizes understanding of grief process and responses
- Shares feelings with professionals and other members of the family
- Performs parental tasks/care to child
- Accepts and uses coping skills that support grieving
- Makes decisions regarding placement and care of dying child
- Contacts and utilizes support services of clergy, social services and hospice as appropriate
- Maintains a presence of parent or family member and privacy to be with child

Anxiety

Related to: Diagnosis, tests, treatments, pain, side effects of medication and prognosis

Defining characteristics: Increased apprehension and fear of death, loss of control, loneliness; increased feelings of helplessness and hopelessness; poor prognosis of terminal illness

Outcome Criteria

Reduced anxiety and fear
Increased comfort of parent(s) and child in expression of feelings

Interventions	Rationales
Assess anxiety level, fears and concerns, ability to express needs, and how anxiety is manifested	Reveals information needed for interventions to relieve anxiety and increased comfort

Interventions	Rationales
Allow family member to stay with child or remain with child during stressful periods if family not able to be there	Promotes comfort of child and provides support during anxious and fearful times
Allow expressions of fears and concerns about terminal stage of illness, answer all questions honestly based on what family has been told about prognosis	Provides opportunity to vent feelings and fears to reduce anxiety
Provide appropriate pain control and preparation prior to invasive procedures (i.e., application of EMLA cream before bone marrow aspiration, or before restarting IV sites)	Promotes comfort and minimizes emotional distress related to invasive procedures
Provide calm reassurance and kindness, be available to child at all times as needed for support	Promotes comfort and love of child to reduce anxiety
Involve child and parent(s) in as much planning and care as possible without forcing participation	Promotes interactions and attitude of caring within family

Information, Instruction, Demonstration

Interventions	Rationales
Inform child and parent(s) of all anticipated care and activities up to death	Promotes understanding of physical needs of dying child, limiting activities to those that are essential
Inform family members, with honesty and openness, of physical changes in child as death nears	Prepares them for the changes and assists in the recognition of impending death
Inform child and parent(s) that they are not to blame for illness and its consequences	Reduces fear and guilt caused by terminal nature of the illness
Inform parent(s) to avoid talking about diagnosis or condition in the child's presence, to talk to the child and sit or lie near the child as desired	Reduces possibility of additional stress for child; reduces child's fear of what is happening or of being alone

Interventions	Rationales
Inform parent(s) and family members of telephone numbers and methods of acquiring information about the child	Provides a source of communication about the child's condition

Discharge or Maintenance Evaluation

- Expresses and exhibits a reduction in anxiety, fear of loneliness
- States sources of anxiety and measures to reduce it
- Utilizes support systems and open visitation, remains with child whether parent or family member
- Promotes accepting, nonjudgmental, calm environment
- Provides comfort measures for child and family to reduce anxiety and concerns

Dying Child

Life threatening illness   Congenital anomaly   Trauma from accident
                                                                or violence

Complete physical dependency

Pain relief
Airway patency
Skin integrity
Rest promotion
Nutritional maintenance
Elimination maintenance
Medication administration

Hospitalized Child

Hospitalization of the child, whether it involves a short-term hospital admission, surgery, a follow-up evaluation, or repeated hospitalizations for a chronic illness or episode, creates a crisis for the child, parent(s), and family members. Responses to hospitalization are related to the age of the child but generally include fear of separation, loss of control, injury, and pain. The ease of transition from home to the hospital depends on how well the child has been prepared for it and how the child's physical and emotional needs have been met. Supporting the parents and family, providing them with information, and encouraging their participation in the child's care contributes to the adjustment and well-being of all concerned.

MEDICAL CARE

Laboratory tests and diagnostic procedures related to illness and treatment regimen.

NURSING CARE PLANS

Essential nursing diagnoses and plans associated with this condition:

Sleep pattern disturbance (114)

Related to: Physiological factors related to illness and psychological stress, external factors of environmental changes
Defining characteristics: Interrupted sleep, irritability, restlessness, lethargy, disorientation, fatigue, pain, separation anxiety, side effects of medication (nausea, vomiting, diarrhea)

Impaired physical mobility (278)

Related to: Intolerance to activity, pain and discomfort, neuro or musculoskeletal impairment
Defining characteristics: Imposed restrictions of movement or activity, imposed bedrest, limited strength, endurance, weakness, fatigue, drainage tubes and IV catheters; disturbances in gait, vision, equilibrium

Altered nutrition: less than body requirements (168)

Related to: Loss of appetite, lack of interest in food, alteration in taste buds, inability to ingest, digest or absorb nutrients, nausea, vomiting, diarrhea, constipation, abdominal pain, oral ulcers
Defining characteristics: Weakness, fatigue, anxiety, anorexia, illness, lack of interest in eating

Altered growth and development (419)

Related to: Separation from significant others, environmental and stimulation deficiencies, effects of repeated hospitalizations, social isolation, sensory and/or motor delays
Defining characteristics: Inability to perform self-care or self-control activities appropriate for age, regressive behavior, fear or unfamiliar environment and treatments, feelings of inferiority, low self-esteem, or alterations to body image

SPECIFIC DIAGNOSES AND CARE PLANS

Anxiety

Related to: Change in health status, change in environment, threat to self-concept, situational crisis
Defining characteristics: Increased apprehension; fear; helplessness; uncertainty; distress over hospitalization; restlessness; expressed concern over procedures, pain, loss of control, separation from significant others; crying; clinging; refusal to interact with staff changes in VS, financial stresses due to required absence from employment

Outcome Criteria

Reduced anxiety expressed by child or noted in child as information and measures given about hospitalization, treatments, and prognosis
Recognition of anxiety by child, parent(s), and family members

Interventions	Rationales
Assess child's parental and family level of anxiety, developmental level, understanding of illness and reason for hospitalization, responses to this and previous hospitalizations	Provides information about sources and level of anxiety related to illness and hospitalization; sources of anxiety and responses vary with age of child and include separation, pain and bodily injury, loss of control, enforced dependence, fear of unknown, fear of equipment, unfamiliar environment and routines, guilt, fear and concern for child's recovery, feelings of powerlessness
Assess social and emotional history of child, parent(s), and family for strengths and successful coping ability	Provides information about strengths and about weaknesses to draw upon to cope with hospitalization
Allow expression of feelings and concerns about illness and procedures and listen individually to child, parent(s), and family	Provides opportunity to vent feelings and fears to reduce anxiety and promote adaptation to hospitalization
Provide a calm, accepting environment and avoid rushing through interactions and care	Assists child and family in establishing trust and obtaining emotional stability
Provide orientation to hospital environment and room, routines, meal and play time, introduction to staff members, forms to sign and hospital policies	Familiarizes child and family with environment, promotes secure feeling, and reduces fear of unknown
Have same personnel following written care plan, care for child; schedule personal contact with child within work day	Promotes continuity and consistency of care to support trusting relationship
Encourage involvement of child and parent(s) in planning and interventions of care; allow parents to remain with child or have open visitations; allow to hold and cuddle the child	Promotes participation in and adaptation to hospitalization, reduces anxiety; allows demonstration of love and affection for child

Interventions	Rationales
Allow child and parent(s) to incorporate home routines as much as possible; bring toys, tapes, photographs and favorite foods from home as appropriate	Promotes security and reduces anxiety associated with new experiences
Maintain a quiet environment, control visitors and interactions	Decreases stimuli that increase anxiety
Allow child to play out feelings, accept feelings and responses expressed by the child	Permits child to express feelings without fear of punishment
Approach child in a positive way; use child's proper name; avoid communicating, either verbally or nonverbally, any rejection, judgments, or negativism	Promotes rapport and trust and maintains identity
Identify and recognize regressive behavior as a part of the illness and assist child in dealing with dependency associated with the hospitalization	Allows for behaviors common to hospitalizations and loss of control
Provide support to child during any procedures or distressing features associated with care, including intrusive procedures, exposure of body parts, need for personal privacy and privacy of others	Reduces anxiety and fear caused by possible bodily injury

Information, Instruction, Demonstration

Interventions	Rationales
Inform and explain all treatments and procedures in simple, understandable language to child and parent(s) according to their intellectual level and age; pace information according to child/parental needs	Provides easily understood information, which decreases anxiety
Inform parent(s) and child that behavior caused by anxiety and fear is normal and expected	Prevents feeling of inadequacy and fear of punishment

Interventions	Rationales
Use therapeutic play to explain and prepare child for procedures; repeat any teaching as needed	Permits child to understand and become familiar with articles used for care or procedure
If surgery planned, instruct in preoperative and postoperative care, surgical procedure to be done, reason for surgery, and length of hospitalization; answer questions about surgery	Prepares child for surgical intervention with minimal anxiety

Discharge or Maintenance Evaluation

- Expression of reduction in anxiety by child, parent(s), and family
- Expresses feelings and fears about hospitalization
- Modifies hospital environment to include home routines
- Prepares child and family for procedures and treatments
- Verbalizes pre- and post-operative procedures and expectations
- Participates in decision making, planning, and implementing care
- Minimizes fear of bodily injury, pain, separation anxiety, loss of control and independence
- Visits or stays with child
- Interacts with staff and develops trust and rapport
- Exhibits understanding of instructions and information given

Self-care deficit, bathing/ hygiene, dressing/grooming, feeding, toileting

Related to: Impaired ability to perform ADL, intolerance to activity, pain and discomfort
Defining characteristics: Inability to wash body, take off or put on clothing, feed self, positioning or mechanical restrictions, weakness, fatigue, imposed bedrest, inability to carry out toileting with use of bedpan or go to bathroom

Outcome Criteria

Maximum self-care capability with or without use of aids

Interventions	Rationales
Assess physical tolerance and abilities to perform ADL, and play activities and restrictions imposed by the illness and medical protocol	Provides information about amount of energy and effect of illness on activity level
Anticipate child's personal needs for toileting, feeding, brushing teeth, bathing and other care if unable to manage on own; allow child to do as much as possible	Prevents embarrassing experiences with toileting and maintain comfort with personal cleanliness and appearance
Provide personal care for infant and small child; assist child and encourage parent(s) to assist child that needs help with ADL, and adjust times and methods to fit home routine	Provides needed assistance where using patterns and articles that child is accustomed to using and doing
Praise child for participation in own care according to age, developmental level, and energy	Promotes self-esteem and independence
Provide assistive aids or devices to perform ADL, allow choices when possible	Assists child in performing self-care for ADL
Balance activities with rest as needed; place needed articles and call light within reach	Prevents fatigue by conserving energy and promoting rest

Information, Instruction, Demonstration

Interventions	Rationales
Instruct child in toileting, feeding, bathing, hygiene, dressing while in hospital environment and inform of differences from home care and methods as needed	Promotes performance of ADL skills already known by child
Inform to rest when tired and to request quiet times	Ensures proper rest and prevents fatigue

Interventions	Rationales
Inform parent(s) to assist child in ADL but to allow child as much independence as condition permits; inform parent(s) that a place is provided for their personal needs in order to allow them to remain with the child	Promotes independence and some control by the child without separating child from parent(s)
Instruct parent(s) to interpret child's needs if child too young to talk	Provides anticipatory care for child

Discharge or Maintenance Evaluation

- Anticipates child's needs
- Helps child to remain as independent as possible in ADL
- Provides aids and devices to assist child in performance of ADL and self-care
- Promotes rest periods before and after activity
- Promotes independence in self-care activities

Diversionary activity deficit

Related to: Environmental lack of diversionary activity, long-term hospitalization
Defining characteristics: Boredom, desire for something to do because usual hobbies and activities cannot be undertaken in hospital

Outcome Criteria

Participation in age-appropriate activities within limitations imposed by illness

Interventions	Rationales
Assess type of activities allowed and desired and amount of motor activity needed; check medical protocol for bedrest or limitations imposed by illness	Provides information about type of activities and play to suggest
Show play room to child and introduce child and family to other children and families with similar illness	Provides a familiar environment for child

Interventions	Rationales
Place child in a room with another child of same age if possible	Promotes interaction and diversion while hospitalized
Schedule care and treatments to allow for play activities	Provides opportunity for play and diversion
Provide age-appropriate play activities according to amount of energy of child and activity allowed, including quiet play with games, television, reading, soft toys, favorite toy	Prevents fatigue resulting from over-activity while ill and in need of rest and quiet
Encourage family to play with child or interact with child	Promotes diversion for child
Provide play activities that include educational needs for schoolage child; bring schoolwork from home if appropriate	Promotes therapy that includes educational needs
Provide a play therapist for assistance in planning activities and assessing child's play needs	Promotes age-appropriate diversionary activities

Information, Instruction, Demonstration

Interventions	Rationales
Inform parent(s) to bring to hospital child's favorite toys or articles for play	Promotes diversionary activity
Inform parent(s) and child of need to monitor activities and rest although still allowing for play and interactions with others	Prevents fatigue during acute phase of illness

Discharge or Maintenance Evaluation

- Schedules play and diversionary activities in care plan
- Provides diversionary activities for child according to abilities and age
- Engages in activities appropriate for age, desires and limitations imposed by illness

- Provides play therapist or child life worker to plan and assist with diversionary activities

Powerlessness

Related to: Health care environment, illness-related regimen

Defining characteristics: Expression of loss of control over situation, expression or behavior indicating dissatisfaction with inability to perform activities and dependence on others, reluctance to express true feelings, fear of alienation from others in the hospital environment

Outcome Criteria

Gains sense of control over situation

Interventions	Rationales
Encourage parent(s) and child to verbalize feelings in an accepting environment	Allows for venting of feelings about loss of control and frustrations over loss of ability to perform activities
Allow for input from child and parent(s) in care goals, care plan, and scheduling of activities, and integrate this input into routines as much as possible	Allows for as much control as possible for child and family
Encourage parent(s) to participate in child's care as much as desired; and to visit or remain with child continuously	Promotes support of child and allows family some control over the situation
Provide encouragement and praise to child and parent(s) for their participation; encourage and defend expression of their true feelings	Promotes positive feedback and reduces fear of rejection by staff because of their behavior
Allow child to perform simple tasks in hospital unit and for own care, such as pouring own water and marking amounts on record at bedside	Promotes independence and control of the environment

Information, Instruction, Demonstration

Interventions	Rationales
Inform parent(s) and child of tasks that they can perform in care plan	Accommodates need for sense of control

Discharge or Maintenance Evaluation

- Visits or remains with child as able
- Participates in goal development, care, and scheduling of treatments
- Incorporates suggestions of child and parent(s) in care
- Verbalizes increase in control over situation and decreased feelings of powerlessness and helplessness
- Accepts responsibility for actions, behaviors that contribute to adaptation to hospitalization
- Complies with medical protocol while hospitalized

Hospitalized Child

Exacerbation of chronic
illness

Acute illness

Surgical/Diagnostic
procedures

Hospitalization (long-term or short-term)

Separation from parent(s)
Loss of control
Unfamiliar environment
Fear of pain

Anxiety/Fear
Protest/Crying
Withdrawal
Denial

Support coping behaviors
Relieve physical and emotional discomforts
Allow as much autonomy as possible
Individualize care dependent on age and abilities
Prepare properly for any procedure/treatment
Provide developmental activities

Play/Therapeutic Play

Play has been recognized as a significant coping strategy by various child developmental theorists. For example: play is the child's way of self expression; play is an expression of the child's understanding of their world and attempts to master the environment; or play provides the child with a measure of control of their environment. The play activities of a child also provide a developmental and a social tool, providing a mechanism to promote their social, cognitive and physical abilities. The effects of illness, treatments, and hospitalization has been identified as a source of emotional distress to the well child's usual coping strategies. Some of the reactions of children to these effects include: crying, clinging to parents, decreased communication, loss of sleep, regressive behaviors. Child developmental theorists have documented the benefits of providing structured play activities/medical play to enable the child to preserve usual coping strategies and emotional health. Therapeutic or structured medical play has been identified as an effective intervention to help children prepare for, cope with, assimilate, and master painful procedures and the stress of hospitalizations. A significant nursing intervention is to provide the child with a pleasurable play experience at the onset of hospitalization which may ease the emotional distress associated with invasive procedures or with the hospitalization process.

NURSING CARE PLANS

Essential nursing diagnoses and plans associated with this condition:

Altered growth and development (419)

Related to: Environmental and stimulation difficulties, effects of physical disability
Defining characteristics: Delay or difficulty in performing skills (motor, social, or expressive) typical of age group, listlessness, decreased responses, inability to perform play activities appropriate for age, fatigue, pain, cognitive/visual/hearing impairment; regressive behaviors

SPECIFIC DIAGNOSES AND CARE PLANS

Risk for trauma

Related to: Developmental age, knowledge deficit and cognitive immaturity predisposing the child to safety hazards in the environment
Defining characteristics: Developmental age, developmental delays, disturbances in gait, vision, hearing, perceptual or cognitive functioning

Outcome Criteria

Therapeutic and normal play activities which foster the child's normal development; adaptation to illness, treatments, and hospitalization; and in reaching their optimum level of functioning

Interventions	Rationales
Assess age of child and reason for particular selection of type and article of play, and intended purpose of play (enjoyment, development, therapy)	Provides information needed to select appropriate toy or activity for play based on age: infants grasp and hold articles and stuffed toys; young child plays with replicas of adult tools and other toys, plays pretend, and later moves from toys to games, hobbies, sports; older child continues with games and sports and begins to daydream; play provides fun, diversion, and learning about procedures for the child who is hospitalized
Select safe toys appropriate for age and amount of activity allowed (active or passive play) and that suit the skills and interest of the child	Provides guidelines for quiet play or play that involves motor activity
Encourage play and allow parent(s) to bring favorite toy, game or other play materials from home	Promotes learning and skill development, and facilitates expression of feelings

Interventions	Rationales
In a quiet environment, plan and implement an age-appropriate play activity to prepare the child for all invasive procedures, to observe child's behavior, or to allow child to reveal fears and concerns with or without someone in attendance	Promotes therapeutic play with a selection of toys and articles that include dolls or puppets (nurse, doctor, child, family members); hospital supplies (syringe, dressings, tape, tubes); paper, crayons, and paints; stuffed toys, toy telephone; prepares the child emotionally and cognitively for invasive procedures; fosters appropriate coping strategies
Remove all unsafe, sharp, broken toys, toys with small parts that can be swallowed, toys inappropriate for age	Prevents trauma or injury to the child
Allow child to communicate type of toy desired and to assist in the selection of toys and play activities	Promotes independence and control over play situation

Information, Instruction, Demonstration

Interventions	Rationales
Inform parent(s) to select toys, play equipment, and supplies that are labeled for intended age group; nontoxic and flame resistant with directions for use; that are durable and do not have sharp edges or points; that do not have small parts that can be swallowed; that do not contain any parts to be ejected; and that are not broken, rusted, or weak and need repairs	Promotes safe play for the child
Inform parent(s) to store play materials meant for older children away from young child to provide a safe place for toys, to discard or repair broken toys	Prevents accidents caused by toys in pathways or by toys meant for older, more mature play

Interventions	Rationales
Inform parent(s) to select play activity based on child's energy and tolerance level during an illness, and to evaluate toys given as gifts to the child	Provides the enjoyment of active or passive play that is geared to child's condition

Discharge or Maintenance Evaluation

- Provides environment for safe play
- Selects play materials related to age and individual needs
- Verbalizes criteria for safe toys and play activities
- Absence of trauma or injury resulting from play
- Utilizes therapeutic play when needed

Play/Therapeutic Play

Play activity
↓
Selected by child purely
for enjoyment
↓
Exploration
Pleasure
Imitation
Socialization
Group games

Passive   Active
↓   ↓
Television   Motor activity
Radio   ↓
Board games   Riding tricycle
Cards   Swimming
Music   Climbing
Puzzles   Skating
Crafts   Sports
Toys

Therapeutic play
↓
Selected to stimulate growth
and development
Express emotions
Releases tension/stress
Communication of fears/needs

↓

Sensorimotor development
Intellectual development
Self-awareness
Moral development

Teaching   Diversional   Expressive
activities   activities   activities
↓   ↓   ↓
Hospital   Toys   Creative drawing
equipment   Games   and painting
Anatomically   Books   Making cards or
correct dolls   Radio, TV, tapes   gifts
Play telephone   Weaving   Dramatic play
Drawings   Crayons and   Puppets
Models   coloring books   Dolls
                                     Clay modeling

References

BOOKS

Barker, E. (Ed.). (1994). *Neuroscience Nursing*. St. Louis: Mosby-Year Book.

Betx, C.L., & Poster, E.C. (1989). *Pediatric nursing reference*. St. Louis: C.V. Mosby.

Burns, C., Barber, N., Brady, M., & Dunn, A. (1996). *Pediatric primary care: A handbook for nurse practitioners*. Philadelphia: W.B. Saunders.

Cammermeyer, M., & Appledorn, C. (Eds.). (1993). *Core curriculum for neuroscience nursing*. (3rd ed.). Chicago: American Association of Neuroscience Nurses.

Foley, G.V., Fochtman, D., & Mooney, K.H. (1993). *Nursing care of the child with cancer* (2nd ed.). Philadelphia: W.B. Saunders.

Govani, L.E., & Hayes, J.E. (1988). *Drugs and nursing implications* (6th ed.). Norwalk: Appleton & Lange.

Hazinski, M.F. (1992). *Nursing care of the critically ill child* (2nd ed.). St. Louis: Mosby Year Book.

Hilgartner, M. W., & Corrigan, J. J. (1995). Coagulation disorders. In R. L. Baehner, D. R. Miller, & L. P. Miller (Eds.), *Blood disorders of infancy and childhood* (pp. 932-953). St. Louis: Mosby.

Jackson, P.L., & Vessey, J.A. (1992). *Primary care of the child with a chronic condition*. St. Louis: Mosby.

Kathleen, K.W., & Armstrong-Dailey, A. (1997). Care of the dying child. In P.A. Pizzo & D.G. Poplack (Eds.), *Principals and practice of pediatric oncology* (pp. 1343-1355). Philadelphia: Lippincott-Raven.

Kee, Joyce LeFever. (1987). Laboratory and diagnostic tests with nursing implications (2nd ed.). Norwalk: Appleton & Lange. North American Nursing Diagnosis Association (1990). Taxonomy I Revised with official nursing diagnoses. St. Louis.

Lewandowski, L.A. (1992). Psychosocial aspects of pediatric critical care. In M.F. Hazinski (Ed.), *Nursing care of the critically ill child* (2nd ed.), (pp. 19-78). St. Louis: Mosby-Year Book.

Ludington, S. M., & Golant, S. K. (1993). *Kangaroo care: The best you can do to help your preterm infant*. New York: Bantam Books.

Lukens, J. N. Iron metabolism and iron deficiency. In R.L. Baehner, D. R. Miller, and L. P. Miller (Eds.), *Blood disorders of infancy and childhood* (pp. 193-219). St. Louis: Mosby.

Mankad, V.N. (1995). Sickle cell anemia and other disorders of abnormal hemoglobin. In R. L. Baehner, D. R. Miller, & L. P. Miller (Eds.)., *Blood disorders of infancy and childhood* (pp. 415-450). St. Louis: Mosby.

Miller, D. R., & O'Reilly, R. J. (1995). Aplastic anemia. In R. L. Baehner, D. R. Miller, & L. P. Miller (Eds.), *Blood disorders of infancy and childhood* (pp. 499-525). St. Louis: Mosby.

Mueller, B. U., & Pizzo, P. A. (1997). Pediatric AIDS and childhood cancer. In P. A. Pizzo & D. G. Poplack (Eds.), *Principles and Practice of Pediatric Oncology* (pp. 1005-1019). Philadelphia: Lippincott-Raven.

National Association of Neonatal Nurses. (1993). *Infant Developmental Care Guidelines*.

Pillitteri, A. (1995). *Maternal and child health nursing: Care of the childbearing family* (2nd ed.). Philadelphia: J. B. Lippincott.

Porth, Carol M. (1986). Pathophysiology. *Concepts of altered health states* (2nd ed.). Philadelphia: J. B. Lippincott.

Richtman, D., & Mooney, K. H. (1993). *Nursing care of the child with cancer* (2nd ed.). Philadelphia: W. B. Saunders.

Sandlund, J. T., Hutchinson, R. C., & Crist, W. M. (1991). Non-Hodgkin's lymphoma. In D. J. Fernbach, & T. J. Vietti (Eds.), *Clinical pediatric oncology* (4th ed.). St. Louis: Mosby.

Schafer, P. S. et al. (1988). *Nursing care plans for the child: A nursing diagnosis approach*. Norwalk: Appleton & Lange.

Selelman, Janice. (1988). *Pediatric nursing: A study and learning tool*. Springhouse: Springhouse Publishing.

Skidmore-Roth, Linda. (1992) *Nursing drug reference*. St. Louis: Mosby-Year Book.

Speer, K. M. (1990). *Pediatric care plans.* Springhouse: Springhouse Publishing.

Whaley, L. F., & Wong, D. L. (1991). *Nursing care of infants and infants and children* (4th ed.). St. Louis: Mosby Year Book.

Wong, D. (1995). *Whaley and Wong's nursing care of infants and children* (5th ed.). St. Louis: Mosby Year Book.

PERIODICALS

Agamalian, B. (1986). Pediatric cardiac catheterization. *Journal of Pediatric Nursing,* 1 (2), 73-79.

Ahern, J., & Grey, M. (1996). New developments in treating children with insulin-dependent diabetes mellitus. *Journal of Pediatric Health Care,* 10 (4), 161-166.

Almekinders, L. C. (1994). Osteomylitis: Essentials of diagnosis and treatment. *Journal of Musculoskeletal Medicine,* 11 (11), 31-32.

Als, H. & Gilkerson, L. (1995). Developmentally supportive care in the neonatal intensive care unit. *Zero to Three,* 15 (6), 44ccc-44jjj.

American Academy of Pediatrics, (1993). Committee on infectious diseases: Use of ribavirin in the treatment of RSV infection. *Pediatrics,* 92 (3), 501-504.

Armstrong-Dailey, A. (1990). Children's hospice care. *Pediatric Nursing,* 16 (4), 337-339, 409.

Avery, M., & Snyder, J. (1990). Oral therapy for acute diarrhea: The underused simple solution. *New England Journal of Medicine,* 323, 891-894.

Bacigaulup, A., Broccia, G., Corda, W. et al. (1995). Antilymphocyte globulin, cyclosporin, and granulocyte colony stimulating factor in patients with acquired aplastic anemia. *Blood,* 85, 1348-1353.

Bali, B. et al. (1986). Diabetes and the school-aged child. *American Journal of Maternal Child Nursing,* 11 (5), 324-330.

Balistereri, W. (1988). Viral hepatitis. *Pediatric Clinics of North America,* 35 (3), 637.

Bellanti, J. A. (Ed.). (1990). Pediatrics vaccination: Update 1990. *Pediatric Clinics of North America,* 37 (3), 513-784.

Berde, C. B. et al. (1988). Pediatric pain management. *Hospital Practices,* 23 (5), 83-94.

Berti, L. C. (1996). Childhood tuberculosis. *Journal of Pediatric Health Care,* 10, 106-114.

Berube, M. (1997). Gastroesophogeal reflux. *Journal of the Society of Pediatric Nurses,* 2, 43-46.

Birmingham, P.K. (1995). Recent advances in acute pain management. *Current Problems in Pediatrics,* 3, 99-112.

Bowden, V.R. Children's literature: The death experience. *Pediatric Nursing,* 19, 17-21.

Breaux, C. et al. (1988). Changing patterns in the diagnosis of hypertrophic pyloric stenosis. *Pediatrics,* 81 (2), 213.

Breitzer, G. M. (1989). Practical approach to the treatment of otitis media in infants and children. *Pediatric Basics,* 51, 11-16.

Buchanan, G. R. (1993). Sickle cell disease: Recent advances: *Current Problems in Pediatrics,* 7, 219-227.

Cahill, M. (1996). Hematologic problems in pediatric patients. *Seminars in Oncology Patients,* 12, 38-50.

Castiglia, P. (1996). Adjusting to childhood asthma. *Journal of Pediatric Health Care,* 10, 82-84.

Castiglia, P. T. (1996). Kawasaki disease. *Journal of Pediatric Health Care,* 10 (3), 124-126.

Charron-Prochownik, D. C., Kovacs, M., Obrosky, D. S., & Ho, V. (1995). Illness characteristics and psychosocial and demographic correlates of illness severity at onset of insulin-dependent diabetes mellitus among school-age children. *Journal of Pediatric Nursing,* 10 (6), 354-359.

Clarke, D., MacKenzie, B., Stutzer, C., Connaughty, S., & McCormick, J. (1996). Caring for dying children: Nurse's experiences. *Pediatric Nursing,* 22, 500-507.

Coody, D. K., Yetman, R. J., & Portman, R. J. (1995). Hypertension in children. *Journal of Pediatric Health Care,* 9, 3-11.

Curry, D. M., & Dulby, J. C. (1994). Developmental surveillance by pediatric nurses. *Pediatric Nursing, 20*, 40-44.

Davidhizar, R. (1997). Disability does not have to be the grief that never ends: Helping patients cope. *Rehabilitation Nursing, 22* (1), 101-112.

Davies, B., & Eng, B. (1993). Factors influencing nursing care of children who are terminally ill: A selective review. *Pediatric Nursing, 19*, 9-14.

Davies, B., Cook, K., O'Loane, M., Clarke, D., MacKenzie, B., Stutzer, C., Connaughty, S., & McCormick, J. (1996). Caring for dying children: Nurse's experiences. *Pediatric Nursing, 22*, 500-507.

Davis, N., & Sweeney, L. (1989). Infantile apnea monitoring and SIDS. *Journal of Pediatric Health Care, 3* (2), 67-75.

Demers, D. M., Vincent, J. M., & Bass, J. W. (1993). Group A streptococcal disease. *Current Opinion in Infectious Diseases, 6* (4), 565-569, 605.

DiMickele, D. (1996). Hemophilia 1996: New approach to an old disease. *Pediatric Clinics of North America, 43*, 709-736.

Dolgin, M. et al. (1989). Behavioral distress in pediatric patients with cancer receiving chemotherapy. *Pediatrics, 84* (1), 103-110.

Dunst, R. M. (1990). Legg-Calve-Perthes disease. *Orthopaedic Nursing, 9* (2), 18-36.

El-Sayyad, M., & Conine, T. A. (1994). Effect of exercise, bracing and electrical surface stimulation on idiopathic scoliosis: A preliminary study. *International Journal of Rehabilitation Research, 17* (1), 70-74.

Epstein, S., & Reilly, J. S. (1989). Sensorineural hearing loss. Pediatric Clinics of North America, 36 (6), 1501-1520.

Falloon, J. et al. (1989). Human immunodeficiency virus infection in children. *Journal of Pediatrics, 114* (1), 1.

Faulkner, M. S. (1996). Family responses to children with diabetes and their influence on self-care. *Journal of Pediatric Nursing, 11* (2), 82-92.

Feber, R. (1988). Sleep disorders in children. *Pediatric Consultant, 7* (2), 1-12.

Foreman, J.W., & Chan, J.C.M. (1988). Chronic renal failure in infants and children. *Journal of Pediatrics, 113*, 793-800.

Francis, E. (1987). Lateral electrical surface stimulation treatment for scoliosis. *Pediatric Nursing, 13* (3), 157.

Freund, B. D., Scacco-Neumann, A., Pisanelli, A. S., & Benchot, R. (1993). Acute rheumatic fever revisited. *Journal of Pediatric Nursing, 8* (3), 167-175.

Fuller, A. K. (1989). Child molestation and pedophilia. *Journal of the American Medical Association, 261* (4), 602-606.

Futcher, J. (1988). Chronic illness and family dynamics. *Pediatric Nursing, 14* (5), 381-385.

Gale, R. O. (1989). The management of acute leukemias. *Clinical Advances in Oncologic Nursing, 1* (3), 1-9.

Gerdes, J. E. (1990). An ambulatory approach to outpatient pediatric cardiac catheterization. *Journal of Post Anesthesia Nursing, 5* (6), 407- 410.

Gibbons, D., Kurdahi, L., & Opas, S. R. (1995). Nursing management of children with sickle cell disease: An update. *Journal of Pediatric Nursing, 10*, 232-242.

Goldberg, C. J., Dowling, F. E., Fogarty, E. E., & Moore, D. P. (1995). School scoliosis screening and the United States preventative services task force. *Spine, 20*, 1368-1374.

Griffiths, S. P. (1993). Acute rheumatic fever: Diagnostic considerations. *Emergency Pediatrics, 6* (2), 24-27.

Hahn, K. (1987). Therapeutic storytelling: Helping children learn and cope. *Pediatric Nursing, 13* (3), 175-178.

Harris, J. et al. (1992). Respiratory syncytial virus: A pediatric nursing plan of care. *Journal of Pediatric Nursing, 7* (2), 128-132.

Hartsell, M. (1987). Chest physiotherapy and mechanical vibration. *Journal of Pediatric Nursing, 2* (2), 135.

Heremia, N. A. (1990). Cytogenic abnormalities and molecular markers of acute lyphoblastic leukemia. *Hematology Clinics of North America, 4*, 795-820.

Herman-Staab, B. (1992). Antecedents to nonorganic failure-to-thrive. *Pediatric Nursing, 18*, 579- 583.

Hidrtz, D. G. (1989). Generalized tonic-clonic and febrile seizures. *Pediatric Clinics of North America, 36*, 365-382.

Hilgartner, M. W. (1994) The prophylactic use of porcine factor VIII. *Seminars in Hematology, 31*, 65-66. (Suppl 4)

Huckstadt, A. (1986). Hemophilia: The person, family, and nurse. *Rehabilitation Nursing, 11* (3), 25-28.

Kaufman, R. et al. (1988). Aspirin use and Reye's Syndrome. *Pediatric Clinics of North America, 35*, 89-208.

Keiser, H. D. (1993). Acute rheumatic fever. *Hospital Medicine, 29* (4), 60, 65-68.

Keller, V. (1995). Management of nausea and vomiting in children. *Journal of Pediatric Nursing, 10*, 280-286.

Kirk, E. A., White, C., & Freeman, S. (1992). Aspects of a nursing education intervention on parents' knowledge of hydrocephalus and shunts. *Journal of Neuroscience Nursing, 24* (2), 99-103.

Kramer, S. J., & Williams, D. R. (1993). The hearing-impaired infant and toddler: Identification, assessment, and intervention. *Infants and Young Children, 6* (1), 35-49.

Krengel, W. F., & King, H. A. (1995). Scoliosis: Diagnostic basics and therapeutic choices. *Journal of Musculoskeletal Medicine, 12* (9), 54-69.

Krowchuk, D. et al. (1990). Pediatric dermatology update. *Pediatrics, 86* (1), 128.

Kunta, N., Adams, J.A., Zahr, L., Killen, R., Cameron, K., & Wasson, H. (1996). Therapeutic play and bone marrow transplantation. *Journal of Pediatric Nursing, 11*, 359-367.

Labelle, H., Dansereau, J., Bellefleur, C., & Poitras, B. (1995). Three-dimensional effect of the Boston brace on the thoracic spine and rib cage. *Spine, 21* (1), 59-64.

Lamontagne, L. L., Johnson, B. D., & Hepworth, J. T. (1995). Evolution of parental stress and coping processes: A framework for critical care practice. *Journal of Pediatric Nursing, 10*, 212-218.

Lane, P.A. (1996). Sickle cell disease. *Pediatric Clinics of North America, 43*, 639-664.

Ledbetter, E. O. (1988). The many faces of pneumococcal pneumonia. *Contemporary Pediatrics, 5* (11), 50-72.

LeVieux-Anglin, L., & Sawyer, E. H. (1993). Incorporating play interventions into nursing care. *Pediatric Nursing, 19*, 459-462.

Lilleyman, J. S. (1994). Intracranial haemorrhage in idiopathic thrombocytopenic purpura. *Archives of Disease in Childhood, 71*, 251-253.

Longjohn, D. B., Zionts, L. E., & Stott, N. S. (1995). Acute hematogenous osteomyelitis of the epiphysis. *Clinical Orthopaedics and Related Research, 316*, 227-234.

Lonstein, J. E. (1994). Adolescent idiopathic scoliosis. *Lancet, 344* (8934), 1407-1412.

Loranger, N. (1992). Play intervention strategies for the Hispanic toddler with separation anxiety. *Pediatric Nursing, 18*, 571-575.

Mader, J. T., & Calhoun, J. (1994). Long-bone osteomyelitis diagnosis and management. *Hospital Practice, 29* (10), 71-74.

McClowry, S. G. (1993). Pediatric nursing psychosocial care: A vision beyond hospitalization. *Pediatric Nursing, 19*, 146-148.

McClowry, S. G., & McLeod, S. M. (1990). The psychosocial responses of school-age children to hospitalization. *Children Health Care, 19* (3), 55-161.

McCullough, F. L. (1989). Skeletal trauma in children. *Orthopedic Nursing, 8* (2), 41-50.

McFarland, K. (1988). Pediatric peritoneal dialysis. *Pediatric Nursing, 14* (5), 426.

Melkoman, G. (1987). Congenital hip dysplasia. *Orthopedic Nursing, 6* (3), 47.

Molter, M. (1993). Working with visually impaired children and their families. *Pediatric Clinics of North America, 4*, 881-890.

Monett, Z. J., & Roberts, P. J. (1995). Patient care for interventional cardiac catheterization. *Nursing Clinics of North America,* 30 (2), 333-345.

Moushey, R. et al. (1988). A perioperative teaching program: A collaborative process for children and their families. *Journal of Pediatric Nursing,* 3 (1), 40-45.

Nemes, J. et al. (1988). Epiglottitis: ED nursing management. *Journal of Emergency Nursing,* 14 (2), 70.

Norinkovich, K. M., Howie, G., & Cariofiles, P. (1995). Quality improvement study of day surgery for tonsillectomy and adenoidectomy patients. *Pediatric Nursing,* 21 (4), 341-343.

O'Donnell, J. K., & Gaedeke, M. K. (1995). Sudden infant death syndrome. *Critical Care Nursing Clinics of North America,* 7 (3), 473-481.

Ozsoylu, S., & Onat, N. (1992). Idiopathic thrombocytopenic purpura in infants under 6 months of age. *Clinical Pediatrics,* 10, 626-628.

Pederson, C., & Harbaugh, B. L. (1995). Children's and adolescent's experiences while undergoing cardiac catheterization. *Maternal-Child Nursing Journal,* 23 (1), 15-25.

Philips, S., & Hartley, J. T. (1988). Developmental differences and interventions for blind children. *Pediatric Nursing,* 14 (3), 201-204.

Pinto, W. C., Avanzi, O., & Dezen, E. (1994). Common sense in the management of adolescent idiopathic scoliosis. *Orthopedic Clinics of North America,* 25 (2), 215-223.

Rang, M. (1996). Management of Legg-Calve-Perthes disease varies with severity. *Journal of Musculoskeletal Medicine,* 4, 10-11.

Reidy, S. J., O'Hara, P. A., & O'Brien, P. (1989). Streptokinase use in children undergoing cardiac catheterization. *Journal of Cardiovascular Nursing,* 4 (1), 46-56.

Roberts, H. R., & Eberst, M. E. (1993). Current management of hemophilia B. *Hematology Oncology of Clinics of North America,* 7, 1269-1281.

Roberts, P. J. (1989). Caring for patients undergoing therapeutic cardiac catheterization. *Critical Care Nursing Clinics of North America,* 1 (2), 275-288.

Rosenberg, A. M. (1989). Advanced drug therapy for juvenile rheumatoid arthritis. *Journal of Pediatrics,* 114, 171-178.

Rudy, C. (1996). Developmental dysplasia of the hip: What's new in the 1990's? *Journal of Pediatric Health Care,* 10, 94-96.

Runton, N. (1988). Congenital cardiac anomalies: A reference guide for nurses. *Journal of Cardiovascular Nursing,* 2 (3), 56-70.

Santosham, M., & Greenough, W. (1991). Oral rehydration therapy: A global perspective. *Journal of Pediatrics,* 118 (4), S44-S51.

Sardegna, K. M., & Loggie, J. M. H. (1996). Hypertension in teens. *Contemporary Pediatrics,* 13 (8), 96-112.

Seligman, S. (1989). Emotional and social development in infancy and early childhood. *Early Childhood Update,* 5 (4), 1-2.

Smith, M. D. (1994). Congenital scoliosis of the cervical or cervicothoracic spine. *Orthopedic Clinics of North America,* 25 (2), 301-310.

Snider, D. E. et al. (1988). Tuberculosis in children. *Pediatric Infectious Disease Journal,* 7, 271-278.

Sorenson, E. (1990), Children's coping responses. *Journal of Pediatric Nursing,* 5 (4), 259-267.

Stevens, B., Stockwell, M., Browne, G., Dent, P., Gafni, A., Martin, R., & Anderson, M. (1995). Evaluation of a homebased traction program for children with congenital dislocated hips and Legg-Perthes disease. *Canadian Journal of Nursing Research,* 4, 133-150.

Svavarsdottir, E. K., & McCubbin, M. (1996). Parenthood transition for parents of an infant diagnosed with a congenital heart condition. *Journal of Pediatric Nursing,* 11, (4), 207-215.

Thomas, G. et al. (1987). Idiopathic thrombocytopenic purpura in children. *Nurse Practitioner,* 12 (4), 24.

Ungerer, J. et al. (1988). Psychosocial functioning in children and young adults with juvenile arthritis. *Pediatrics,* 81 (2), 195.

Upadhyay, S. S., Nelson, I. W., Ho, E. K. W., Hsu, L. C. S., & Leong, J. C. Y. (1995). New prognostic factors to predict the final outcome of brace treatment in adolescent idiopathic scoliosis. *Spine,* 20 (5), 537-545.

Vessey, J. et al. (1990). Teaching children about their internal bodies. *Pediatric Nurse,* 16 (1), 29-33.

Vogt, B. A. (1997). Identifying kidney disease: Simple steps can make a difference. *Contemporary Pediatrics,* 14 (3), 115-127.

Waidley, E. K. (1985). Show and tell: Preparing children for invasive procedures. *American Journal of Nursing,* 85 (7), 811-812.

Wakley, C. (1989). Cardiac catheterization, *Nursing,* 3 (36), 20-23.

Walker, C. (1989). Use of art and play therapy in pediatric oncology. *Journal of Pediatric Oncology Nursing,* 6 (4), 121-126.

Winkelstein, M. (1989). Fostering positive self-concept in the school-age child. *Pediatric Nursing,* 15 (3), 229-233.

Winter, H., & Chang, T. L. (1996). Gastrointestinal and nutritional problems in children with immunodeficiency and AIDS. *Pediatric Clinics of North America,* 43, 573-591.

Winter, R. B. (1994). The pendulum has swung too far: Bracing for adolescent idiopathic scoliosis in the 1990's. *Orthopedic Clinics of North America,* 25 (2), 195-204.

Wynn, S. et al. (1988). Long-term prognosis for children with nephrotic syndrome. *Clinical Pediatrics,* 27 (2), 63.

Young, J. A. et al. (1989). Radiation treatment for the child with cancer. *Issues in Contemporary Pediatric Nursing,* 12 (2/3), 159-170.

Zahr, L. K et al. (1989). Assessment and management of the child with asthma. *Pediatric Nursing,* 15, 109-114.

Ziegler, D. B. & Prior, M. M. (1994). Preparation for surgery and adjustment to hospitalization. *Pediatric Surgical Nursing,* 29, 655-668.

SKIDMORE-ROTH PUBLISHING, INC.

400 Inverness Drive South, Suite 260, Englewood, CO 80112

Ph. 1-800-825-3150

title	code	isbn #	price	qty
INSTANT INSTRUCTOR SERIES				
AIDS HIV, Bradley-Springer 1995	ADIN01	1-57930-010-0	$9.95	
C.C.U., Randall 1995	CCINC1	1-56930-022-4	$9.95	
Geriatric, Jaffe 1992	GRN01	0-944132-68-5	$9.95	
Hemodialysis, Fowlds 1994	DLN01	1-56930-020-8	$9.95	
I.C.U., Randall 1995	ICUI01	1-56930-021-6	$9.95	
IV	IVI01	1-56930-043-7	$9.95	
Obstetric, Jaffe 1992	OBIN01	0-944132-67-7	$9.95	
Oncology, Gale 1994	ONIN01	1-56930-023-2	$9.95	
Pediatric, Keller 1992	PDIN01	0-944132-66-9	$9.95	
Psychiatric, Yard 1992	PSYI01	0-944132-69-3	$9.95	
NURSING CARE PLANS SERIES				
Critical Care, Comer 1998	CNCP01	1-56930-035-6	$38.95	
Geriatric (2nd ed.), Jaffe 1996	GNCP02	1-56933-052-6	$38.95	
HIV/AIDS (2nd ed.), Bradley-Springer 1998	ADSC02	1-56930-097-6	$38.95	
Oncology, Gale 1996	ONCP01	1-56930-004-6	$38.95	
Pediatric (2nd ed.), Jaffe 1998	PNOP02	1-56930-057-7	$38.95	
SURVIVAL SERIES				
Geriatric Survival Handbook (3rd ed.), Acello 1997	G8G001	1-56930-061-5	$26.95	
Nurse's Survival Handbook (3rd ed.), Acello 1998	NSGD03	1-56930-040-2	$39.95	
Obstetric Survival Handbook (2nd ed.), Masten 1998	OBSG01	1-56930-083-6	$35.95	
Pediatric Nurse's Survival Guide, Rebeschi 1996	PNGD01	1-56930-018-6	$29.95	
NURSING/OTHER				
Body in Brief (3rd ed.), Rayman 1997	BBRF03	1-56930-055-0	$35.95	
Diagnostic and Lab Cards (3rd ed.), Skidmore-Roth, 1998	DLC03	1-56930-065-8	$28.95	
Drug Comparison Handbook (2nd ed.), Reilly 1995	DRUG02	1-56930-16-x	$35.95	
Essential Laboratory Mathematics, Johnson & Timmons, 1997	ELM01	1-56930-056-9	$29.95	
Geriatric Long-Term Procedures & Treatments (2nd ed.), Jaffe 1994	GLTP02	1-56930-045-3	$34.95	
Geriatric Nutrition and Diet (3rd ed.), Jaffe 1998	NUT03	1-56930-096-8	$25.95	
Handbook of Long-Term Care (2nd ed.), Vitale 1997	HLTC02	1-56930-068-6	$28.95	
Handbook for Nurse Assistants (2nd ed), Nurse Asst. Consort. 1997	HNA02	1-56930-059-3	$23.95	
I.C.U. Quick Reference (2nd ed.), Comer 1998	ICQU02	1-56930-071-2	$35.95	
Infection Control, Palmer 1996	INFO01	1-56930-061-8	$94.95	
Nursing Diagnosis Cards (2nd ed.), Weber 1997	NDC02	1-56930-060-7	$29.95	

title	code	isbn #	price	qty
Nurse's Trivia Calendar, Rayman	NTC98	1-56930-073-9	$11.95	
OBRA (3rd ed.), Jaffe 1998	OBRA03	1-56930-047-X	$119.95	
OSHA Book (2nd ed.), Goodner 1997	OSHA	1-56930-069-0	$119.95	
Procedure Cards (3rd ed.), Jaffe 1996	PCCU03	1-56930-054-2	$24.95	
Pharmacy Tech, Reilly 1994	PHAR01	1-56930-005-4	$25.95	
Spanish for Medical Personnel, Meizel 1993	SPAN01	1-56930-001-1	$21.95	
Staff Development for the Psych Nurse, Finkelman 1992	STDEV0	0-944132-78-2	$59.95	
OUTLINE SERIES				
Diabetes Outline, Barnwell 1995	DBOL01	1-56930-031-3	$23.95	
Fundamentals of Nursing Outline, Chin 1995	FUND01	1-56930-029-1	$23.95	
Geriatric Outline, Morice 1995	GER01	1-56930-050-x	$23.95	
Hemodynamic Monitoring Outline, Schactman 1995	HDMO01	1-56930-034-8	$23.95	
High Acuity Outline, Reynolds 1995	HAT001	1-56930-028-3	$23.95	
Med-Surgical Nursing Outline (2nd ed.), Reynolds 1998	MSN02	1-56930-068-2	$23.95	
Obstetric Nursing Outline (2nd ed.), Masten 1997	OBS02	1-56930-070-4	$23.95	
Pediatric Nursing Outline, Froese-Fretz <u>et al</u> 1998	PN02	1-56930-067-4	$23.95	
RN NCLEX REVIEW SERIES				
PN/VN Review Cards (3rd ed.), Goodner 1998	PNRC03	1-56930-093-3	$32.95	
RN Review Cards (3rd ed.), Goodner 1998	RNRC03	1-56930-092-5	$32.95	

Name_____

Address_____

City_____ State_____ Zip_____

Phone (_____)_____

❑ VISA   ❑ MasterCard   ❑ American Express   ❑ Check/Money Order

Card #_____ Exp. Date_____

Signature (required)_____

Prices subject to change. Please add $6.95 each for postage and handling. Include your local sales tax.

MAIL OR FAX ORDER TO:
SKIDMORE-ROTH PUBLISHING, INC.
400 Inverness Drive South, Suite 260
Englewood, Colorado 80112
1-800-825-3150

Visit our website at: http://www.skidmore-roth.com